The Forgotten and Hidden Facts of

VITAMINS

&

MINERALS

By Dottore Conoscenti Tutti, MD

The Basis of Functional Medicine, Alternative Medicine, and
Complementary Medicine

Disclaimer

This book is intended as a medical reference and historical record only. It is not intended to diagnose and treat any condition. If you have any medical problem, I urge you to find a competent physician and begin the collaborative process of history taking, examination, testing, diagnosis, and the development of a treatment plan. Medical problem solving is a joint effort of patient and doctor. The doctor cannot treat the patient alone—without the patient's participation, the results are often less than optimal. The information in this book is good material to start the conversation and begin the collaboration between patient and doctor.

The author and publisher disclaim liability for any medical outcomes that may occur as a result of applying methods suggested in this book.

The Forgotten and Hidden Facts of Vitamins and Minerals

The Basis of Functional Medicine, Alternative Medicine, and Complementary Medicine

Dottore Conoscenti Tutti, MD

Copyright © 2024 by Caduceus Libri Publishing

All rights reserved, including the right to reproduce this book or portions thereof in any form whatsoever.

Caduceus Libri Publishing, 41 Watchung Plaza, Ste 305, Montclair, NJ 07042

Web page: DrTutti.com

Library of Congress Control Number: 2024912916

ISBN: 979-8-9898609-0-6

Printed in the United States of America

To my parents, wife, and children.

Contents

Vitamins

Vitamin A 4

Vitamin B 31

Vitamin B_2 (Riboflavin) 52

Vitamin B_3 (Niacin) 60

Vitamin B_6 81

Folic Acid 93

Vitamin B_{12} 109

Biotin 136

Vitamin C 142

Vitamin D 193

Vitamin E 214

Vitamin K 247

Vitamin P 263

Minerals

Boron 272

Calcium 288

Copper 301

Iodine 314

Iron 334

Lithium 347

Magnesium 354

Potassium 371

Selenium 378

Sodium	392
Strontium	402
Zinc	408

Appendix

Water	424
Vitamin C and Cancer	440
Patient Handouts	457
Berberine	457
Bone Health	462
DHEA Hormone Replacement	465
Estrogen Metabolite Ratios	472
Fish Oils	475

Vitamins

The Origin of the Word *Vitamin*

In the late 1800s, a new interest was developing in the area of nutrition. Such diseases as scurvy, beriberi, pellagra, and rickets did not align with the germ theory that had become popular. These were diseases you did not catch. You could not get them from someone close to you. But you could get them from not taking in the proper nutrients. It was becoming accepted that elements such as iron, copper, sodium, and potassium were needed for good health, but organic compounds such as proteins, fats, and carbohydrates were more difficult to understand.

If animals were fed purified protein, carbohydrates, and fats, they did not thrive. Their diets lacked an essential substance. It was only when milk, which contained some unknown essential ingredient, was added that a new understanding of nutrition began to bud.

Through the work of men like the Dutch physician Christiaan Eijkman and his collaborator Grijns, who discovered the cause of beriberi, nutritional diseases were beginning to gain recognition. The Swiss biochemist Lunin, in 1881, established the idea of an essential missing compound despite the diet containing pure basic fats, proteins, carbohydrates, and minerals such as sodium, potassium, and calcium.

In the sphere of scientific study, it was recognized that something missing from—and not something added to—the diet caused these diseases. In fact, in 1911, the Polish biochemist Casimir Funk, working at the Lister Institute of London, published his theory of **vitamines**. He believed from his studies that there were substances that were essential to life and that these substances contained nitrogen in the form of a group of proteins called amines. So, from the Latin word for "life," **vita**, and the term **amine**, denoting a protein or nitrogen product, he coined the word **vitamine**. On further study he learned that not all essential substances contain nitrogen and dropped the final *e*, and the word in now spelled as we know it: **vitamin**.

Eating food to become strong and healthy is simple enough, but then comes the selection process. Selecting the right food is not intuitive. We do not know which foods to eat to promote and maintain health. What we need is not always readily available. Cravings are a guide to what we should eat, but they are not always directed by need. A pregnant woman may have a craving for a particular food as her body directs her to particular nutrients—or to a taste that may or may not be a nutritious selection. This may be our more primitive instincts kicking in, but often today, with food so readily available, our intuitive selection is guided by taste, the texture of the food in our mouths, or simply social pressures. Dining out in our modern society is a form of entertainment, a social event, and even a demonstration of good fortune and social standing. Even where you eat can better your social position in the community, but it may not promote good nutrition and better health.

Vitamin A

Benefits of Vitamin A

- Reduces complications and mortality in measles cases
- Effective in treating gastritis and stomach erosion and ulcers
- Supports healthy skin, preventing blemishes
- Topical treatment for cervical cancer
- May reduce menorrhagia (heavy menstrual bleeding)
- Promotes healthy breast tissue
- Protects epithelial and mucosal surfaces
- Protects against the development of preeclampsia
- Prevents night blindness
- Prevents dry eyes and supports corneal health
- Critical in preventing interstitial cystitis
- Reduces actinic keratosis
- Prevents and treats macular degeneration

History of Vitamin A

The first recorded uses of vitamin A relate to eye conditions. Vitamin A affects two parts of the eye: the anterior structures of the cornea and conjunctiva, and the posterior retinal nervous tissue, which receives images and transfers them into electrical impulses that are transmitted to the brain by the optic nerve. The cornea gets most of its nutrients from local tissues and effusion through tears. The retina gets its nutrients through the blood.

The use of vitamin A in medicine dates back 3,500 years to ancient Egypt, where it was known as a cure for a deficiency rather than as a substance. It was used as a treatment for *sharew*, which was probably a corneal condition characterized by thinning or discoloration. The Ebers Papyrus of 1500 B.C. reports a treatment involving the application of ox liver to the eye to preserve vision. This would be an effective treatment only for conditions of the cornea or conjunctiva.

If ox liver had been used to treat night blindness, the patient would have had to ingest the liver to treat the rhodopsin or iodopsin involved in night blindness. The Greeks recorded night blindness for the first time, using the word *nyktos* (night) or *nyktalopia* (night blindness), and the treatment was eating raw beef liver and honey or eating goat's liver. In the Middle Ages, the Dutch recorded eating goat's liver to assist night vision. In 1859, Edward Schwarz, an Austrian physician, reported 75 cases of poor night vision on a world trip from Cape Horn to Gibraltar. He treated his patients with boiled ox liver and reported that this was a permanent cure. He was the first to call night blindness a nutritional disease.[1]

In 1907, S. V. McCollum at Wisconsin College of Agriculture, while working with cows fed wheat, oats, or maize, showed that the wheat-fed cows did not thrive, became blind, and produced only premature dead calves. Oat-fed cows did better but were not completely healthy. Cattle fed with yellow maize did not show any ill health. The yellow substance provided protection. For convenience and to obtain research results faster, he switched from cattle to rats. Through his experiments, he showed that there is a fat-soluble factor in both butter and egg yolk that is required for growth and development as well as vision and the health of the cornea. This he called the "fat-soluble factor A." This is in contrast to the water-soluble B substances that were being studied at the same time.

---

[1] Wolf, G., "Discovery of Vitamin A," Wiley, April 19, 2001, https://doi.org/10.1038/npg.els.0003419.

Shortly thereafter, it was discovered that cod-liver oil has that same "**fat-soluble factor A**," and it was noted that it also prevents dry eye, medically referred to as xerophthalmia. The researchers found that some of the "fat-soluble factor A" was yellow and some was clear and colorless. Eventually, the clear, colorless form could be separated from the yellow pigment. The clear, colorless, fatty substance is the active molecule of retinol or Vitamin A. The yellow, inactive substance is beta-carotene. In 1930, T. Moore showed, through animal studies, that beta-carotene is a provitamin (a substance that can be converted to a vitamin in the body) that is converted to retinol—that is, vitamin A. This conversion of beta-carotene to retinol occurs at the intestinal mucosa, and the retinol is stored in the liver.

In the 1930s, Karrer et al. isolated the molecule and defined the chemical structure of both beta-carotene and retinol. Isler et al. were the first to do a total synthesis of the molecule of retinol, in 1947.

Functions of Vitamin A and Vitamin A Compounds

Vitamin A, or retinol, is needed for the support of the immune system, vision, growth and development, red blood cell production, the skin, and mucus membranes. It can aid in preventing conditions such as acne, psoriasis, gastric ulcers, and inflammatory bowel disease, and it promotes wound healing. Vitamin A is fat soluble and acts more like a hormone than a nutrient. Fish, egg yolks, butter, and liver are direct sources of this vitamin. It is rarely included in multivitamins; instead, as a supplement, it is usually offered as retinol, retinal, and retinoic acid.

Retinol

Retinal

Retinoic Acid

Retinol, retinal, and retinoic acid are vitamin A compounds, not to be confused with beta-carotene, which is made up of two retinol molecules attached together. The body will cleave or separate the beta-carotene into two retinol molecules. The cleavage point will be at the bond indicated by the arrow.

Beta-Carotene

Beta-carotene is in the group of plant-derived carotenoids that are antioxidants and that include alpha-carotene, beta-carotene, gamma-carotene, cryptoxanthin, zeaxanthin, and lutein. These are all good for vision and generally derived from green, yellow, red, and orange fruits and vegetables. Astaxanthin, another related antioxidant, derives from algae. Carotenoids have antiaging properties and properties that inhibit cognitive decline, coronary artery disease, and macular degeneration. Beta-carotene is the only one that is converted to retinol, and that conversion requires sufficient zinc, copper, magnesium, and thyroid hormone.

The term **vitamin A** refers to a group of molecules that, through chemical reactions, are related to each other. The term is used especially in commercial products, academic papers, and studies reported in the news. The best advice I can give you when looking at the supplement facts on a vitamin package or reading a report on the benefits or dangers of vitamin A is know which molecule they are talking about. You do not have to be a pharmacist or a doctor to read these ingredients. You just have to know a few words to go from confusion to understanding.

There are two functional groups of molecules in the vitamin A family. The first is a group called provitamins. These minimally active molecules effect little change at the cellular level and function as a storage form of molecules that will become the active retinols of vitamin A. In medical literature, the retinols of vitamin A have a narrow therapeutic range of benefit. In other words, the range between enough and too much is limited. We discuss dosing later in this section, but too much vitamin A supplementation is reported to lead to dry and itchy skin, headaches, increased intracranial pressure, and vomiting.

I must say, I have never seen this in my practice or have seen a reported case. Provitamin A molecules can be taken in large quantities without concern. The body will store carotenoids and zeaxanthins without harming tissues, even though the skin may take on a yellow or orange coloring on the soles of the feet or palms of the hands. It does not deposit in the sclera—that is, the whites of the eyes. The provitamins are safe to eat, as most of them are in foods: red and yellow peppers, pumpkin, and sweet potatoes. The body will regulate the conversion of the provitamins to the active vitamins as needed, and toxicity will not occur.

The conversion of the provitamin beta-carotene is dependent on the amount of retinol the body has, not the amount of beta-carotene that is available for conversion. Three molecules comprise vitamin A: **retinol** is an alcohol, **retinal** is an aldehyde, and **retinoic acid** is an oxidized form of retinol. These molecules convert back and forth as the forms are needed, except for the production of retinoic acid, which is a one-way reaction to the acid form.

Retinoic acid is not talked about much, but it is a hormone growth factor for epithelia. This is fundamental to understanding vitamin A. My definition of a hormone is a chemical, or messenger molecule, that is transmitted from one cell to other cells and that tells them how to behave or function. A good example is estradiol, the most significant female hormone produced in the ovaries and sent to tissues such as the breasts, uterus, and vagina and that tells those cells how to behave, be it regarding structure or producing secretions that are needed for milk production or mucus production for lubrication. A lack of hormones implies that the cells of the end organ will have no direction and will not produce the proper secretions; hence, the cells do not mature as they should. Cells without proper direction will do as they will and may deviate and become cancerous. I liken it to a kid who needs adult supervision but is without direction and who, as a result, misbehaves and becomes something undesirable.

Retinoic acid is a hormone growth factor for epithelial cells. Retinoic acid is a hormone that tells epithelial cells how to structure themselves, how many mucous cells or sweat cells to have in their structure, how elastic the cells are to be placed about muscle cells, and how this is all coordinated. This is a significant fact considering that epithelial cells are the surface of the gastrointestinal system. They line the mouth, esophagus, stomach, small intestine, and the large bowel. These same cells, epithelia, cover the cervix and the vaginal surface and even line the bladder. This includes the airway from the nasal lining, down the trachea and into the airways and the surface of the lung that exchanges air. Epithelial tissue seems to be everywhere. The conjunctiva of the eye and the outer surface of the cornea are specialized epithelial cells. And to be healthy, all these cells need retinoic acid.

Years ago, I was talking to a renowned gastroenterologist discussing a patient with a peptic ulcer who we had in common. I asked him what the cause might be. He was straightforward and direct. I expected him to say it was stress, spicy food, too much aspirin, or a sign of cancer. But no, he said, "Who cares? Just take the drugs—they work." So much for the oracle.

I did not think this was a good answer, and I kept wondering why peptic ulcers develop. I began to ask the question of what was missing that caused the ulcer to develop in the first place. In looking over my physiology books, I remembered learning something about vitamin A and support of the lining of the intestines in medical school. Physiology books are a good source of information about healthy systems; medical books usually talk about the sick or about diseases.

I went back to the books and started using vitamin A in my practice, giving 10,000 or 20,000 units to everyone who was taking proton pump inhibitors or antiulcer drugs. I asked anyone who was taking Tagamet, Zantac, Prilosec, Nexium, or Protonix to take vitamin A every day. What I found was that at least half of these patients could give up the antiulcer medication in a month.

Knowing how safe the vitamin is, I have now moved my recommendation up to 40,000 to 50,000 units daily.

I get many complaints of dry eyes from mostly older women. Usually, an accompanying complaint is hypothyroidism, and if they are the chatty type, they will also talk about vaginal dryness. So how are eyeballs and vaginas connected? As you can see, epithelial cells all need vitamin A to restore health and vigor. In fact, Tori Hudson, a naturopath in Washington State, treats cervical aplasia and cervical cancer by painting the cervix with vitamin A.

The skin is also an epithelial cell, and drug companies looking for a better skin care product developed tretinoin, a derivative of vitamin A, to treat wrinkles and acne. This is a synthetic rather than a natural form of vitamin A. Another form is isotretinoin (Accutane), and it does not fit into the chemistry of the body. It can also cause birth defects if taken during pregnancy.

The *Merck Manual* reports that in the past, vitamin A was used to treat measles. There is maybe a relationship between the measles vaccine and autism. The explosive number of new cases of autism parallels the use of the MMR—measles, mumps, and rubella—vaccine. Mary Megson has studied autism, and her research shows a total deficiency of vitamin A in children with autism. Maybe there is a link between the two. The MMR vaccine depletes the body of vitamin A. I suggest that this is not the only cause of autism, but maybe premedicating children with vitamin A, monitoring it with blood tests, and supplementing it might help ameliorate or prevent autism. Remember that retinol, vitamin A, is usually not in multivitamins. The medical literature has frightened people so much regarding the side effects of vitamin A that it is even difficult to find it in the pure form.

Beta-Carotene

Sometimes even natural products can become harmful. Beta-carotene is the only vitamin supplement I am aware of that can promote cancer. It is seldom harmful to healthy people whose bodies can convert it to retinol by being cleaved or broken into two identical molecules. However, sometimes the beta-carotene molecule is not cut into two molecules of retinol. If given beta-carotene supplements, patients with chronic obstructive pulmonary disease (COPD), especially those with chronic bronchitis, smokers, and those with asbestosis, have a higher incidence of lung cancer.[2] This does not occur in disease-free people who ingest beta-carotene or eat foods that contain beta-carotene. The current explanation is that in the diseased lung of someone who has chronic bronchitis, with all the production of mucus, the increased trapping of bacteria, toxic pollutants, and free oxygen radicals of oxidation may produce other molecules, or these molecules themselves cleave or cut the beta-carotene molecule not in the middle but at random locations, producing harmful cancer-inducing substances.[3]

Beta-carotene is a provitamin to vitamin A. That is, it is not vitamin A but a compound that must be converted to vitamin A. This conversion is dependent not on how much beta-carotene is available but on the body's need for retinol. Beta-carotene can be taken in large quantities and still not be converted to vitamin A, or retinol. Large quantities of beta-carotene and the other carotenoids can be taken in amounts where the yellow pigment will appear to color the palms and soles, as is seen in primates. This is harmless and is not toxic. A change of diet will cause the coloring to fade.

---

[2] Goodman, G., et al., "The Beta-Carotene and Retinol Efficacy Trial: Incidence of Lung Cancer and Cardiovascular Disease Mortality during 6-Year Follow-Up after Stopping Beta-Carotene and Retinol Supplements," *Journal of the National Cancer Institute*, 2004, *96*(23), 1743–1750, https://doi.org/10.1093/jnci/djh320.
[3] Higdon, J., et al., "Vitamin A," Linus Pauling Institute, Oregon State University, last updated January 2024, https://lpi.oregonstate.edu/mic/vitamins/vitamin-A.

On a personal note, when my children were infants, my wife prepared all their food from scratch, passing all vegetables through the food processor. One day while feeding my daughter, Lauren, my wife became upset that the tip of Lauren's nose was orange. Even the tips of her ears looked like they were changing color. My wife became upset, and maybe even panicky. How could a baby that ate no commercially prepared foods get so sick? Fortunately, after rereading the stack of baby books, we found the answer. Fresh carrots eaten every day often causes a nice orange color that will fade in about two weeks if carrots are eliminated from the diet.

The labels on vitamin bottles will often state that the product is "vitamin A in the form of beta-carotene." What that means is that there is no vitamin A in the product. Beta-carotene and vitamin A are different molecules, and vitamin A is not necessarily converted from beta-carotene. For the conversion to occur, the body must have enough vitamin C, protein, thyroid hormone, copper, and zinc. Vitamin E is necessary for the storage and utilization of vitamin A. Vitamin A requires proper absorption of preformed vitamin A, or beta-carotene and the proper conditions for the conversion.

Beta-carotene is helpful with vitamin A for improving the immune response in all epithelial cells, including the vaginal mucosa and the wall of the bladder, and in preventing cystic breast disease. The glandular tissue of the breast is derived from epithelial tissue embryologically. Cysts are trapped islands of epithelial tissue with no duct to transport milk to the nipple. Beta-carotene affects the immune system by lowering *IL-6*, a proinflammatory cell mediator, increasing T cell levels, and promoting phagocytosis, or the white cells eating or consuming debris or pathogens. Beta-carotene has a much stronger effect on the immune system than vitamin A has, and vitamin A has more of a growth and health effect on epithelial cells—that is, all mucosal cells in the gastrointestinal tract, the vaginal and bladder wall surfaces, and specialized forms such as the unique tissue of the conjunctiva of the eye and the surface of the cornea. Vitamin A supports the structure of the mucosa, promoting healthy cell growth, and the function of the goblet cells that produce the mucus that coat the surface of the mucosa. This mucus barrier prevents direct irritation from foreign substances that might damage the epithelium. In the stomach, the mucus protects the wall of the stomach from being attacked by stomach acid. Without mucus, the stomach becomes irritated, which can cause gastritis or even a gastric ulcer.

Research on the Benefits of Vitamins

Much of what I report in this book is not taken from obscure magazines, out-of-date books, or Sunday supplements. In fact, a quick perusal of the footnotes demonstrates that much of the information was taken from mainstream medical periodicals and respected textbooks. This information is hidden in plain sight, often overlooked or ignored by many doctors. Big Pharma has an interest in promoting its own synthetic or adulterated products. It never puts its chemicals and biologic preparations in a true head-to-head comparison to the products of Mother Nature. The practitioners of medicine have been negligent in not reviewing and promoting their own clinical work, but sometimes good, reliable information is published. However, it does not gain the attention it deserves.

Skin Cancer

In 2019, an authoritative American Medical Association publication, *JAMA Dermatology*, published a significant article on skin cancer and vitamin A. The authors reported on two studies comprising 123,000 men and women over 28 years that showed consumption of retinol, vitamin A, and carotenoids that lowered the occurrence of cutaneous squamous cell carcinoma. This cancer was found to be 17% less common in the top 20% of those who consumed the most vitamin A versus the 20% who consumed the least.[4] This article also confirms that vitamin A is not a poison but a true nutrient.

Measles

Measles mortality is reduced in children under the age of two if they are given 200,000 units of vitamin A two days in a row. Treatment for one day has little effect on the course of the disease, but two days of treatment reduced the mortality rate to 48% if the oil-based vitamin was used, and the mortality rate was 81% for the water-based preparation.[5] Both the World Health Organization and UNICEF recommend treating children with vitamin A.[6]

Absorption of Iron

Iron is absorbed better if vitamin A levels are sufficient than if they are not.[7] It is better to use an organic iron than a salt for better absorption and utilization.

Stomach Ulcers and Intestinal Problems

Stomach ulcers and intestinal problems can be diminished with 20,000 to 40,000 units of vitamin A, such as retinol palmitate, taken orally daily. The intestinal lining, which includes the stomach and esophagus, contains receptors for vitamin A. That means this vitamin is also a hormone that can stimulate the epithelial lining to

---

[4] Life Extension, "In the News: December 2019," "Greater Vitamin A and Carotenoid Intake Linked with Lower Risk of Skin Cancer," 2019, https://www.lifeextension.com/magazine/2019/12/in-the-news; see also Kim, J., et al., "Association of Vitamin A Intake with Cutaneous Squamous Cell Carcinoma Risk in the United States," *JAMA Dermatology*, 2019, *155*(11), 1260–1268.

[5] D'Souza, R. M., and D'Souza, R., "Vitamin A for Treating Measles in Children," *Cochrane Database of Systematic Reviews*, 2002, 1, CD001479.

[6] D'Souza, R. M., and D'Souza, R., "Vitamin A for the Treatment of Children with Measles—A Systematic Review," *Journal of Tropical Pediatrics*, 2002, *48*(6), 323–327.

[7] Suharno, D., et al., "Supplementation with Vitamin A and Iron for Nutritional Anemia in Pregnant Women in West Java, Indonesia," *Lancet*, 1993, *342*(8883), 1325–1328.

grow properly and repair if injured. Vitamin A will stimulate the lining of the stomach to produce the proper cells that make up the surface of the stomach. This includes the parietal cells that produce stomach acid, the goblet cells that produce the mucus that coats the inner surface of the stomach, and the epithelial cells that make up the bulk of the inner lining.

Vitamin A affects the entire lining of the gastrointestinal tract from the lips to the anus. This important vitamin/hormone is necessary for the health of the epithelial tissue. This includes easing such conditions as ulcerative colitis and irritable bowel syndrome.

The Bladder

The bladder is lined with epithelial cells. Vitamin A is necessary for the health and integrity of the mucosal lining, protecting it from infection and irritants. D-mannose at 500 mg twice a day is often prescribed to protect the mucosal lining of the bladder and to keep bacteria from sticking to it. I feel vitamin A is a better choice in that it supports the mucosal lining in both its structure and the production of mucus. No harm would be done if both were used at the same time.

The Female Reproductive System

Vaginal health is dependent on vitamin A, as is all epithelial-derived tissue. It supports both the structures of the vaginal wall and the cervix of the uterus. Again, it is required for the proper support of the wall structures of elastic, muscular, and mucus-producing cells. Vitamin A, applied locally or taken orally, is a convenient way to treat dryness.

Dysplasia of the cervix is influenced by both carotenoids and retinoic acid. Dysplasia is defined as the premalignant transformation of cells. While this condition is abnormal, it is not cancer—the tissue is starting to take on some of the characteristics of cancer. In fact, it has been shown that women with a diet rich in vitamin A have less dysplasia, and if they do, it may not progress to cancer. A diet low in carotenoids and vitamin A tends to progress to cancer at a faster rate.[8] The best source of protection is from yellow-orange vegetables and fruits such as cantaloupe, orange-flesh honeydew melon, yellow squash, peaches, carrots, and red and yellow peppers.

Carcinoma In Situ

Carcinoma in situ is a pathological term applied to the epithelium in its evolution from normal to cancerous. This term is applied to epithelia of the cervix, vagina, endometrium, epidermis of the skin, bronchial epithelium, and intestinal and bladder epithelial lining that exhibit "the cytological features similar to those of invasive cancer but no demonstrable penetration into the sub epithelial stroma."[9] Carcinoma in situ is confined to the local epithelial tissue and does not penetrate into the surrounding tissues such as elastic or muscular supporting tissues, does not cross the basement membrane, and does not travel to other parts of the body or metastasize.

The progression of epithelia tissue from normal to cancerous involves two stages between normal and cancerous. The first is dysplasia, where some of the cells show premalignant changes of multiple nuclei and mitotic figures, including tripolar mitoses. These changes do not involve the entire thickness of the epithelium from the growth area to the surface. One can think of it as islands of abnormal cells scattered among normal cells, and it is not found in areas where epithelium should not be found.

Carcinoma in situ is a more prolific change of the epithelium, with variation in the size and number of the nuclei. It involves the full depth of the epithelium but does not invade the surrounding

---

[8] Nagata C, et al., "Serum Carotenoids and Vitamins and Risk of Cervical Dysplasia from a Case-Control Study in Japan," *British Journal of Cancer*, 1999, *81*(7), 1234–1237.

[9] Anderson, W. A. D., and Scotti, T. M., *Synopsis of Pathology*, C.V. Mosby Company, 1972, 309–310.

tissue. It is not metastatic. It does not involve the local tissue or stroma, including the local blood vessels.

The progression of tissue changes from best to worst, starting with normal and then the first abnormal and least involved change, is dysplasia that has scattered abnormal cells with normal cells. The next is carcinoma in situ, where the entire epithelial layer shows mitotic changes, but this is not found beyond the bounds of where the normal tissue is found. It may be thicker and bulkier than normal, but it does not invade the local surrounding tissue. Cancer is tissue that has changed, with little resemblance to normal tissue. It is characterized by microscopic changes of multiple nuclei and many mitotic changes, and it grows, invading local and distant areas of the body.

The pathologist may see the above changes as a progression from normal tissue to cancer, where one form goes from one to the next. Some studies have shown little progression, such as carcinoma in situ of the breast. Little to no dysplasia is found, and no progression to cancer is observed. This is referred to as stage zero. To treat, or not to treat, is controversial. All allopathic treatments—chemotherapy, radiation, and surgery—have potential downsides, including death. If you are diagnosed with stage-zero changes, take time to consider your options. Treatment options should include nutrition changes; lifestyle changes; stress reduction; the resolution of personal conflicts, including forgiveness; exercise; detoxing; and spiritual fulfillment.

Vitamins Related to Skin Care

Skin care is the condition most related to vitamin A. It is found in many products that are intended to rejuvenate the skin: antiwrinkle cream, antiaging retinol cream, age-defying retinol moisturizer, and the list goes on. Most of these creams and serums contain retinol, but they also contain 15 to 20 other chemicals that act as vehicles, stabilizers, fragrances, and moisturizers. Most of these you do not want or need. Moisturizers, after repeated use, keep your skin from producing its own oils, making it dryer than when you started applying the product. Fragrances are other chemicals that you may not need, and ditto for vehicles and stabilizers—all of these will be absorbed into your body through the skin.

The skin renews itself every 42 days, from the basal layer to the sloughing off of dead skin. The peel process that is used in the esthetic field uses retinol at high concentrations that cause the skin to sustain a chemical burn and fall off. There is an inflammatory process with redness, tenderness, and hopefully repair from the basal layer. Peels were first started years ago using phenol, and that process was harsh until the chemical was switched to Retin-A, which is essentially a high concentration of retinol. Retinol is vitamin A, but the applied concentration of Retin-A is 10,000 times the concentration found in the body. Some of the preparations may even be synthetic. At these levels, what was a nutrient and hormone becomes a toxic substance and destroys the skin, causing it to peel and slough off.

I recommend for skin rejuvenation of the face, the back of the hands, or any areas of roughness that a weak serum of retinol be applied nightly. The best preparation of retinol is a 2.5% encapsulated solution. This is a low dose, near the normal physiological concentration, acting as a nutrient and a hormone to stimulate the basal layer of cells. At this level of concentration, the retinol can get into the nucleus of the basal cell and direct it to proliferate normally, developing healthy cells. It will take at least one skin cycle of 42 days for the new cells to reach the surface. Results are usually reported in 10 to 14 days but continue for the full cycle. There is much improvement in the first cycle, but as the treatment is continued, better results are experienced after two or three cycles (84 to 126 days).

To me, the lower 2.5% concentration of the retinol serum is more natural, is more physiological, and does not damage the skin. It does this entire repair without increased redness, excessive exfoliation, and pain. It works well on dry patches of skin and areas of discoloration and reduces the depth of wrinkles. In my opinion, it gets you to a healthy state and looks better than a peel in less time, and you don't have to hide during the period of reconstruction.

Longevity

Longevity is given a boost by vitamin A. In studies conducted by the Institute of Functional Medicine in 2009, it was demonstrated that healthy centenarians had vitamin A levels comparable to healthy young adults. Typically, vitamin A level falls with age, as is found in the majority of older people. It is believed that vitamin A helps to reduce inflammation. Aging is associated with inflammation, increasing as one ages. Researchers of aging have recently coined the term **"inflammaging"** to tie aging and inflammation into a new concept.[10]

It is now known that the immune system is dependent on vitamin A. It is required for the development of the T cells and B cells of the cellular immune system and antibodies of the humoral immune system. Your ability to mount a response to an infection is very much dependent on vitamin A. Vitamin C and vitamin D have long been known to help you fight infections, and now there is a better understanding that vitamin A should be supplemented to counteract infections.

Actinic Keratosis

Actinic keratosis can be reduced in size or totally removed with topical retinol. These are the exuberant raised lesions that present anywhere on the head, body, or extremities, appearing alone or in clusters as rough, scaly, reddish to gray bumps or macula, measuring from 2 to 15 mm. They often appear dry, do not itch, and do not bleed. They accentuate your age, and they are ugly.

---

[10] Pizzorno, L., "Vitamin A—Tolerance Extends Longevity," Longevity Medicine Review, July 15, 2009.

The usual treatment for them is to shave them off or cut them out, leaving a scar. The only thing that remains from this ugly growth is an ugly scar.

From my personal experience and observation, the best treatment is the nightly application of a 2.5% encapsulated retinol solution. This is a weak but physiological concentration of retinol that can penetrate the epidermis, get down to the basal layer (the area of new skin growth), and stimulate the growth of new normal keratinocytes. It may take only one keratinocyte maturation cycle of 42 days to replace a small lesion. New normal cells develop in the basal area as keratinocytes and mature and transform into corneocytes, replacing this rough, ugly blemish into flat, normal skin. The lesion essentially rises to the surface and exfoliates, leaving normal tissue.

I discovered this by applying retinol to my own face for a general antiwrinkle and rejuvenation treatment. My patients have reported similar results. The bonus is that your friends will notice and comment on how well you look. I find that this is a sophisticated, nutritional, and hormonal rejuvenation of the skin—helping your body to repair itself.

Vitamin A Toxicity

It is difficult to ingest excessive doses of vitamin A from natural sources, as high concentrations of the vitamin are not present in typical foods. However, toxicity is possible in extreme situations, which I doubt any of us would be in. It has been reported that Arctic explorers ate polar bear or seal liver and that shortly after, some developed irritability, headaches, drowsiness, and even peeling of the skin, some with discoloration. No deaths were ever reported, and the condition rapidly disappeared after not eating the organs.[11] This does not even happen after eating cod liver, another naturally occurring food with a high concentration of vitamin A.

Vitamin A toxicity is related to manufactured high concentrations and synthetic forms that have been developed to treat skin conditions. Toxicity from these sources tend to stem from massive doses—in excess of 300,000 units—given to infants or children or from the ingestion of synthetic compounds of 13-cis-retinoic acid, also known as isotretinoin. **Isotretinoin** (Accutane) is used orally for the treatment of acne. Unfortunately, it promotes birth defects if the mother uses it during the fetal development stage of pregnancy.

Retin-A is the brand name of the topical form of tretinoin. It is used for topical peels of the facial skin to remove the older upper layer of skin, allowing the younger, deeper skin to come to the surface sooner, making the skin look younger. This is a harsh procedure: During the peeling process, the skin becomes red, inflamed, and tender as the older upper layer sloughs off. You certainly do not want to be seen in public during this stage of the process.

There are many derivatives of natural retinol, called ***retinoids***. The suffix *–oid* means "like" or "having a resemblance to." A retinoid has similar effects as retinol, but it is not retinol—and the effect of a retinoid is not the same as that of retinol. Your body will not metabolize it the same, and in the long term, you will not get the natural effect. A retinoid might have a less desirable outcome, may be toxic, or may even cause cancer.

Retinol has two natural derivatives: retinal and retinoic acid. These are three molecules that are not toxic at concentrations that are found in the body. I do not find any need for the synthetic

---

[11] Beers, M. H., and Berkow, R. (eds.), "Vitamin A," *The Merck Manual of Diagnosis and Therapy*, 17th edition, 1999, 35.

retinoids. Your body will have a tough time metabolizing them. Retinol will give you what you need without any inflammation, side effects, or unforeseen consequences.

To avoid overuse and overconsumption of vitamin A, many over-the-counter multivitamins contain little or no vitamin A and small amounts of provitamin A, known as carotenoids.

Vitamin A Deficiency

Fat-soluble vitamins act more like hormones than nutrients, so a deficiency of a fat-soluble vitamin is more serious than a deficiency of a water-soluble vitamin. Fat-soluble vitamins interact with the cell contents, and cells even have specific receptor sites for turning genes on and off. Therefore, optimal daily consumption is important!

Children who are deficient in vitamin A more frequently suffer from diarrhea, respiratory diseases, and measles. Severe infectious diseases are also more deadly with vitamin A deficiencies. The recommended dietary allowance (RDA) for children one to three years old is 1,000 units per day; for children four to eight years old, 1,333 units per day; and for adolescents and adults, 2,333 units per day.

Vitamin A deficiencies have three main causes, and understanding these causes can be helpful in investigating the reason for the deficiency and how one should go about correcting it. First, vitamin A deficiency can be caused by a lack of vitamin A or provitamin A (beta-carotene) in the diet. In the case of infants, being weaned too early may contribute to the problem. Second, deficiencies may be caused by too little to no absorption. Vitamin A is a fat and is best absorbed if it is first dissolved in oils such as animal fat or vegetable fat (for example, olive oil, coconut oil, or avocado oil). Vegans have trouble absorbing vitamin A by itself. If the biliary system is not functioning well and not putting out bile to dissolve fats, or the small intestine is impaired by a disease such as Crohn's disease or celiac disease or malabsorption of any type, the vitamin will not be taken in.

The third cause is when the provitamin, beta-carotene, can enter the body and be absorbed, but cannot be converted to retinol or vitamin A. There can be an abundance of beta-carotene and little to no conversion to retinol. This conversion is dependent on several factors, the first being an adequate amount of the enzyme 15-15'-dioxygenase to cleave one molecule of beta-carotene into two molecules of retinol. Refer to the molecular structure of beta-carotene and note where the arrow points to the bond to be broken. Not only must this enzyme be present, but other substances are necessary in sufficient amounts for the enzyme to function. Normal thyroid function is necessary to support the conversion, as are the proper levels of zinc and copper.

Healthy levels of vitamin A depend on enough of the vitamin or provitamin in the diet, absorption, and then conversion to retinol, retinal, and retinoic acid.

Vitamin A refers to a group of molecules that often function in similar reactions and fit the vitamin A receptors. This is interesting in that the body has receptors for a substance that is formed outside of it and that basically functions as a hormone. Vitamin D is another fat-soluble vitamin that is known to have receptors in many tissues, including the brain, and that influences depression and mood. Vitamin E and vitamin K are the two other fat-soluble vitamins that influence fertility, blood hemostasis, and bone growth. It is because of this that I have started to think of the fat-soluble vitamins as exogenous hormones. They are substances that stimulate specific cells and tissues to behave in particular ways. Hormones are the directors of cells, and they tell them how to behave. Without them, cells do as they want—they are uncoordinated, organ function and structure are lost, and, I believe, low hormone levels invite the development of cancer. I am not saying that a lack of vitamins causes cancer, but it does create an environment for it to develop.

Some of the carotenoid compounds can be converted to retinol easily, some with more effort, and some not at all. The easiest to convert is beta-carotene. Alpha-carotene and beta-cryptoxanthin produce less retinol in comparison to beta-carotene. Lutein and zeaxanthin remain as carotenoid forms of vitamin A and help prevent macular degeneration.

Measuring Vitamin A Levels

The evaluation of proper body stores of retinol is difficult. Vitamin A levels can be measured from two sources: blood and tissue. Blood levels are easily measured from a blood sample, but these measurements do not reflect the tissue levels, which are more important, as it is in the tissues where vitamin A has its effect. Vitamin A is stored mostly in the liver. Blood levels do not correlate with the liver levels. The best evaluation of storage levels is measuring the amount in the liver. However, this is impractical, as it requires a liver biopsy—a risky procedure. A large hypodermic needle must be inserted into the upper right abdomen and a sample of liver tissue extracted for assay. Bleeding is a possible complication, and infection another possibility.

Thus, blood level is the preferred measurement of vitamin A, but a more practical approach is evaluating the eye. When storage levels of vitamin A become low, all the indicators are ophthalmic. Presentations include dry eye, night blindness, delayed dark adaptation, Bitot's spots, and abnormal conjunctival cytology smears.[12] It is interesting that delayed dark adaptation is the best

---

[12] Tanumihardjo, S. A., "Assessing Vitamin A Status: Past, Present, and Future," *Journal of Nutrition*, 2004, *134*(1), 290S–293S, https://doi.org/10.1093/jn/134.1.290s.

predictor of macular degeneration. Bitot's spots are brownish discolorations of epithelial cell debris located in the conjunctiva that overlies the white of the eye. These are found during prolonged periods of low vitamin A levels.

Plasma retinol level	
Range	Measurement in micrograms per deciliter (mcg/dL)
Normal	20–50
Low	10–19
Deficient	<10

Zinc is required for the metabolism of vitamin A in its production from beta-carotene and the release of retinol from its storage form, retinyl palmitate, in the liver. Moreover, vitamin A helps in the absorption of iron in either oral or intravenous form. If there is difficulty in raising iron serum levels, consider adding 20,000 to 40,000 units of vitamin A daily.

Sources of Vitamin A

Natural versus Synthetic Vitamin A

With so many forms of vitamin A, which ones are the most suitable? Vitamin A occurs naturally preformed, as provitamins, and as synthetic vitamins that are formed in the laboratory and not found in nature. I do not recommend the latter. Preformed vitamins and provitamins are made by Mother Nature, and your body can metabolize them. Synthesized vitamins are made with commercial value in mind. If someone synthesizes a molecule that is not previously found in nature, this compound can be patented by the inventor or drug company and sold only by them for the length of the patent and one renewal. After that, it becomes a generic drug, and anyone can manufacture and sell it. Part of the task of the manufacturer of a new drug is to show that it is safe, effective, and nontoxic. Sometimes, altering the natural product or attaching a side chain to the molecule makes a new molecule. At other times, an entirely different structure is developed, but the effect it has may or may not be similar to the molecule it is replacing.

The making of new molecules to perform old functions is an excellent idea, and in the short term, they can demonstrate efficacy, safety, and nontoxicity. Unfortunately, the window that is being studied is often not long enough to reveal the deleterious effects of the new drug. It is not uncommon to have a drug on the market for many years, only to learn that after prolonged use, it is harmful. An example is Zantac. It was used for decades to treat hyperacidity that produced gastritis and peptic ulcers. After almost 40 years on the market, the FDA has called it a carcinogen. N-nitrosodimethylamine (NDMA), a breakdown product of Zantac (ranitidine), was found in Zantec capsules.[13]

One issue I have is that these new molecules never existed before. This new arrangement of atoms into a new molecule is new to Mother Nature. She has no method to metabolize this molecule and remove it from the body. The first and second metabolic products may accumulate to toxic levels, alter the natural chemistry, or effect genetic changes that do not appear until the next generation.

Vitamin A has been studied extensively because of its effect on epithelial cells, within which skin is classified. In looking for a

---

[13] Moncivais, K., "Current Status of the Zantac Recall," Consumer Safety, https://www.consumersafety.org/news/current-status-of-the-zantac-recall/, July 28, 2020.

substitute or more potent retinol, chemists have gone on to produce what are called second- and third-generation retinoids that have vitamin A biologic activity. The second-generation retinoids varied by chemical changes of the cyclic end group. The third-generation retinoids are chemicals that interact with the retinoid receptors. Their structures do not even resemble retinol, but they do affect the receptors.[14]

The effects may be chemical, structural, or multigenerational. The more the substituted chemical differs from Mother Nature, the riskier it is.

Vitamin A Supplements

Pure Encapsulations makes a capsule of 10,000 units (3,000 mcg) of vitamin A palmitate in Norwegian cod liver oil. This is a tiny gel capsule that is easy to swallow. For gastritis, stomach and duodenal ulcers, dry eyes, and vaginal dryness, take 10,000 to 50,000 units daily. For colds, flu, and respiratory infections, take the short-term protocol of

- 150,000 units of vitamin A on day one and then 50,000 units for the next two days,
- 2,000 mg of vitamin C twice a day, and
- 15,000 units of vitamin D_3 on the first day, followed by 10,000 units for the next two days.

Topical forms of retinol can be applied to the face. The Organic Pharmacy offers **Retinol Night Serum**, an encapsulated retinol of 2.5% concentration. It is a clear liquid that does not precipitate or layer out, and it has a nonoily base with a pleasant fragrance. It can be purchased directly from the Organic Pharmacy at

---

[14] Burkhart, C., Morell, D., and Goldsmith, L., "Retinoids," In Brunton, L., Chabner, B., and Knollman, B. (eds.), *Goodman & Gilman's the Pharmacological Basis of Therapeutics*, 12th edition, McGraw-Hill Medical, 2011, 1809.

www.theorganicpharmacy.com. Another purveyor of retinol is Julia Hunter, MD, with **Maximal Strength Vitamin A Plus**, which is in a vehicle that sometimes separates and needs to be shaken well prior to use.

Some multivitamin manufacturers are starting to include vitamin A in products. For example, Alive Adult Gummies by Nature's Way contains 5,000 units of vitamin A. Retinyl palmitate is usually a gelcap and is available from Solgar, Nature's Way, and Source Naturals. Neutrogena products also contain retinol, but it is accompanied by oils, solvents, and fragrances that you do not need in your body.

Retinyl palmitate is formed by the combination of two molecules, retinol and palmitic acid, to form an ester. An ester is formed by joining an alcohol and an acid together, with the removal of a water molecule in the process. The new molecule is usually more stable from oxidation and degradation than the alcohol. Another example is retinyl acetate. Retinyl palmitate is a stable preparation and is good for oral intake or topical application.

Dry vitamin A is a trade term that refers to the combination of vitamin A and beta-carotene. Often, you will see the description of "vitamin A as retinyl palmitate and beta-carotene" or "vitamin A as beta-carotene." The former is a mixture of an ester of retinol that must be released in the body to free up the retinol and a provitamin; the latter is not retinol, and the beta-carotene must be cleaved and converted to retinol. A direct source of retinol that does not need conversion is cod liver oil.

To clarify the distinctions between the products we are talking about, remember there are three natural forms of vitamin A: retinol, retinal, and retinoic acid. I do not recommend Retin-A or tretinoin. Both these forms are detrimental to health. Retin-A and tretinoin are synthetic forms of retinoic acid and are used primarily for skin application and skin peels. The words Retin-A and tretinoin usually denote synthetically produced retinoic acid that is used at concentrations of 100 to 10,000 times the strength that would be found in the body and naturally produced from retinol. These higher concentrations can burn the skin and cause structural damage. I do not recommend that anyone use either of these two preparations.

Vitamin B

Vitamin B1 (Thiamine)

Benefits of Thiamine

- Cure for beriberi
- Helps break down carbohydrates and produce energy
- Required for proper fetal development
- Treats some forms of dementia
- A long-forgotten nutrient related to heart failure and rhythm control
- An essential ingredient with other B vitamins for the treatment of neuropathies
- Prevents diabetic retinopathy
- Decreases nighttime bathroom trips
- Is essential to control sleep apnea
- Repairs the autonomic nervous system

History of Thiamine

Thiamine was reported to have been discovered in 1910, but the search for the cause of beriberi, a disease of peripheral neuropathy, started long before then. A general surgeon in the Japanese Navy, Dr. Takaki Kanehiro, in 1884 hypothesized that beriberi was due to dietary insufficiencies and not an unidentified germ, a theory that was popular in the 19th century. He removed white rice from the ship's diet to add vegetables, barley, milk, meat, and bread and incorrectly attributed the crew's improved health to increased protein. The Japanese Navy did not support the more expensive diet and rejected the concept for more than 20 years, despite continued death from beriberi. In 1905, it was demonstrated that the antiberiberi factor was washed away by removing the outer covering of the rice, a process referred to as polishing. In that outer layer of rice is the husk, the bran, the germ, and even a nutrient of the rice itself called **aleurone**, which is lost in the milling process. The remaining white rice is called the grain. Aleurone is an earlier name for a substance we now call thiamine. Dr. Takaki's effort was not forgotten. He was later given the honorary title of baron in Japan for his efforts.[15] He enjoyed the title of Barley Baron.

In 1897, another military doctor in the Dutch Indies (now known as Indonesia), Dr. Christiaan Eijkman, observed that chickens fed polished rice developed paralysis. He thought that the rice contained a carbohydrate that was toxic. The paralysis improved when the diet was changed. In 1901, his associate, Gerrit Grijns, put forward the idea that the removal of the polishings removed the nutrients from the diet, causing beriberi. Grijns had the concept right, but Eijkman received the Noble Prize in Physiology and Medicine in 1929 for the discovery of vitamins.[16]

Real progress was made in 1910 by Umetaro Suzuki, a Japanese chemist at the Tokyo Imperial University. He isolated a compound from rice bran that he initially named **aberic acid**. He claimed it had anti-beriberi action. Later, the name aberic acid was changed by Suzuki to **orizanin** to reflect its origin from rice bran. Suzuki is credited with the concept of vitamins—nutrients that the body cannot manufacture but must come from outside sources. Shortly thereafter in 1911, a Polish biochemist, Casimir Funk, also isolated from rice bran an **antineuritic** substance. Funk is credited with the development of the word **vitamin**. **Vita** refers to life, and the **amino**

---

[15] McCollum, E. V., *A History of Nutrition*, Houghton Mifflin, 1957.
[16] Carpenter, K. J., "The Nobel Prize and the Discovery of Vitamins," The Nobel Prize, June 22, 2004, https://www.nobelprize.org/prizes/themes/the-nobel-prize-and-the-discovery-of-vitamins/.

group within thiamine is essential for life or the essential amino group. Putting the words together, ***vita + amine***, resulted in **vitamine**. The *e* was dropped because not all vitamins contain the amino group, the example being vitamin C, which does not contain any amino groups.

Funk did not isolate the structure, but he knew it was in the husk of the rice. It took another 16 years before the team of Barend Coenraad Petrus Jansen and Willem Frederik Donath, two Dutch chemists, isolated and crystallized thiamine in 1926. The structure of thiamine was demonstrated by Robert Runnels Williams in 1934 and finally synthesized by Williams in 1936.

Overall, it took 53 years from 1884, from suspecting a nutrient deficiency to defining the defect, to produce the molecule that was responsible for beriberi.

Vitamin B1 (Thiamine) and Benfotiamine

The study of vitamins is a study of deficiencies. Vitamins are substances that, if lacking in one's diet, allow certain conditions to develop that are not compatible with life. Through the observation of dietary practices, foods eliminated, and foods that relieved diseases, the search for the active substance was found in the foods that restored health.

Thiamine, or Vitamin B_1

Thiamine is constructed of an aminopyrimidine, a six-member ring, and a thiazolium, a five-member ring joined with a carbon atom known as a methylene bridge. It is positively charged and usually presented as a chloride salt, -Cl⁻.

Benfotiamine

Benfotiamine is a synthetic molecule that can be easily absorbed and metabolized by the body into thiamine. It was developed in the 1950s in Japan. It was found not to have any toxicity and to be easily converted to thiamine, and unlike thiamine, it is fat soluble. It is considered a precursor to thiamine, but it is not a natural molecule. It is produced in the laboratory, and then the body converts it to thiamine.

Functions of Thiamine

Thiamine is concerned with the metabolism of carbohydrates. It is required as a cofactor to assist in the catabolism of sugars into the production of energy. This process of breaking down sugar to energy in plants and animals was identified and elucidated by chemists from 1897 to 1940. To give this process a cryptogenic name or the semblance of being based in antiquity, obscuring the understanding from most people, it was called ***glycolysis***.

Put two Greek words together—*glykys* (sweet) and *lysis* (dissolution or breakdown)—and then pronounce the new word by running the two words together. There you go! We lost half of the audience. I prefer to accent both the first two syllables and the last two syllables, pausing in the middle, allowing the listener to visualize the concept. It irks me to try and anglicize every word, only to lose the audience in the selection of pronunciation. I prefer ***glycol lysis***.

Thiamine, to be active, joins with other molecules, the most significant of which is phosphate. The two most important forms are **thiamine monophosphate (TMP)** and **thiamine diphosphate**, also called **thiamine pyrophosphate (TPP)**. For our discussion, thiamine is mostly inert until it is coupled with one or two phosphates. At that point, it can participate in the breakdown of carbohydrates and the production of **cellular energy (ATP)**.

Just for informational completeness, there are other forms of thiamine: thiamine triphosphate, adenosine thiamine diphosphate, and adenosine thiamine triphosphate. Does this sound like too much information? It is. I only present it for advanced students so that they are aware that I am simplifying the subject for my audience, my patients. The takeaway is that thiamine is essentially inert and must be activated to thiamine diphosphate to be of value.

Thiamine is not only needed for the metabolism of carbohydrates but also for the function of the brain, the heart, and the kidneys and the control of diabetes. It is helpful in alleviating sepsis. It touches many conditions of life, and more is being understood every day.

Newly Discovered Functions of Thiamine

It has been more than 100 years since the discovery of thiamine, and we are still discovering more about this vitamin. This book is not the final word on our knowledge of vitamins; instead, it is a record of what we know up to this point. Astute observers and doctors are still adding information to our knowledge of vitamins and minerals.

Recent advances in the effects of thiamine have taught us more about energy production, central and peripheral nervous systems, cardiac function, and intestinal function. But thiamine is the first vitamin, and it will not be the only vitamin, to demonstrate support and repair of the autonomic nervous system. The autonomic system monitors and controls functions in our bodies, such as regulating body temperature, sweating, breathing, digestion, and elimination. Together with other vitamins and minerals, medical conditions will be better understood and better treated as an appreciation and concern for the nutrition of the autonomic nervous system comes about.

In 2013, an Italian doctor, Antonio Costantini, published a case study with his coinvestigators about a 47-year-old man who had severe imbalance, slurred speech, high blood pressure, heart failure, sleep apnea, and depression.[17] He was treated with intramuscular injections of thiamine that reversed nearly all his problems despite him having normal thiamine levels prior to the injections. This man had many symptoms similar to those of Parkinson's disease, and many of these were reversed with high levels of thiamine. The daily requirement of thiamine is about 1 mg. The 100 mg dose that he received is certainly a high daily dose in quantity, but it was given intramuscularly, thus avoiding issues of absorption.

It was learned that even with a normal blood level of thiamine, thiamine must be transported across the blood-brain barrier with a transporter protein. If there is little to no transporter protein, thiamine will not reach the brain. The problem of no transporter molecule can be circumvented by giving large doses of thiamine,

---

[17] Costantini, A., et al., "High-Dose Thiamine as Initial Treatment for Parkinson's Disease," *BMJ Case Reports*, 2013, 1, https://doi.org/10.1136/bcr-2013-009289.

essentially flooding the brain with thiamine, and through diffusion, getting enough thiamine to the brain to return function.

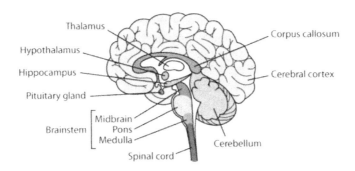

To this day, the diagnosis of Parkinson's disease is purely a clinical judgement call, with no laboratory blood analysis or imaging by X-ray or CT scan to confirm it. It is a condition of rapid aging from loss of dopamine, a brain chemical that promotes motor movement. It is characterized by the loss of facial expression, swallowing, and the ability to walk, tremors, slowness of movement, stiffness, and cognitive impairment. Dopamine is produced in the substantia nigra of the midbrain, and it supports motor movement. In Parkinson's disease, lower levels of thiamine are found in the midbrain, and in dementia, the frontal cortex of the brain that controls cognitive function is deficient of thiamine.

Relying on the blood level of thiamine to determine the vitamin's sufficiency is not a proper evaluation. Evaluating motor skills, physiologic functions, and cognition is more effective. It is apparent that brain tissue levels are more important than blood levels of thiamine when we are discussing issues that involve the brain. However, it is not practical to biopsy the brain for thiamine levels with these conditions, so the evaluation is best made by measuring performance following high-dose thiamine treatment.

Dr. Costantini demonstrated that there is selective neuronal damage in the centers that are typically involved with Parkinson's disease and that the injection of high doses of thiamine was effective in reversing symptoms.[18] Similarly, spinocerebellar ataxia type 2 with degeneration of the cerebellum, some brainstem areas, and the connections between the two partially responds to high-dose thiamine injections. Weekly intramuscular injections of 100 mg of thiamine improved fatigue initially, and three months later, improvement was observed in motor function.[19]

Benfotiamine is a synthetic, fat-soluble, oral form of vitamin B_1 that can pass through the blood-brain barrier, and once in the brain, it can break down into thiamine. This helps to avoid the need for high-dose injections of thiamine. A group of US and German scientists have found that benfotiamine can prevent diabetic retinopathy by blocking the formation of **advanced glycation of end products (AGEs)**.[20] This is the process during which high levels of sugar attach to proteins or nervous tissue, deteriorating its function and structure. This process causes retinal detachment, bleeding in the eye, and blindness.

Thiamine is critical to prevent and treat neuromuscular problems such as Parkinson's disease, diabetic retinopathy, and all forms of ataxia—that is, impaired coordination. Now that we are aware that thiamine can boost dopamine production in the substantia nigra in the early stages of Parkinson's disease and that high doses of thiamine (500 mg administered intravenously three times a day) are necessary to treat **Korsakoff's psychosis**, a dementia produced by alcohol abuse, it begs the question: Is what the medical literature refers to as nonalcoholic Korsakoff's psychosis any different from Alzheimer's disease?

The neurological problems of thiamine deficiency and Alzheimer's disease are similar, with cognitive deficits, reduced brain

---

[18] Costantini et al., "High-Dose Thiamine."
[19] Costantini, A., et al., "Thiamine Spinocerebellar Ataxia Type 2," *BMJ Case Reports*, 2013, 1, http://dx.doi.org/10.1136/bcr-2012-007302.
[20] Obrenovich, M. E, and Monnier, V. M., "Vitamin B1 Blocks Damage Caused by Hyperglycemia," *Science of Aging Knowledge Environment*, 2003, 10, PE6, https://doi.org/10.1126/sageke.2003.10.pe6.

glucose metabolism, memory deficits, neuritic plaques, and tau protein deposits on nerve tissue. Early treatment with thiamine reverses many of these problems, including plaque and tau formation, features formerly only associated to Alzheimer's disease.[21]

Benfotiamine is the best product to avoid cognitive decline within the brain. As a fat-soluble product, it freely permeates the blood-brain barrier. It can be taken orally in capsule or tablet form, and it breaks down into thiamine. It does not become an analog of thiamine—it becomes thiamine. Benfotiamine is also a safe product for Alzheimer's disease. It decreases beta-amyloid plaques, neurofibrillary tangles, oxidative stress, inflammation, and advanced glycation end products. Clinically, there is less cognitive decline.[22] The treatment dosage for any cerebral, cerebellar, brain stem, or midbrain deficiency, including the spinal cord and peripheral nerves, should be 400 mg per day. This may be given in a single dose or divided into 200 mg twice a day.

New information is showing that when many areas of the brain are deficient in thiamine, it presents as dementia, impaired coordination, and loss of bodily functions. I am sure that as we study the contribution of thiamine to the functions of the brain, many other conditions will be solved.

Frequent trips to the bathroom at night can be avoided with thiamine. It all starts in your head. The urge to urinate is an autonomic function coordinated in the **periaqueductal gray matter** of the mid brain, an area of the brain stem. The brain stem connects your brain to the spinal cord and is responsible for many

---

[21] Gibson, G. E., et al., "Vitamin B1 (Thiamine) and Dementia," *Annals of the New York Academy of Sciences*, 2016, *1367*(1), 21–30, https://doi.org/10.1111/nyas.13031.

[22] Gibson, G. E., et al., "Benfotiamine and Cognitive Decline in Alzheimer's Disease: Results of a Randomized Placebo-Controlled Phase IIa Clinical Trial," *Journal of Alzheimer's Disease*, 2020, *78*(3), 898–1010, https://doi.org/10.3233/jad-200896.

involuntary functions such as urinating, breathing, some involuntary portions of swallowing, peristaltic movement of the intestines, and the heartbeat. The periaqueductal gray matter is in the pons of the brain stem. It surrounds the aqueduct of Silvius that connects the third and fourth ventricles of the brain. Lateral to this is the **substantia nigra**, a structure whose function is also sensitive to thiamine deficiency. In fact, the functioning of many areas of the midbrain is dependent on adequate thiamine.

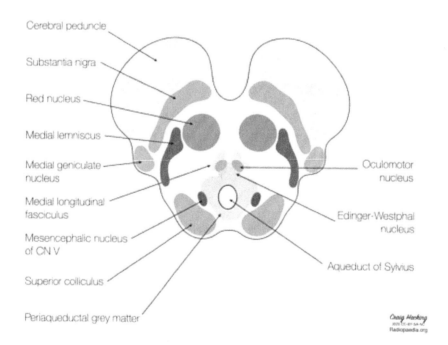

Midbrain (Case courtesy of Craig Hacking, Radiopaedia.org)

Voluntary micturition is controlled by the cerebral cortex communicating with the periaqueductal gray matter at the Pontine micturition center (PMC). The bladder wall has two sensors that can send signals of urgency to the PMC. The first sensor detects stretching of the bladder wall from the bladder filling with urine; the second sensor detects a high concentration of urine. The PMC shares this information with the cerebral cortex to make you aware of the situation, and then the PMC coordinates the release of urine at both the voluntary sphincter and the involuntary sphincter.

This all works well if there is sufficient thiamine in the periaqueductal gray matter and the PMC. Insufficient thiamine will cause poor coordination of urine retention or release, awareness or unawareness to void, and the most annoying symptom: having to void every two hours at night, only to pee one or two ounces. This interrupts sleep, increasing fatigue, and decreases mental acuity. Many drugs have been tried, and they have all failed because this is not a drug issue but a vitamin deficiency.

Remember, this is a deficiency of thiamin in the brain. Blood levels will most likely be normal. Replenishment of vitamin B_1 should be by intramuscular injection of 100 mg of thiamine once or twice a week, or benfotiamine, 200 to 400 mg a day orally.

The region of the midbrain, pons, and medulla oblongata is where many autonomic functions are controlled. It is a structure that requires thiamine to support its many chemical reactions. Breathing has four centers in the pons to monitor respirations and to control the diaphragm, accessory respiratory muscles, and the internal and external intercostal muscles between the ribs. The airway must remain open and unobstructed. The phrenic nerve is the only nerve that connects to the diaphragm, the major muscle of breathing. The hypoglossal nerve that elevates the soft palate and pushes the tongue forward originates from the medulla oblongata. If this nerve center is deprived of thiamine, a condition called sleep apnea develops.

Initially, a mechanical treatment was developed using a **CPAP** or **continuous positive airway pressure** machine to keep the airway open. This was followed by Inspire, a device that stimulates the hypoglossal nerve on one side to elevate the soft palate to keep the airway open. I suggest treating a malnourished brain stem with thiamine would be a more effective and natural approach to wellness.

Peripheral neuropathy is a common condition in the hands, but more frequent in the feet and legs, that presents with tingling, loss of sensation, numbness, loss of function, and pain. It is often found following chemotherapy and with severe diabetes, malnutrition, and alcohol use. Injury to the spine can also provoke peripheral neuropathy. This condition arises from damage to the axon or long arm of the nerve cell. The axons of fast-conducting nerves, such as nerves that carry information of touch and pressure, and nerves that activate skeletal muscles are covered with a myelin sheath.

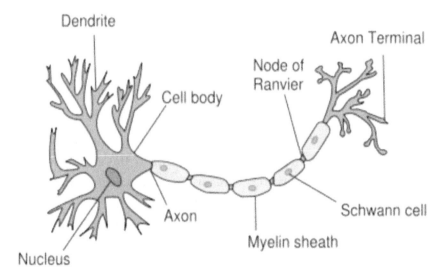

Structure of a Simplified Neuron in the Peripheral Nervous System (From "Anatomy and Physiology" by the US National Cancer Institute's Surveillance, Epidemiology and End Results [SEER] Program)

The myelin sheath is a lipid structure that surrounds the axon produced by the Schwann cell, permitting the nerve impulse to jump quickly along the axon, faster than an axon without the lipid covering. B vitamins are required to maintain the sheath and the nerve. The most important vitamin in this group is thiamine. It is necessary to repair and support the peripheral nerves. Proper repair of the nerve cell body and axon also requires additional nutrients, such as vitamins B_6 and B_{12} and alpha lipoic acid. Alpha lipoic acid is an antioxidant produced in the mitochondria that assists thiamine in converting glucose into energy, and it restores structure and function to nerve tissue.

A good starting point to treat peripheral neuropathy is with both forms of vitamin B_1: 100 mg of water-soluble thiamine, orally or by injection, and 400 mg of fat-soluble benfotiamine orally. Add to this 100 mg of pyridoxamine (B_6), 1,000 to 2,000 micrograms of cyanocobalamin (B_{12}), and 100 mg to 600 mg of alpha lipoic acid orally per day. A Myers's cocktail given once or twice a week would certainly have a strong effect on peripheral neuropathy and avoid issues of poor absorption of the vitamins.

Thiamine Deficiency

Causes of Thiamine Deficiency

In 1998, the Food and Nutrition Board of the Institute of Medicine presented the recommended dietary allowance (RDA) for thiamine as follows:

Recommended Dietary Allowance (RDA) for Thiamine			
Life stage	Age	Male (mg/day)	Female (mg/day)
Infant	0–6 months	0.2	0.2
	7–12 months	0.3	0.3
Child	1–3 years	0.5	0.5
	4–8 years	0.6	0.6
	9–13 years	0.9	0.9
Adolescent	14–18 years	1.2	1.0
Adult	19 years and older	1.2	1.1
Pregnant	All ages	–	1.4
Breastfeeding	All ages	–	1.4

Thiamine deficiency starts with inadequate intake, the body's increased consumption of thiamine, excessive loss of thiamine, and the consumption or neutralization of thiamine from food or immunologic factors. The RDA is not very high, but if diet is a poor source of thiamine or the diet is high in carbohydrates, this will develop into a deficiency. Interestingly, the priority of thiamine is the fetus or the nursing infant. In a pregnant or nursing mother, thiamine will go to the baby even if it means that the mother develops a deficiency. Thiamine is necessary for the developing nervous system and cardiovascular system.

General plant-based sources of thiamine include black beans, lentils, green peas, acorn squash, cauliflower, and asparagus; protein-based sources include eggs, brewer's yeast, trout, pork products, and mussels. Processed foods such as breakfast cereals, commercial bread, macaroni, and cakes are also fortified with thiamine. All these foods contain about 1 mg per serving, and according to the table above, this is about what is needed daily.

Thiamin supplements are usually available as tablets and capsules of 50 mg, 100 mg, and 200 mg. B-complex formulations generally contain 50 mg or 100 mg of thiamine in addition to the other B vitamins.

Inadequate thiamine intake is a source of deficiency, especially in low-income populations that have diets high in carbohydrates. Women who are breastfeeding and have a thiamine deficiency may pass on the deficiency to their infants. People with alcohol use disorder may not eat properly or eat too little, and excessive alcohol consumption with a higher fluid intake will wash away what little thiamine is available in the diet of a person with alcohol use disorder. Those who suffer from anorexia nervosa or who have had bariatric surgery may also eat too little, leading to thiamine deficiency. Patients with malabsorption, those with severe vomiting during pregnancy, and those receiving intravenous nutrition after undergoing bowel surgery may not be provided with enough thiamine. People with alcohol use disorder also develop impaired intestinal absorption of thiamine.

Deficiencies can also occur because of increases in thiamine utilization. For example, the body's consumption of thiamine increases with fever, adolescent growth spurts, increased physical activity, pregnancy, and breastfeeding.

Excessive thiamine loss is a major cause of deficiency. This can happen when a person's attention is diverted to other problems. It can insidiously creep into their health during the treatment of hypertension, kidney disease, diabetes, or Alzheimer's disease. Thiamine deficiency may not be present when they started treatment for these problems, but over time, neuropathies, heart failure, cardiac rhythm abnormalities, and poor blood glucose control develops during the course of treatment. I stress that in this modern age of medical interventions, this is more likely to be the cause of thiamine deficiency than inadequate intake or decreased consumption of thiamine.

Diuretics for the treatment of fluid retention, hypertension, and heart failure prevent the reabsorption of thiamine in the kidneys. Hemodialysis, a treatment for renal insufficiency or kidney failure, removes too much thiamine in the process of cleansing the blood. Furthermore, diabetic medications have a major effect on thiamine deficiency. All **three forms of diabetes, type 1, type 2**, and **gestational diabetes**, exacerbate the loss of thiamine, and low thiamine levels have a deleterious effect on diabetes. This opens the door for neuropathies, mental deficiencies, poor carbohydrate handling, heart failure, and vascular issues.

All these problems are considered part of the diabetic presentation, but I say they are provoked by the loss of thiamine due to diabetes. If this is true, these secondary diabetic issues can be correctable with additional thiamine. In fact, I have noticed a significant improvement in my diabetic patients due to the Myers's cocktail that I administer in my office. They do not develop the secondary issues as readily as the general diabetic population. The Myers's cocktail provides 100 mg of thiamine intravenously with magnesium, B_5, B_6, B_{12}, and vitamin C.

Excessive thiamine loss is a modern-day problem, often unrecognized and contributing to the initial problems, insidiously, over time. The normal serum range of thiamine is 2.7–13.3 nanograms per milliliter (ng/ml).[23]

Anti-thiamine factors **(ATF)** are substances in foods that react with thiamine to oxidize it and make it inactive. In this situation, the best course of action is to not measure the thiamine but to measure the **transketolase enzyme**, a product of thiamine that decreases early in thiamine deficiency. Examples of anti-thiamine factors are coffee, tea, decaffeinated drinks, and some raw fish. Many of the ATFs in fish are destroyed by the process of cooking.

Some drugs that cause excessive thiamine loss are diuretics, furosemide (Lasix), hydrochlorothiazide, diabetic medication (metformin), antiulcer medications, famotidine (Pepcid), fluroquinolone antibiotics (Levaqiun, Cipro, and Avelox), anticonvulsive medications (Dilantin), birth control pills, and cardiac glycosides of digoxin (Lanoxin). The binge drinking of alcohol also causes excessive thiamine loss.[24]

Symptoms that may develop with a thiamine deficiency are confusion, a staggering walk called ataxia, ophthalmoplegia presenting as an inability to focus the eye or uncontrolled horizontal or vertical rapid eye movements, seizures, papilledema or swelling in the back of the eye causing double vision in one eye, short-term memory loss, a fast heart rate (called tachycardia), mood changes, shortness of breath, and sensory-motor neuropathy with numbness or poor movement in the extremities. Any of these symptoms can develop from reduced thiamine from the drugs you take for other conditions that you are treating. You may feel that your condition is worsening—and it is, from the medications you are taking for

---

[23] BioReference Laboratories, Inc., May 2022.
[24] Arthur, M., "12 Signs You Might Have a Thiamine Deficiency," Baylor Scott & White Health, October 7, 2019, https://www.bswhealth.com/blog/12-signs-you-might-have-a-thiamine-deficiency.

hypertension, heart failure, diabetes, seizures, and kidney failure. And I did not even mention the most dangerous class of drugs: chemotherapy. The most common chemotherapeutic agent that removes thiamine is 5-fluorouracil (Adrucil).

If any of these symptoms sound familiar to you, either on or off these drugs, have your thiamine level tested. I would start with the blood-level test, and even if that is normal and the symptoms continue, start a therapeutic trial of 100 mg of thiamine or B-complex 100 daily, and monitor yourself for improvement. It has been my experience that injectable thiamine works best.

Classic Presentations of Thiamine Deficiency

Historically, thiamine deficiency presented as beriberi, Wernicke–Korsakoff syndrome, excessive alcohol consumption, complications of diabetes, and, recently, Alzheimer's disease.

Beriberi has two distinct and sometimes overlapping presentations related to the nervous system and the cardiovascular system. The effects on the nervous system start in the peripheral nerves with a sense of heaviness and weakness, progressing to hypersensitivity or numbness, and resulting in aching and burning. This can progress to loss of muscle strength to the point of foot drop or wrist drop. Usually, the lower extremities are affected first and then the symptoms progress to the upper extremities. Cardiovascular symptoms start with shortness of breath on exertion, rapid rhythm, palpitations, bounding pulses, enlarged heart, and high-output cardiac failure because the arteries are significantly dilated, offering little resistance to blood flow. The EKG shows inversion of the T wave and prolongation of the Q-T interval—in short, severe heart failure that can be fatal. A third form of beriberi involves the intestinal tract, with symptoms of nausea, vomiting, and severe abdominal pain caused by enzymes lacking thiamine and causing the buildup of pyruvic acid and lactic acid, a condition called lactic acidosis.

In the brain, there is a two-stage mental incapacity related to a low thiamine level and alcohol abuse. The initial stage is Wernicke's encephalopathy, characterized by abnormal eye movement, abnormal gait, and cognitive impairment. The second stage is called Korsakoff's dementia, which is characterized by amnesia, confabulation, and loss of recent memory. If both conditions occur together, it is referred to as Wernicke–Korsakoff syndrome or cerebral beriberi.

Recent studies on dementia have shown a deficiency in the brain of thiamine in its two active forms: thiamine monophosphate and thiamine diphosphate. The deficiency of thiamine is found in several types of dementias—Korsakoff's and Alzheimer's dementia—that are clinically indistinguishable from diabetic dementia. Perhaps the commonality of these dementias is that they all have demonstrated low thiamine diphosphate and reduced glucose metabolism, which can be seen on a **positron-emission tomography (PET)** scan.

Using PET scanning, Langbaum and his group showed that brain glucose utilization can predict the progression of normal to mild cognitive impairment (MCI) to Alzheimer's over a nine-year period. His study consisted of 882 participants over the age of 55: 229 healthy people, 405 with mild cognitive impairment, and 188 with mild Alzheimer's disease.[25]

Remember that the only source of energy for the brain and peripheral nerves is glucose. But how does this glucose become available to the brain and peripheral nerves? Thiamine must be available in the nervous tissue to supply glucose from food. Thiamine is necessary to correct all neurologic problems. It is necessary for treating multiple sclerosis, dementia, neuropathy, seizure, spasm, autonomic dysfunction, uncontrolled micturition,

---

[25] Langbaum, J. B., et al., "Categorical and Correlational Analysis of Baseline Fluorodeoxyglucose Positron Emission Tomography Images from the Alzheimer's Disease Neuroimaging Initiative (ADNI)," *Neuroimaging*, 2009, *45*(4), 1107–1116.

and sleep apnea. For thiamine to be effective, it must get into the brain. A normal blood level does not indicate sufficient thiamine in the brain or nervous tissue.

Thiamine Supplements

Thiamine is produced as tablets, capsules, liquids, and sterile injectable preparations for intermuscular and intravenous administration. The manufactured injectable preparations are produced with a preservative. Compounding pharmacies produce injectables with no preservatives, but they usually have a short shelf life.

Thiamine is readily available over the counter and does not require a prescription. Only the injectable form requires a prescription. Most major brands of supplements supply thiamine in 50 mg, 100 mg, 200 mg, and 500 mg tablets and capsules. I prefer capsules because some manufacturers stamp out or compress the tablets during manufacture with so much pressure that it is difficult to dissolve the tablet.

Another source of thiamine is B complex. Thiamine is packaged in the same capsule with other B vitamins such as vitamins B_2, B_3, B_5, B_6, B_9 (folate), and B_{12}. The vitamins work better together and are usually sold as B-50 or B-100. B-50 means 50 mg each of B_1, B_2, B_3, and so on; B-100 means 100 mg each of B_1, B_2, B_3, and so on. Folate may be 400 micrograms, and B_{12} may be 500 to 1,000 micrograms. This helps to reduce the number of pills to take daily.

Recently, the FDA has stopped the manufacture of injectable forms of thiamine by compounding pharmacies if a similar product is available from commercial producers. It gets worse. The FDA has at the same time put limitations on how much thiamine can be produced through one regulation or another. This has caused a shortage of thiamine, and suppliers have limited amounts to sell. Currently, in 2022, injectable thiamine is sold on allocation, meaning you can buy only a fraction of the amount you need per week or month. This is not a supply chain problem but has been caused by the government stopping the manufacture and distribution of a vitamin. This vitamin is neither toxic nor dangerous but helps avoid or treat short-term problems such as sepsis and Korsakoff's dementia and long-term problems such as heart failure and diabetes. Who is the FDA serving with actions like this? Certainly not the American people. I believe the FDA is attempting to limit the use of the Marik protocol—intravenous vitamin C, hydrocortisone, and thiamine for septic shock—favoring the more expensive Big Pharma–patented drugs.[26]

The fat-soluble form of B_1 is benfotiamine. It passes through the fatty cell walls of the body before it is converted to thiamine, and it can pass through the blood-brain barrier, giving it easy access to the brain. It might be a better form of thiamine to treat Alzheimer's. It is sold in tablets and capsules. Life Extension sells it in capsules of 100 mg of benfotiamine with 25 mg of thiamine, or a larger size of 300 mg of benfotiamine with 10 mg of thiamine. Swanson sells capsules that contain 300 mg of benfotiamine with 40 mg of leucine. The vitamins and amino acids have been added to ensure that each formulation is unique so that the formula does not infringe on those of similar manufacturers. PureBulk sells both gel caps and veggie caps of 200 mg and in powder form in bags of 50 mg, 100 mg, 250 mg, 500 mg, and 1 kg. The oral forms are readily available for purchase; the intravenous form is much less widely available.

Thiamine and benfotiamine are also found in multivitamins and prenatal preparations. Foods are fortified with thiamine. It is difficult to avoid it. But poor food and lifestyle choices, various medical conditions, and personal behavior can cause a thiamine deficiency. You are responsible for your own health.

---

[26] See "The Semmelweis Reflex" in the chapter on vitamin C.

Vitamin B2 (Riboflavin)

Benefits of Riboflavin

- Prevents or delays the development of cataracts
- Reduces the severity and development of migraine headaches
- Improves the skin blemishes associated with rosacea
- Reduces preeclampsia in pregnancy
- Found with lower levels of homocysteine
- Enhances iron absorption in iron-deficiency anemia

History of Riboflavin

Riboflavin was the second B vitamin to be discovered, earning it the designation of B_2. It was first seen under the microscope in 1872 as a florescent yellow-green substance in milk called **lactochrome** by the English chemist Alexander Wynter Blyth. It was eventually referred to as **lactoflavin**, and American chemists called it vitamin G but then adopted the English designation of B_2. Sixty years later, lactochrome was identified as **riboflavin**.

Riboflavin

Functions of Riboflavin

In conjunction with other B vitamins, riboflavin helps transform proteins, carbohydrates, and fats into energy. The most abundant source of riboflavin is milk and milk products such as cheese and yogurt. Lower amounts are found in liver, beef, fish, mushrooms, and eggs. It does directly help with some health issues such as eye health, pregnancy, skin conditions, iron-deficiency anemia, and migraine headaches.

The most important function of riboflavin is that it is converted to the coenzymes **flavin adenine dinucleotide (FAD)** and **flavin mononucleotide (FMN).** These coenzymes are involved with oxidation-reduction, or redox, reactions—transferring electrons by attaching or removing molecular groups to another molecule. The subject of coenzymes and metabolism by riboflavin is much deeper than needs to be discussed in this book, so I will focus on the benefits of riboflavin and how it can be utilized for better health.

Riboflavin also plays an important role in the metabolism of drugs and toxins and in protecting us from oxidative stress. It helps by lowering homocysteine by converting it to methionine. It enhances both iron and folic acid absorption. It aids in the conversion of B_6 pyridoxine, transforming the inactive form of B_6 to the active form, pyridoxine 5'- phosphate, and tryptophan to niacin.

Regeneration of Glutathione

Glutathione is an antioxidant that is produced in the liver, and it has the ability to remove metabolic waste products from the body and the brain. The first evidence of this is in acute bronchitis and pneumonia. The sputum will become yellow, and as the situation worsens, it becomes green in color. This green coloring is from the glutathione as it helps to remove waste products. It not only is an antioxidant but can also detox the body of some organic free radicals and metals.

My experience is primarily with Parkinson's disease. Glutathione improves fluid movement of the extremities, promotes higher levels of energy, and stimulates better facial expressions. I generally inject a 3 g solution, intravenously, as a show push. You can expect the best outcome when the injection causes the person to become sleepy or fall asleep, usually for about five minutes. There is no loss of blood pressure, pulse, or respirations. If the person falls asleep, this is a good predictor that metabolic waste products are being pulled from the brain and that you will see clinical improvement. With continued injections, you will see little to no sleeping and more clinical improvement.

Glutathione consists of three amino acids: glycine, cysteine, and glutamic acid. As an antioxidant, it is consumed in reactions with other substances, but it can be regenerated to its antioxidant potential with riboflavin.

The production of glutathione falls with age. The lower the glutathione level is in age-matched patients, the more prevalent cataract formation becomes.[27] This is not the only cause of cataracts, but it appears as significant as a robust vitamin C level in cataract prevention.

Homocysteine Levels and Hypertension

Elevated levels of homocysteine have been related to cardiovascular disease, specifically the buildup of plaque on arterial walls. The usual treatment to convert homocysteine to methionine was to add a methyl **group (-CH$_3$)** to homocysteine. This is usually treated by giving a combination of vitamins: B$_{12}$, folic acid, and pyridoxine (i.e., B$_6$).

Some patients are resistant to this vitamin treatment, and their homocysteine levels do not drop below 10.0. Recently, it has been learned that a genotype that affects up to 26% of people with

---

[27]. Leske, M.C., et al., "Biochemical Factors in Lens Opacities. Case-Control Study," *Archives of Ophthalmology*, 1995, *113*(9), 1113–1119.

European ancestry could be the cause. People with this genotype do not have **5-methyltetrahydrofolate (5-MTHF)**, which is necessary for the methylation of homocysteine to methionine. The **homozygous genotype MTHFR 677TT**, 5,10-methylenetetrahydrofolate can be assisted with riboflavin as a cofactor to convert it to 5-MTHF, reducing the homocysteine level and cardiovascular disease. The results of the JINGO Project indicate that the homozygous genotype of MTHFR 667TT contributes to 12% of all persons with hypertension.[28]

Migraine Headaches

Migraine headaches are characterized by pain and a throbbing or pounding sensation on one side of the head, accompanied by nausea, vomiting, or sensitivity to light or sounds. They generally occur several times a month. They are preceded by hormonal changes, and menstruation, excessive fatigue, exercise, stress, and even certain smells can provoke a migraine headache. Traditionally, treatment has been to place the patient in a quiet, darkened room and to avoid unnecessary stimulation. Medications used to manage pain include aspirin and ibuprofen, escalating to sumatriptan (Imitrex) and even controlled substances.

Fortunately, the management of migraine headaches has turned to prevention to avoid having headaches or to lower their frequency. Riboflavin does not completely eliminate migraines, but a dose of 400 mg daily can reduce the intensity of the pain and the frequency of the headaches.[29] Riboflavin is a vitamin, not a prescription drug, so it is readily available to anyone from the local vitamin store. It is essentially nontoxic, very tolerable, and cheap. It can be found in

---

[28] Ward, M., et al., "Impact of the Common MTHFR 677C→T Polymorphism on Blood Pressure in Adulthood and Role of Riboflavin in Modifying the Genetic Risk of Hypertension: Evidence from the JINGO Project," *BMC Medicine*, 2020, *18*(31), https://doi.org/10.1186/s12916-020-01780-x.

[29] Schoenen, J., Jacquy, J., and Lenaerts, M., "Effectiveness of High-Dose Riboflavin in Migraine Prophylaxis. A Randomized Controlled Trial," *Neurology*, 1998, *50*(2), 466–470, https://doi.org/10.1212/wnl.50.2.466.

tablets or capsules of 25 mg, 50 mg, 100 mg, and 400 mg. Because the daily dosage is 400 mg, if only 100 mg capsules can be found, four capsules should be taken daily.

Riboflavin Deficiency

There is no classical disease or poor health condition that is emblematic of riboflavin deficiency. Riboflavin fulfills a supportive role for the other B vitamins. Low riboflavin levels may lead to dandruff, skin lesions and cracks in the corners of the mouth, an inflamed tongue and swollen throat and mouth, sensitivity to light, hormonal imbalance, and nerve degeneration that produces tingling, pain, fatigue, and numbness, but other vitamin deficiencies also produce these symptoms. It is supportive of the epithelial tissues of the skin, eye, and mucous membranes, but its effect is not as pronounced as that of vitamin A.

An association between low riboflavin and preeclampsia, also called toxemia of pregnancy, and eclampsia has been shown, but riboflavin does not correct it, again showing it plays a supportive role rather than the lead role.

Riboflavin, even at low doses, will give a yellow color to the urine that is not harmful, even though the color may be quite intense and bright. The table below lists the recommended dietary allowance, as per the Food and Nutrition Board of the Institute of Medicine.[30]

---

[30] Food and Nutrition Board, Institute of Medicine, "Riboflavin," 1998, 87–122.

Recommended Dietary Allowance (RDA) for Riboflavin			
Life stage	Age	Male (mg/day)	Female (mg/day)
Infant	0–6 months	0.3	0.3
	7–12 months	0.4	0.4
Child	1–3 years	0.5	0.5
	4–8 years	0.6	0.6
	9–13 years	0.9	0.9
Adolescent	14–18 years	1.3	1.0
Adult	19 years and older	1.3	1.1
Pregnant	All ages	–	1.4
Breastfeeding	All ages	–	1.6

Conditions and Drugs That Limit the Absorption of Riboflavin

Conditions that limit the absorption of riboflavin are primarily gut issues: celiac disease, Crohn's disease, ulcerative colitis, and inflammatory bowel disease. Additional inhibitors of absorption include kidney disease, rheumatoid arthritis, and alcohol use.

Drugs that limit riboflavin absorption include the following:

- Sulfa drugs, specifically trimethoprim-sulfamethoxazole, sold under the brand names Bactrim and Septra; sulfasalazine (Azulfidine and Sulfazine); and sulfonamide antibiotics (Gantrisin)[31]
- The antibiotic group of macrolides, namely azithromycin and erythromycin
- Penicillin derivatives such as amoxicillin and clavulanate
- The quinolone group, namely ciprofloxacin and levofloxacin
- The tetracycline group, namely doxycycline, minocycline, and tetracycline.
- Cephalosporins
- Tricyclic antidepressants
- Birth control medications
- Psychotherapeutic medications

Riboflavin Supplements

Riboflavin can be bought as an individual vitamin in dosages of 25 mg, 50 mg, 100 mg, and 400 mg from producers such as NOW Foods, Solgar, Nature's Bounty, and Biotech Pharmaceutical. Riboflavin is also sold in the active form that does not have to be converted in your body to **riboflavin 5'-phosphate (R5P).**

---

[31] Complementary and Alternative Medicine, St. Luke's Hospital, Chesterfield, MO, 2022.

Vendors of the active form are Thorne, Natural Factors, and Swanson. Swanson sells the molecule riboflavin, the active molecule of R5P, and the activated molecule R5P in a B-complex formulation. These are forms that might be useful for migraine headaches and restoring glutathione.

For general health, remember that vitamin B_2 is also a component of the B-complex formulation. Considering that the eight B vitamins work together to produce energy and convert homocysteine to methionine, the best choice would be a B-complex supplement. B-complex formulations contain B_1 (thiamine), B_2 (riboflavin), B_3 (niacin, or forms of it), B_5 (pantothenic acid), B_6 (pyridoxine), B_7 (biotin), B_9 (folic acid), and B_{12} (cobalamin). This combination holds many benefits, such as promoting cell health, red blood cell growth, energy, vision, brain health, digestion, appetite, nerve function, cholesterol and hormone production, cardiovascular health, and muscular health.

Vitamin B3 (Niacin)

Benefits of Vitamin B$_3$

- Lowers cholesterol
- Moderates arthritis, asthma, diabetes, heart disease, stress, and stroke
- Is an antiaging nutrient
- Treats pellagra (rough skin)
- Reduces the pain of arthritis
- Reduces the risk for cancer and inhibits cancer growth
- Detoxes silicone after exposure to leaky breast implants
- May help to avoid glaucoma

History of Niacin

Niacin, one of the molecules of vitamin B$_3$, is also known as **nicotinic acid, nicotinate,** and **pyridine-3-carboxylic acid**. It was the third B vitamin to be discovered, giving it the B$_3$ designation. Previously, in America, it was designated as vitamin G, but that designation was dropped for the British designation of B$_3$. Today, it is famous for its cholesterol-lowering effect.

Most of the B vitamins are involved with energy production, as well as catabolic and anabolic activity. The feature that brought niacin to vitamin classification was that it prevented death from pellagra. The story of niacin is about pellagra.

Pelle agra means "rough skin" in Italian. This term was first used by Frappoli in 1771, as he was studying the development of rough brown or red patches of skin that developed around the neck, known as Casal's necklace, with sharp margins on the sun-exposed areas of the arms and dorsum of the hands. This is not a minor rash, but one that is angry looking with significantly dry, sharp demarcations and patches that would separate from the deeper skin. For centuries, the condition was lethal and frequently mistaken for leprosy.

The condition was first recorded in Spain in 1735, by Gasper Casal y Julian. It is characterized by the four Ds: dermatitis, diarrhea, dementia, and death. It was endemic in Southern Europe until the early 1900s. In Italy, Dr. Gaetano Strambio established a hospital for treating *pellagrins* in Legnago, Italy, and authored a three-volume work, *De Pellagra* (1786–1789), describing his findings. He believed pellagra was caused by spoiled bread and polenta. Cesare Lombroso proposed the possibility of toxins from rotten maize. It was neither.

Pellagra was not limited to Europe. It appeared in the United States in 1912, in Spartanburg, South Carolina. By that time, 30,000 cases of pellagra had been recorded, and 40% of them would be lethal. In America, too, the privately endowed Thompson-McFadden Pellagra Commission erroneously thought it was an infectious disease.

A fresh look was necessary to investigate the etiology of pellagra, and the US Public Health Service, at the direction of the surgeon general, sent one of its own physicians, Dr. Joseph Goldberger, to investigate. Dr. Goldberger developed a reputation as an epidemiologist through his previous work on yellow fever, typhus, dengue fever, and typhoid. His experience with infectious diseases led him to observe that in mental hospitals and orphanages, the disease did not spread from the patients or the children to adult staffers. Instead, the disease was limited to the inmates and children, who ate a different, more limited, diet than the staff. Dr. Goldberger, as an officer of the Public Health Service, was able to order better quality food from the federal government. This was done to improve the quality of the food, which previously was limited to small amounts of animal protein, corn, and protein foods: milk, eggs, beans, and peas. This experiment was controversial, if not insulting to the people of Louisiana, Mississippi, and North Carolina, as it implied that the diets of the South were insufficient.

In three to six months, he was able to reduce the incidence of pellagra. He conducted the studies repeatedly over two years in both psychiatric hospitals and orphanages. Each time, the analysis pointed to a deficiency. He eventually knew what foods were missing, but the exact substance, niacin, would not be isolated and defined for another 20 years.

Functions of Niacin

Niacin is another name for **nicotinic acid**, invented to avoid confusion with **nicotine** found in tobacco. Someone not accustomed to reading names of chemical substances or hearing the pronunciation of two similar-sounding words may not discern accurately between the two chemicals.

Niacin, or Nicotinic Acid

Niacin is the first form of vitamin B_3 that comes to mind, and often the only one most people know. This compound, when taken orally, sometimes as a dose as low as 100 mg, may cause uncomfortable flushing, redness of the skin, and burning from capillary dilatation as it brings the internal heat of the body to the surface with the release of histamine. This is also the first chemical known to lower total cholesterol and raise high-density lipid (HDL) cholesterol. There are other effective forms of B_3 that do not have such uncomfortable side effects.

Nicotinamide, or Niacinamide

Nicotinamide is also known as **niacinamide**. It is like niacin in that it has the same pyridine ring—the six-member ring where one of the carbons is replaced with nitrogen—but the carboxyl group (COOH) on the right side of the molecule is replaced with the amide (COH_2N) side chain, so ingesting it causes no uncomfortable symptoms. It performs many of the same reactions as niacin, yet it has a few uncomfortable characteristics of its own.

This form of vitamin B_3 is attracting more attention because of its antiaging properties. Nicotinamide promotes longevity by affecting a gene through the production of silent information regulator 2 (Sir2). Sir2 then increases silent information regulator 2 protein (Sir2p), which increases cell longevity. It controls the rate of cell aging by regulating the production of genetic waste material and the accumulation of genetic waste, and it ages the cell. Nicotinamide is now considered a first-line antiaging vitamin. This vitamin will become part of **nicotinamide adenine dinucleotide (NAD)**, which participates in over 400 reactions related to the metabolism of food, the production of energy, and the building of anatomical structures and regulates metabolism and energy.

Inositol nicotinate, also known more precisely as **inositol hexanicotinate**, is a sugar carbohydrate with six niacin molecules attached. This product is constructed first with the central wheel of inositol, and then an ester is formed by combining the –OH portion of the hydroxyl group and the carboxyl acid, COOH, to join the two molecules and producing water, H_2O, as a by-product in the process. This inositol nicotinate can deliver six molecules of niacin into the body slowly, as the niacin molecules are released over time without the harsh symptoms of plain niacin that is reactive in the tissues when it is delivered in the raw state.

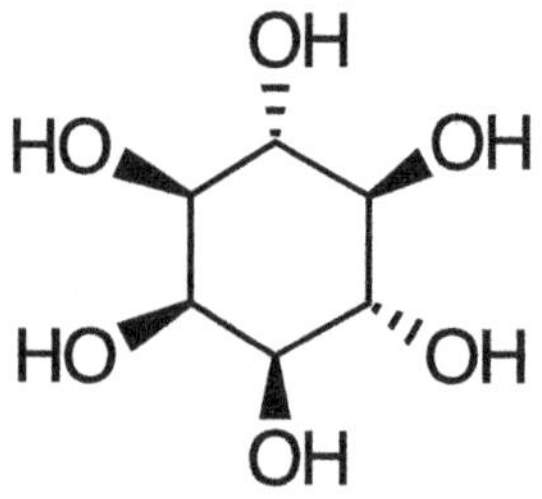

Inositol

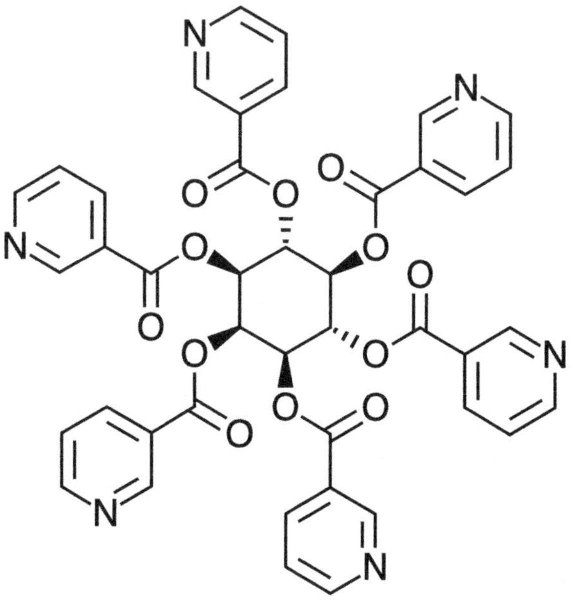

Inositol Hexanicotinate

Inositol nicotinate will dilate small arterioles and capillaries, but it has less of an effect on cholesterol levels than niacin does. It is also known as no-flush niacin and has been described as sustained release, timed release, and extended release. Different purveyors of niacin liberally use these terms, having different definitions of what they mean. These terms may refer to attaching other molecules, or radicals, to the niacin molecule or to the physical packaging of the niacin. The latter includes placing it in a wax matrix that is difficult to digest, thus slowly liberating the niacin, or in a nondissolvable plastic capsule with a microscopic hole so that the product can slowly ooze out over time to lessen the flush that occurs from niacin. No two manufacturers use the same terms to describe what they sell. The one thing that is clear is that the release forms are all confusing.

Big Pharma introduced a new invention that contains niacin and, reportedly, inactive ingredients: Niaspan. It contained, in addition to niacin, hypromellose, polyethylene glycol, fillers, and coloring compounds. It had many contraindications, including kidney disease, angina, stomach ulcers, diabetes, gout, conflicting with statin drugs, and muscle disorders. It provoked many symptoms, such as severe flushing, upset stomach, muscle cramps, shortness of breath, light-headedness, dizziness, and liver toxicity. It was around for a few years, but the short-acting form was discontinued on June 30, 2017. This was not a safe product, nor very effective. It was a failed attempt to commercially repackage niacin.

There are many molecules known as B_3, but our attention will be on the three significant molecules: niacin, the new name for nicotinic acid; nicotinamide, also called niacinamide; and inositol nicotinate, or inositol hexanicotinate.

Niacin is concerned with the basic metabolism of the body. It is directly involved with the production of energy from oxidative and reductive, or redox, reactions. These redox reactions either accept or donate electrons. This is performed by niacin becoming part of coenzymes that facilitate either catabolic or anabolic reactions. The catabolic reactions start with macronutrients such as proteins, fats, and carbohydrates, converting them to simple molecules of carbon dioxide, urea, ammonia, amino acids, nitrogenous bases, sugars, and fatty acids. The anabolic reactions start with small molecules such as nitrogenous bases, sugars, fatty acids, ammonia, and urea, producing larger molecules of proteins, fats, polysaccharides, and nucleic acids.

The **coenzymes of niacin** are involved with **nicotinamide adenine dinucleotide (NAD)**. NAD works with the help of **NADH**, the reduced form; **NADP**, the phosphorylated form; and **NADPH**, the reduced phosphorylated form. Nicotinamide is integral to all these enzymes, and without it, there could be no life. It is a molecule that is necessary but needed in only small amounts. It is reused in the process and not consumed to any great extent. It can be converted to niacin, but niacin cannot be converted to nicotinamide. This molecule has the ability to improve diabetes, reduce stress and anxiety, reduce stroke size, inhibit cancer, promote longevity, and calm inflammation of arthritis. In the skin it helps build collagen; this causes lightening of the skin and better regulates sebaceous gland output, resulting in reduced pore size and less acne. Nicotinamide can help maintain moisture by helping to produce a lipid (fatty) ceramide barrier. This is beneficial to eczema, dry skin, and fine lines and wrinkles.

Nicotinamide and the Treatment of Arthritis

Another function of vitamin B_3 that has been forgotten is its ability to treat arthritis. In *The Common Form of Joint Dysfunction: Its Incidence and Treatment*, published in 1949, William Kaufman, MD, PhD, details how he analyzed and characterized arthritis and gave patients niacinamide (nicotinamide) in frequent small doses to give relief. "Small doses" in this case refers not to dosing three or four times a day but to dosing at intervals of one to two hours—not an easy regimen to follow. His work has been mostly ignored by the medical community, in favor of patented manufactured drugs. I do not think it should be ignored; it deserves another look, especially for anyone who has arthritis. His technique may be helpful for someone with arthritis. I feel it has some take-home value and can be used today. It appears safe and easy to implement.

Dr. Kaufman's approach to arthritis starts with his view that considered not only the pathologic changes in the joint but also external factors. He pointed out four complicating syndromes found with arthritis: physical and psychological stresses, allergies, obesity, and posture. In addition to treating the joint, niacinamide has an affinity for the benzodiazepine receptors in the brain that promotes a calming effect. It increases maximal muscle strength and relieves fatigue. It repairs broken DNA strains. He recognized that one vitamin was not the answer. Most things in nature are a blend of multiple factors, and to his credit, he also added vitamin C, thiamine, and riboflavin to the treatment of arthritis.[32]

Dr. Kaufman's book came out in 1949, and from my perspective, this was the beginning of the transformation of drug companies to Big Pharma. Originally, drug companies refined natural products, for example, delivering good-quality codeine from the poppy and producing a consistent homogenous calamine lotion. This was before they began to take a natural substance like a hormone, add a unique side chain, and demonstrate that this new molecule had similar qualities to the natural substance, despite never having existed in nature before. Because it was a new structure, it was considered an invention and could be patented. Consequently, the drug company owned the new molecule, no one else could produce it, and they could charge as much money as they could get away with. And that is the genesis of Big Pharma.

At the time Kaufman proposed and demonstrated that vitamins were effective for arthritis, Big Pharma was busy producing analog and patented synthetic drugs. This newfound method of wealth production transformed the drug industry in direction and purpose. With the new wealth and protection of the patent laws for their products, they moved away from natural and proven methods to synthetic products that in most instances are not effective and often have negative and harmful effects. Dr. William Kaufman's work was ignored and buried under massive amounts of advertising and the promotional efforts of Big Pharma to promote their brand of

---

[32] Hoffer, A., Saul, A W, and Foster, H., *Niacin: The Real Story*, 2012, Basic Health Publications, 81–88.

medicine. What we have lost are natural, compatible-with-life therapies that are the least damaging and more health promoting than anything the synthetic world can produce.

Vioxx (rofecoxib), a drug produced by Merck & Co. to treat arthritis, caused some 70,000 deaths before it was taken off the market. Niacinamide, according to Poison Control, has not caused any deaths. Kaufman and his work is an example of what has been hidden and lost in the field of modern pharmacology and medicine.

Niacin Deficiency

Niacin plays a role in pellagra, schizophrenia, and cancer.

Pellagra

In 1914, Dr. Joseph Goldberger demonstrated that pellagra was due to a nutritional deficiency. In 1930, it killed 30,000 Americans. Fortunately, in the mid-1930s, Dr. Conrad Elvehjem in Wisconsin discovered that niacin and niacinamide was the anti-pellagra vitamin. Once this vitamin was discovered, it was not long after, in 1942, that the mandatory fortification of wheat products eliminated pellagra and the death that came to nearly half its victims.[33]

Pellagra encompasses all the symptoms of the four Ds, but even a deficiency in niacin can still cause one or two of the symptoms, such as delusion, diarrhea, or dermatitis. Not having all the symptoms makes it difficult to diagnose. In fact, today, the deficiency is so rare that most doctors would not recognize it.

I had a patient, Ronnie, who had been diagnosed with schizophrenia and had frequent delusional events that would provoke him to beat up his roommate in the group home he was living in. Because he had been diagnosed with schizophrenia, after a violent emotional outburst, he was often taken to the hospital for

---

[33] Hoffer, Saul, and Foster, *Niacin: The Real Story*, 13.

care instead of to jail for assault. Ronnie had additional symptoms of headaches, gastritis, fine sores and cuts on his hands, and a reddish discoloration to the neck area. On one of his many visits to the psychiatric unit in the hospital, I asked the head psychiatrist, "What are the lesions on his hands?" The doctor responded that he had seen these lesions before in the psychiatric unit, but he did not know what they were from.

It puzzled me that Ronnie had three of the four Ds: delusional thoughts, gastritis (for which he took Pepcid), and dermatitis of the hands and neck. Finding no help from my colleagues and thinking this may be pellagra, I figured what harm could it do if I gave him a vitamin? I did not think that I would get much support from the pharmacy to dispense niacin, and less encouragement from my doctor friends, so I decided to go it alone. I brought in a bottle of niacin from outside the hospital to treat my patient. How idiotic was this? I was sneaking a bottle of a nutrient into the hospital to treat my patient. Unfortunately, this is modern medicine.

I anticipated the results, but I was amazed to actually see them happen. Within five days of starting the niacin, Ronnie developed clarity of thought and responded to questions appropriately. Within a few days, he reported that he had no gastritis. And in five days, the hand lesions and dermatitis of the neck were gone. It sounds hard to believe, but I have photographs of the skin lesions.

From this example, I wonder how often doctors do not recognize fundamental nutritional deficiencies, thinking they do not exist now or they have all been cured.

Schizophrenia and Niacin

The pioneer in researching the link between schizophrenia and niacin was Abram Hoffer, MD, PhD, from Saskatchewan, Canada. He had proven in the early 1950s, in a double-blind, placebo-controlled study, that niacin improved the symptoms of 90% of the patients in his study with schizophrenia. This is an impressive number of patients treated with excellent results and no toxicity. No patented drug ever came close to its effectiveness and safety.

Fifty percent of schizophrenics will show improvement with compassionate care. Compassionate care was the only treatment available after the Civil War in America until the 1900s. Patients were placed in a care facility, treated with compassion, and taught how to make their bed, wash and fold their clothes, bathe themselves, and conduct themselves with others in the home. Usually, after about a year, they would improve enough that they could be returned to the farm to be a productive family member.

Sigmund Freud ushered in psychotherapy, often referred to as talk therapy. There were mental institutions for housing the "crazies." In the 1900s, **electroconvulsive therapy (ECT)** became a new mode and standard for treating major depression or bipolar disease. Hoffer's niacin treatment was introduced when psychiatry was again changing direction. The popular theory in the 1950s was that the patient had a **"chemical imbalance."** This premise was a handy framework to introduce all sorts of antipsychotic chemicals, and there were many, to balance the chemistry. These were not benign drugs; most had to me monitored, drug levels taken, and if given for too long of a period, an incurable condition such as **tardive dyskinesia** would develop. Tardive dyskinesia is constant, repetitive movement of the extremities with lip-smacking and facial distortions. Even if the previous medication was restarted, the symptoms would not cease.

Advertising, supercharged with an army of drug salesmen from Big Pharma, known as detail agents, visited doctors' offices with journal reports, charts, pens, notepads, keychains, and samples promoting the details of the latest psychiatric drug. Unfortunately, these drugs were effective in only 10% of the population. They were no match for the 50% recovery rate for compassionate care and the 90% recovery rate for niacin.

Abram Hoffer's Research

Abram Hoffer did not have a promotional budget, and niacin, as a natural vitamin of Mother Nature, could not be patented. The drug companies in their studies would not even mention niacin, nor put it in a head-to-head study with their products. This is the usual design of these studies—there is no mention of vitamins, bio-identical hormones, or placing their product in direct head-to-head comparison to the currently used compound.

Nevertheless, Abram Hoffer treated more than 5,000 people with schizophrenia in his lifetime. He developed many concepts for the use of niacin; the following three he found most fundamental:

1. Niacin is involved in the manufacture of nicotinamide adenine dinucleotide (NAD), a coenzyme that is needed for the production of energy. It is one of the critical components of the Krebs cycle to make and recycle adenine triphosphate (ATP), the body's energy stores.
2. It works as an antihistamine against cerebral allergens, which are produced from eating the foods people crave the most—junk food and sugar.
3. It reduces the production of **adrenochrome**, an oxidized form of adrenalin, and its effect is similar to the effect of LSD on the brain. In fact, people under the influence of LSD can be returned to normal with the intravenous administration of 50–100 mg of niacin.[34]

Niacin Synthesis and Niacin Receptors

Two more factors are significant and may change our approach to niacin. First, niacin is not a true vitamin in that the body can produce it, even though most of it comes from our diet. The body can manufacture niacin from tryptophan, but the synthesis is an

---

[34] Agnew, N., and Hoffer, A., "Nicotinic Acid Modified Lysergic Acid Diethylamide Psychosis," *Journal of Mental Science*, 1955, *101*(422), 12–27, https://doi.org/10.1192/bjp.101.422.12.

inefficient process. The body needs at least 60 mg of tryptophan to produce 1 mg of niacin. Clearly, an external source of niacin is needed.

Second, postmortem studies of brain tissue from both patients with schizophrenia and patients with no disorders or conditions have demonstrated that there is a receptor for proteins that contain niacin. Patients with schizophrenia have little to no protein with niacin that attaches to the receptor. The question arises: If there is a receptor, is the protein niacin compound a hormone? This may be the mechanism that transforms a schizophrenic brain to a typical brain. Additionally, is the insufficient production of the protein niacin compound a genetic defect that suggests that schizophrenia is a genetic disease or, at least, a familiar trait?

Besides lack of niacin in the diet, people with schizophrenia are known to have a block between tryptophan and NAD production. It soon becomes apparent that with the internal loss of the production of niacin, reduced intake of nutritious foods, and contemporary foods being less nutrient dense, mental disease will increase. Incidentally, tryptophan is needed to prevent another mental disease: depression. Tryptophan is needed for the production of serotonin; a shortage of this compound invites depression.

Niacin and Cancer

Niacin deficiency is more common in patients with cancer. It is felt that niacin prevents chromosome breakage and maintains the integrity of the telomere lengths.[35] Niacin may or may not prevent cancer, but in those who are supplemented with niacin, cancer progresses at a slower rate.[36] Taking niacin or nicotinamide when cancer is present certainly does not have a downside. Airplane pilots

---

[35] Kirkland, J. B., "Niacin Requirements for Genomic Stability," *Mutation Research*, 2012, *733*(1–2), 14–20, https://doi.org/10.1016/j.mrfmmm.2011.11.008.
[36] Weitberg, A. B., "Effect of Nicotinic Acid Supplementation In Vivo on Oxygen Radical–Induced Genetic Damage in Human Lymphocytes," *Mutation Research*, 1989, *216*(4), 197–201, https://doi.org/10.1016/0165-1161(89)90005-8.

chronically exposed to ionizing radiation, a known human carcinogen, who took niacin at 28.4 mg/day, as compared to 20.5 mg/day, had less chromosome translocations, a measurement of DNA damage.[37] Chromosomal translocations are found as a precursor to many cancers.

Recent studies confirm that niacin deficiency delays DNA repair while promoting DNA strand brakeage, promotes chromosomal translocations and telomere shortening, and increases chances of mutation with mutated cell survival. All patients with cancer are deficient in niacin and need more than the RDA of B_3. The best B_3 supplement for those with cancer is 500 mg of niacinamide three times a day.[38]

Niacin may answer the question of why cancer grows better in some individuals than others. Two people may have similar cell types of cancer, but in one it may thrive and grow robustly, and in another person, it barely advances over many years. This observation lends itself to two approaches to cancer: give someone chemotherapy to poison the cancer and, incidentally, poison the body or nurture the body by giving the proper nutrients, permitting the body to use its own defenses to fight the cancer.

Recommended Dietary Allowance of Niacin

The RDA of niacin is 16 mg for men and 14 mg for women. This was determined by measuring at what level niacin appears in the urine and not the blood level or tissue level. It is reasoned that if the body eliminates niacin, the need must have been satisfied. No deficiencies were found with these recommended levels.

---

[37] Yong, L. C., and Petersen, M. R., "High Dietary Niacin Intake Is Associated with Decreased Chromosome Translocation Frequency in Airline Pilots," *British Journal of Nutrition*, 2011, *105*(4), 496–505, https://doi.org/10.1017/s000711451000379x.

[38] Penberthy, W.T., Saul, A.W., and Smith, R. G., "Niacin and Cancer – How Vitamin B3 Protects and Even Helps Repair Your DNA," Orthomolecular Medicine News Service, *Townsend Letter*, August/September 2022, 64–65.

Recommended Dietary Allowance (RDA) of Niacin[39]			
Life stage	Age	Male (mg/day)	Female (mg/day)
Infant	0–12 months	2–4	2–4
Child	1–8–13 years	6–8–12	6–8–12
Adolescent	14–18 years	16	14
Adult	19 years and older	16	14
Pregnant	All ages	–	18
Breastfeeding	All ages	–	17

Vitamin B_3 is found in eggs, green vegetables, beans, fish, and milk.

Additional Benefits of Niacin

Vitamin B_3 can be beneficial in the treatment of toxicity related to breast implants. Nicotinamide can also aid in the prevention of glaucoma.

---

[39] Higdon, J., et al., "Niacin," Linus Pauling Institute, Oregon State University, last updated October 2018, https://lpi.oregonstate.edu/mic/vitamins/niacin#RDA.

Breast Implants and Vitamin B$_3$

Vitamin B$_3$ can correct some of the toxicities of silicone breast implants. Breast implants have been notorious for causing a myriad of symptoms of allergic reactions, fatigue, muscle aches, chest wall pain, neuropathies, numbing, and conditions similar to rheumatoid arthritis, lupus, chronic fatigue, and dermatitis. The time intervals from receiving the implants to the development of symptoms range anywhere from one month to 12 years, but the usual presentation of symptoms usually occurs within four to eight years. In my experience, any implant can give reactions or deteriorate. This includes titanium hip and knee hardware causing metal toxicities from the components of the amalgams that make up the prostheses.

Silicone breast implants underwent development as problems arose. The initial implants consisted of a silicone or Silastic bag made of a silicone formula used to create a soft, flexible plastic that could be a barrier or wall material. Inside the bag was a more liquid formula of silicone that gave it a weighty and bouncy movement, similar to that of breast tissue. Over time the bag might deteriorate, leaking out the fluid silicone into the local tissues and destroying the integrity and health of the muscles, fat, lymphatic tissue, and nerves. To solve this problem, the fluid in the bags was changed to saline, or saltwater, in the hope of avoiding the issue of silicone toxicity. Unfortunately, the Silastic bags themselves were made of silicone. It just took a little longer for the solid form of silicone to deteriorate and cause destruction.

Silicone is a polymer that is made up of multiple similar molecular units, one attached to another. How long the chain of similar units is made determines whether it is a low molecular weight or a high molecular weight silicone. The molecular weight relates to the physical quality that determines whether it will be a liquid or solid, and if a solid, how flexible or firm it will be.

The silicone can deteriorate in the body to silica. Free forms of silica have been found in the bodies of recipients of silicone implants even though the manufacturers claimed the silicone was inert and unable to react with the tissues.

Silicone from breast implants and injections can be removed with vitamin B_3. The best form of B_3 in this situation is inositol hexanicotinate, 500 mg orally, one to three times a day. This will convert the silicone to silicon chloride:

$$\underset{ClCl}{\overset{H_2}{-Si-}}$$

The silicon chloride will mostly be excreted in the urine. Free silicon can be excreted through the skin.[40] Excretion via the skin is by the sweat glands, and the waste may present as tiny glass beads that look like grains of sand. They feel like small bumps and can be removed by picking at them or using a rough sea sponge when bathing.

I have seen these glass beads in the skin of a patient who was recovering from removal of her breast implants. After seven years, her right implant began to leak, giving her symptoms of toxicity: local breast swelling, lymph gland swelling and tenderness, regional and breast pain, fatigue, and generally feeling sick. The involved areas of toxicity were well documented and followed with thermography. Thermography is an imaging tool, an infrared camera, that detects metabolically active areas on the body that give off more heat than the surrounding tissue. It is used to aid in the location of tumors, infections, and vascular issues.

To learn about breast health, diagnostics, and preventive care, I advise you to read Patricia Bowden-Luccardi's book *Thermography*. Written in terms that inform rather than confuse, the comprehensive book clarifies a topic that will educate anyone who takes the time to inform themself. It is a handbook for women of any age—and for

---

[40] Shanklin, D., *Inositol*, Plastikos Plastic and Reconstructive Surgery, 2009, https://web.archive.org/web/20170308003353/http://www.plastikos.com/doc/articles/silicone/11.pdf.

doctors who need a quick lesson on thermography. They did not teach this in medical school.[41] The technique does not squeeze the breasts with high pressure and does not subject them to radiation like a mammogram does.

Inositol hexanicotinate 500 mg, three times a day, would be a very good maintenance treatment for anyone with silicone implants to prevent, or at least reduce, the toxic exposure and the symptoms of toxicity.

Glaucoma

Glaucoma is a disorder of the eye characterized by increased eyeball pressure called **intraocular pressure**. A small amount of pressure in the eye keeps it in a spherical shape. This is good, but too much pressure within the eye damages the retina and optic nerve. This results in loss of vision and can cause total blindness. Normal eyeball pressure, measured with an instrument called a tonometer, is 20 millimeters of mercury (mmHg), and the heathy range is 15–25 mmHg.

Glaucoma occurs because the normal flow of fluid within the eye is disrupted. There are two distinct fluids in the eye: the **vitreous humor** and the **aqueous humor**. The vitreous humor is jelly like and found behind the lens. The fluid, originating in the ciliary body, flows toward the retina. Some of it is filtered at the retinal vessels; the remainder flows to the anterior chamber, in front of the lens. The aqueous humor is a more fluid solution, also produced in the ciliary body, but it passes between the ligaments of the lens, then through the pupil, and into the anterior chamber. From the anterior chamber, the fluid is removed at a filter known as the **trabeculae**, located at the juncture of the cornea and iris.[42] These two curved surfaces meet each other at an acute angle or a wider angle, and this

---

[41] Bowden-Luccardi, P., *Thermography and the Fibrocystic and Dense Breast: A Radiation-Free Survival Guide for Happy Healthy Breasts*, 2020.
[42] Guyton, A. C., "Intraocular Fluid," *Textbook of Medical Physiology*, 4th edition, Elsevier, 1971, 256.

characteristic is used to categorize the cause of the glaucoma. Whether it is open-angle or closed-angle glaucoma is relevant to the treatment options and methods.

The consensus is that the cause of the increased intraocular pressure may be vasomotor, emotional instability, hereditary, familial, congenital anomalies, traumatic, or a physical block to the drainage system at the trabeculae. But maybe glaucoma is a gradual dysfunction of retinal ganglion cells and their axons. What if it is nutritional and can even be avoided? Alan R. Gaby, MD, penned an article in the *Townsend Letter* worth reading: "Preventing and Treating Glaucoma by Enhancing Mitochondrial Function."[43] According to Gaby, the retina is one of the most metabolically active tissues in the body. It requires energy from the mitochondria in the form of adenosine triphosphate (ATP), coenzyme Q10 (CoQ10), and magnesium (Mg).

Gaby mentions another observation in animal studies. A certain breed of mouse known as DBA/2J develops spontaneous glaucoma. These mice have decreased levels of nicotinamide adenine dinucleotide (NAD) in the retinal cells before glaucoma occurs. Vitamin B_3 (nicotinamide) is required to produce NAD. The effects of nicotinamide on glaucoma in humans has also been studied. Judith Nzoughet and her colleagues reported that in the most common form of glaucoma, the open-angle form, 30% of the patients included in their study were deficient in nicotinamide compared to matched controls.[44] In another study on 57 patients with glaucoma over 12 weeks, participants received 1,500 mg of nicotinamide daily for the first six weeks and then 1,500 mg twice a

---

[43] October 2021, 87–88.
[44] Nzoughet, J. K., et al., "Nicotinamide Deficiency in Open-Angle Glaucoma," *Investigative Ophthalmology & Visual Science*, 2019, 60(7), 2509–2514. https://doi.org/10.1167/iovs.19-27099.

day for the next six weeks. Improvement was measured and found to be significant in retinal function and visual field defects.[45]

Glaucoma is no longer a mysterious disease. It just does not happen on its own. Its treatment is not limited to the ophthalmologist. Prevention and treatment of glaucoma is in your hands. As you can see, there are things you can do to avoid and treat glaucoma. My recommendation is as follows:

- Nicotinamide: 1,500 mg twice a day
- Coenzyme Q-10: 200–400 mg a day
- Magnesium glycinate: 400 mg a day

Niacin Supplements

Niacin, the most basic form of the B_3 vitamin, comes in 100 mg, 250 mg, 300 mg, and 500 mg tablets and capsules sold by Life Extension, Solgar, Pure Encapsulations, Swanson, and Nature's Bounty, to name just a few. Start with the lower dosage, as this is the molecule that will cause flushing and the sensation of heat until you can tolerate more.

Nicotinamide, or niacinamide, is available in 500 mg, 1,000 mg, and 1,500 mg capsules sold by Thorne, Pure Encapsulations, Now Foods, and Source Naturals.

Nicotinamide riboside, a relatively recent discovery, is a form of vitamin B_3. However, this view depends on one's concept of where the beginning is. Is niacin the root molecule, or can it be processed to have another molecule attached to it and still be considered a molecule of B_3? I disagree with some chemists on that question. Let me tell you why.

---

[45] Hui F, et al. "Improvement in Inner Retinal Function with Nicotinamide (Vitamin B_3) Supplementation: A Crossover Randomized Clinical Trial," *Clinical & Experimental Ophthalmology*, 2020, *48*(7), 903–914, https://doi.org/10.1111/ceo.13818.

Nicotinamide Riboside

This form of B$_3$ is derived from cow's milk. It has been noted that nicotinamide riboside is more easily converted into nicotinamide adenine dinucleotide (NAD), but to me, it represents only an intermediate step between niacin and NAD.

Tryptophan is an amino acid that in the body can be converted into niacin. This reaction is limited in the amount that can be converted in an inefficient process. Not enough tryptophan can be converted into niacin to meet the body's needs or prevent pellagra. For practical purposes, all niacin must be obtained from external sources to meet the needs of the body to prevent disease and death. This qualifies niacin to be a vitamin: The body needs it, and only an external source can provide it.

Nevertheless, nicotinamide riboside is being advertised as a new form of niacin under the trade name Tru Niagen in 300 mg and 150 mg capsules, intended for daily consumption to increase energy. Life Extension sells it as NAD$^+$ Cell Regenerator alone and compounded with resveratrol. In my opinion, nicotinamide riboside is an intermediate product between niacin and NAD. It is not a new form of B$_3$.

Vitamin B6

Benefits of Vitamin B$_6$

- Prevents the accumulation of homocysteine and coronary plaque
- Lifts depression
- Improves diabetic control
- Improves neuropathy
- Preserves kidney function
- Relieves painful menses by balancing hormones
- Eases carpal tunnel syndrome

History of Vitamin B6: Pyridoxine, Pyridoxal, and Pyridoxamine

Rudolf Peters, in 1930, brought attention to a condition of acrodynia in rats fed a semisynthetic diet that produced severe cutaneous lesions.[46] In 1934, Paul György discovered that this skin condition, rat acrodynia, as well as convulsions and microcytic anemia in laboratory rats, pigs, and dogs, could be relieved with vitamin B$_6$. In 1936, Birch and György gave it the name vitamin B$_6$ because it was the sixth B vitamin to be discovered. In 1938, Samuel Lepkovsky isolated vitamin B$_6$, and the name pyridoxine was assigned to it by the Council of Pharmacy and Chemistry because of its structure. Esmond Snell, in 1942, characterized the biochemistry

---

[46] Rosenberg, I. H., "A History of the Isolation and Identification of Vitamin B(6)," *Annals of Nutrition and Metabolism*, 2012, *61*(3), 236–238 , https://doi.org/10.1159/000343113.

of both pyridoxamine and pyridoxal, two other forms of vitamin B_6.[47]

Three inactive forms of vitamin B_6 were identified: pyridoxine, pyridoxal, and pyridoxamine. Pyridoxine and pyridoxal are both converted to the active form of pyridoxal phosphate, whereas pyridoxamine is converted to the active form of pyridoxamine phosphate.

Pyridoxine   Pyridoxal   Pyridoxamine

Pyridoxal Phosphate   Pyridoxamine Phosphate

Functions of Vitamin B_6

The general functions of vitamin B_6 are involved with the metabolism of amino acids, detoxification of substances in the liver, skin health, central and peripheral nerve function, and controlling gastrointestinal symptoms of radiation sickness, and it participates in controlling arterial plaque formation. Additionally, vitamin B_6

---

[47] Kaushansky, K., and Kipps, T. J., "Pyridoxine," In Brunton, L., Chabner, B., and Knollman, B. (eds.), *Goodman & Gilman's the Pharmacological Basis of Therapeutics*, 12th edition, McGraw-Hill Medical, 2011, 1086.

participates in more than 100 chemical reactions in cells, forming red blood cells, producing proteins, manufacturing neurotransmitter chemicals in the brain, balancing hormones, processing homocysteine, preventing seizures, lifting depression, and improving diabetic control.

Cardiovascular Disease and Homocysteine

In the mid-1960s, Dr. Kilmer McCully, a young pathology instructor at Harvard University, examined a baby with homocysteine disease who, at the age of one month, died of a heart attack. The coronary arteries were heavy with cholesterol plaque—a very unusual finding for a baby. After the autopsy, he discussed the findings with the family and informed them that the baby had died of a heart attack. It was through this meeting that the family informed him that the baby's uncle, also an infant of one month, had died in that very hospital 20 years earlier.

Dr. McCully's interest was aroused, and he checked the archives in his hospital's basement and found the uncle's autopsy report and pathology slides. The uncle also had homocysteine disease and coronary plaques and had indeed died of a heart attack.[48] This observation that homocysteine may be related to coronary plaques and heart attacks would occupy Dr. McCully for the rest of his professional life.

Initially, he was funded, worked at Harvard, and performed experiments on rabbits, producing coronary plaques and heart attacks in the rabbits by injecting them with homocysteine. Therapeutically, he showed that an elevated homocysteine level could be lowered by treating with 3.5 mg of vitamin B_6, 400 micrograms (mcg) of folic acid, and 15 mcg of vitamin B_{12}. This turned out to be a hard sell in the 1970s, when the American Heart Association and the National Heart, Lung, and Blood Institute were

---

[48] Information from a personal conversation at an ACAM conference, 1997.

pushing the narrative that cholesterol from saturated fats was the only cause of coronary plaques.

McCully proposed an inexpensive cure for atherosclerosis of coronary vessels with vitamins, compared to the up-and-coming treatment with statin drugs developed by Big Pharma. Funding began to dry up at Harvard for McCully, his supervisor retired, he lost administrative support, and he was denied sufficient laboratory access. The big money was on the side of the statins. And McCully, without tenure at Harvard, was dismissed from the faculty. With no job and no respect, he retreated to the Providence, Rhode Island, Veterans Hospital Laboratory until a new generation of investigators took an interest in homocysteine and coronary disease.[49]

In the United States, the Nurses' Health Study, initiated by the National Institutes of Health (NIH) to monitor women's health, looked at the incidence of coronary artery disease and vitamin B_6 levels. The researchers conducted a prospective study with 80,082 women and measured the women's intake of B_6 versus the development of coronary artery disease. They categorized them into five groups, or quintiles, according to vitamin B_6 intake. The highest median intake was 4.6 mg per day for the top 20%. The lowest median intake was 1.1 mg/day for the bottom 20%. The result was 34% less coronary disease for the highest vitamin B_6 intake versus the lowest intake.[50] Similarly, a Japanese prospective study consisting of 40,000 individuals showed a 48% lower risk of heart attack between the quintile with the highest intake versus the lowest intake.[51]

---

[49] Stacey, M. "The Fall and Rise of Kilmer McCully," *New York Times Magazine*, August 10, 1997, 25.

[50] Rimm, E. B., et al., "Folate and Vitamin B_6 from Diet and Supplements in Relation to Risk of Coronary Heart Disease among Women," *JAMA*, 1998, *279*(5), 359–364, https://doi.org/10.1001/jama.279.5.359.

[51] Ishihara, J., et al., "Intake of Folate, Vitamin B6 and Vitamin B12 and the Risk of CHD: The Japan Public Health Center-Based Prospective Study Cohort I," *Journal of the American College of Nutrition*, 2008, *27*(1), 127–136, https://doi.org/10.1080/07315724.2008.10719684.

The form of vitamin B₆ that is most involved with protection from coronary disease is **pyridoxal 5'-phosphate**. This is the form that should be in your B complex, usually at 15 to 20 mg. It is often written as **P5P** when sold as a single ingredient and sold as 50 mg or more per capsule. This is the same P5P that in difficult diabetes and gestational diabetes cases can lower the blood glucose.

Menstrual Relief

Vitamin B₆, **pyridoxine, pyridoxal**, and their phosphate form pyridoxal 5'-phosphate help relieve the symptoms of menses. B₆ taken during the menses reduces the high estradiol level and preserves the progesterone level, giving relief from symptoms.

Protecting Tissues from Excess Sugar

I do not want to leave you with the thought that vitamin B₆ is not healthy. It is very beneficial. In fact, the form of B₆ known as **pyridoxamine** is very beneficial to diabetics. It functions as an antioxidant, preventing advanced glycation end products (AGEs) and preserving renal function. It protects kidney function. The kidneys actively remove creatinine, a waste product, from the blood. This ability deteriorates under conditions of prolonged elevations of blood glucose, such as in poorly controlled diabetes.

Excretion of creatinine by the kidney is a measure of kidney function, which is measured using a test called the **glomerular filtration rate (GFR)**. This test is performed by collecting urine for 24 hours and measuring the volume and the concentration of creatinine to give the rate of removal of creatinine. Normal values range from 60 to 110 ml per minute. There is another test called the **estimated glomerular filtration rate (eGFR)** reported on blood chemistry work that is a calculated number that is used instead of 24-hour urine collection as a quick estimate. It is easier to take one blood sample instead of collecting urine in a jug for a day and then taking it to the laboratory for analysis.

The eGFR gives a quick estimate of kidney function, but the accuracy is poor because the formula to calculate the eGFR requires the patient's age, sex, race, creatinine blood level, height, and weight. The last two, height and weight, are usually not reported with the lab request, and the value reported can vary widely, anywhere from normal to stage-three kidney disease. I have seen samples where the 24-hour urine test is reported as 80 ml/min (normal) and the blood sample, the eGFR, is reported at 45 ml/min, suggesting the person has stage-three kidney disease. This is because the size of the patient, their height and weight, degree of hydration, and muscle mass are not taken into account.

Vitamin B_6 in the form of pyridoxamine preserves kidney function in the setting of high blood sugar (glucose). The medical community has advocated using ACE inhibitors or ACE blockers, blood pressure medications, in diabetics, as they can protect kidney function as well as treat hypertension. Both categories of substances, vitamins and blood pressure medications, will protect kidney function. However, the vitamin is far superior to the blood pressure medications in protecting kidney function. In a head-to-head evaluation, pyridoxamine is much more effective and efficacious than the prescription medications.

This fact has been known for the past two decades but received little attention until 2010, when pyridoxamine was removed from the market. Until then, most vitamin B_6 preparations contained all three forms of B_6—pyridoxal, pyridoxine, and pyridoxamine—plus the phosphate forms of these compounds: pyridoxal phosphate, P5P, and pyridoxamine phosphate. It seems that a company, in doing its research, became aware of the protective effect of pyridoxamine. To develop a product for diabetes, it set about doing clinical trials for FDA-approved indications. The FDA said that no drug in clinical trial can be on the market at the same time. This interpretation, or ruling, required all vitamin purveyors to remove pyridoxamine from their product line. Despite pyridoxamine having been on the market for years and still being found in food (liver, grains, spinach, green beans, and bananas), it was banned as a supplement.

Pyridoxamine is a natural product that belongs to you and me, but the FDA has taken it from us and sold it to private interests. It even has a registered trade name of Pyridorin, which is not yet available as a commercial product. Currently, pyridoxamine is not available in the US from any American supplier, nor can it be bought as Primage from LifeLink, a British company. Its importation has been blocked. Portugal is another country that has pyridoxamine as Pyridox-Pro, which is also not available to Americans.

After Cancer Treatments

Vitamin B_6 is helpful after chemotherapy and radiation therapy. Both modalities destroy normal tissue as much as the tumors. There is no precise formula for when to stop treatment or when to continue. The one thing we do know is that continued treatment destroys normal tissue. A common problem is neuropathy: loss of nerve function and nerve pain that results from treatment. This is where chemotherapy and radiation should be stopped and the B vitamins initiated. In my opinion, they should have been given all along. They are nutrition, and no healing can occur without nutrition.

The most beneficial and effective treatment for nerve pain is neither opioids nor analgesics but nutrition with B complex and the Myers's cocktail.

Contents of the Myers's Cocktail	
Ingredient	Amount
Magnesium	1 g
Vitamin B_1 (thiamine)	100 mg
Vitamin B_5 (dexpanthenol)	200 mg

Vitamin B$_6$ (pyridoxine)	100 mg
Vitamin B$_{12}$ (cyanocobalamin)	2 mg
Vitamin C (ascorbic acid)	2.5 g

This can be given as a slow push or diluted in normal saline, lactated ringers, or dextrose 5% in water (D5W). This combination of nutrients promotes the quickest nerve and nerve function recovery that I know of.

Many oncologists say that giving vitamins interferes with chemotherapy and that they should not be given. I say chemotherapy interferes with life, and do not expect improvement without vitamins.

The addition of vitamin C to any cancer treatment prolongs survival and the person's well-being while they are here. See the appendix for the Cameron and Pauling treatment of cancer performed in the 1970s. Read the study for yourself. This gives you enough information to chart your own path in the treatment of cancer. You should not be a passenger in the treatment of cancer—you should be the captain of the decision team.

Vitamin B$_6$ Deficiency

No single syndrome indicates vitamin B$_6$ deficiency because it is involved in so many processes. It may present as general ill health or the worsening of an already defined condition of depression, diabetes, or premenstrual syndrome. However, as described in the section on the history of vitamin B$_6$, scientists working with lab animals with controlled diets observed some clues of a deficiency. Their attention to detail and persistent experimenting brought new knowledge about vitamin B$_6$, not only as a vitamin but also as a blend of similar compounds that we refer to as vitamin B$_6$.

The Food and Nutrition Board of the Institute of Medicine as of 1998 recommends vitamin B_6 in the form of pyridoxine taken in the doses set out in the table that follows:

Recommended Dietary Allowance (RDA) for Vitamin B_6			
Life stage	Age	Male (mg/day)	Female (mg/day)
Infant	0–6 months	0.1	0.1
	7–12 months	0.3	0.3
Child	1–3 years	0.5	0.5
	4–8 years	0.6	0.6
	9–13 years	1.0	1.0
Adolescent	14–18 years	1.3	1.2
Adult	19–50 years	1.7	1.3
	50 years and older		1.5
Pregnant	All ages	–	1.9
Breastfeeding	All ages	–	2.0

Vitamin B$_6$ Toxicity and Neuropathy

B vitamins are considered safe and relatively toxin free. It is generally believed that if too much of a vitamin is taken, more than the body needs, it will be excreted by way of the urine. It is thought that the fat-soluble vitamins may be toxic and accumulate in the fat or other tissues. I find that this generalization of the fat-soluble vitamins (K, A, D, and E) is not as true as it may seem.

In my practice, I use all the vitamins, and I take them myself. One day, while walking down a hallway, I started to drift toward one side and needed quick corrective action so as not to fall over. I noticed it several times and began to wonder whether I had had a stroke or transient ischemic attack (TIA). I was not dizzy and had no ear or allergy problems. Was I taking too much of a vitamin or too many vitamins? I happened to be researching vitamin B$_6$ at the time and began to look at pyridoxine and pyridoxamine. I try all the vitamins I prescribe to see if what is said about them is true regarding their benefits and their ill effects. I had been taking B$_6$ and on a whim decided to stop taking it for a few weeks.

Within two or three weeks of having stopped the vitamin B$_6$, I could walk without drifting and was back to my old self again. I have never heard of this happening to anyone else, and I have not had any of my patients complain of this or describe similar effects. I have been told by my office staff that I talk too much during the patient visits, but no patients are complaining—or maybe I am misreading their body language.

I administer IV infusions in my office as well as the Myers's cocktail, which may take 5 to 10 minutes as a slow push. One day, while giving an IV Myers's push, I was discussing something with the patient during this process. I was telling my patient, Joe, about the observation I made about B$_6$ and drifting, and that I thought it was due to too much B$_6$. Joe said he experienced the same drifting and that he had wanted to ask me about it for some time. He asked if it could be a stroke or TIA coming on, or was it his age? I told him I did not know if it was coincidental or if it was related. Anyway, I instructed him to stop taking the B complex—this is usually how most people take B vitamins—and see if he gets similar results. Likewise, he experienced freedom from the drifting and was feeling much better in a few weeks.

I thought I would put this in my book as a personal observation. Recently, I started to read the book *The End of Alzheimer's* by Dale E. Bredesen, MD, and was pleased that he reported neuropathy from too much vitamin B_6. This was the first I ever saw this or any similar description of this neuropathy. Bredesen reported that toxic levels above 110 nanomoles per liter (nmol/L) of B_6 can be "toxic to your peripheral nerves, specifically the nerves that carry the sensations of touch and pressure and are critical for gauging where your arms and legs are in space."[52] I believe I discovered this before him, but he reported it first. I will give him credit for that, but more than that, this adds to our understanding and proper use of vitamins.

Vitamin B_6 Supplements

Vitamin B_6 is sold in liquid form to be dispensed in drops for oral administration or in a sterile liquid, usually for intravenous administration. A powder form, the most common delivery, is dispensed in tablet or capsule form. It can be found in a multivitamin or as a single component.

Life Extension sells vitamin B_6 as pyridoxine 250 mg and pyridoxal as pyridoxal 5'-phosphate in 100 mg. The latter preparation, P5P, is the metabolically active form. Pyridoxine must conjugate with phosphate in the body to make it active. Now Foods sells vitamin B_6 as P-5-P Nervous System Health, with 33 mg of B_6 from 50 mg of the coenzyme P5P and with 25 mg of magnesium bisglycinate.

---

[52] 2017, 121.

Thorne's Pyridoxal 5'-Phosphate capsules contain 33.8 mg. Pure Encapsulations offers several B_6 supplements. Its P_5P 50 contains 50 mg activated vitamin B_6. Its B_6 Complex capsules contain 200 mg of vitamin B_6 as pyridoxine and 5% pyridoxal 5'-phosphate with additional B vitamins: 100 mg of B_1 (thiamine), 15 mg of B_2 (riboflavin), 110 mg of B_3 (niacin) as nicotinamide and 9% inositol, folate as 667 mcg of DFE and 400 mcg of MTHF, 1,000 mcg of vitamin B_{12}, 400 mcg of biotin, 100 mcg of pantothenic acid, 12 mg of choline, and 25 mg of inositol.

Not all molecular forms of B_6 are available in the United States. The most important molecule, pyridoxamine, cannot be manufactured or imported because of its potential health benefits and pharmaceutical value, as discussed in "Protecting Tissues from Excess Sugar" in the "Functions of Vitamin B_6" section. This vitamin should be reclassified as "generally safe" and returned to the marketplace for everyone's benefit. This is like charging you for how much sunlight you are consuming.

If you travel to a foreign country, especially England or Portugal, purchase Primage, Pridox-Pro, or generic pyridoxamine or pyridoxamine phosphate. Do not accept the switch and bait if when you ask for pyridoxamine they give you pyridoxal or pyridoxine. Likewise, if you search the internet for pyridoxamine, you will be shown pyridoxal or pyridoxine, *not* pyridoxamine. These are not the same molecules, and they do not have similar functions. Pyridoxamine can be one of the best gifts you can give yourself to preserve kidney and neurologic function, preventing glucose from attaching to proteins, ruining these structures, and advancing aging.

Folic Acid

Benefits of Folic Acid

- Prevents and treats anemia
- Prevents birth defects of the nervous system
- Maintains the intestinal tract and promotes absorption
- Prevents cleft lip
- Increases alertness and memory
- Reduces the risk of Alzheimer's disease
- Treats the symptoms of menopause
- Reduces cardiovascular disease
- Reduces the complications of pregnancy
- With vitamins B_{12} and B_6, treats homocysteine
- Reduces tingling pain and numbness in the arms and legs
- Improves psoriasis and vitiligo

History of Folic Acid

The story of folic acid starts in India in 1931, with a simple observation that a form of tropical macrocytic anemia responds to crude liver extracts and extracts of yeast. Vitamin B_{12} macrocytic anemia, similar in appearance to folate macrocytic anemia, responds to pure extracts of liver. Hematologically, under the microscope both anemias look the same, and the anemia of one vitamin can be treated with the other vitamin.[53] Lucy Wills, a British physician doing research in Bombay, India, on pernicious anemia of pregnancy noted

---

[53] But a point of caution: Folic acid cannot be used to treat the neurologic problems of vitamin B_{12} deficiency. Folic acid doses are limited to 400 mcg so that its use will not mask a vitamin B_{12} deficiency. It is not because folic acid is harmful.

that this macrocytic anemia did not respond to pure extract of liver, but it did respond to Marmite, a commercial yeast extract available in stores. Wills demonstrated her findings in both rats and monkeys. Later, the effective, crude liver extract was used and named the **Wills factor**. Folic acid was also referred to as **vitamin M**, possibly from its source in Marmite.

Folic acid had many names as it was becoming known as a nutrient and then a vitamin. Manning and Stokstad, in 1938, identified folic acid as **Factor U** in yeast, because it corrected an anemia and growth failure in chickens. Hogan and Parrott identified the same substance in 1939 but called it **vitamin Bc**.

Folate was recognized as a growth factor in bacterial cultures, especially *Lactobacillus casei,* where it became known as the ***L. Casei* factor** and as the **norite eluate factor** because it would adhere to charcoal filters used in the process of its extraction. **SLR** factor was folic acid found in streptococcus bacteria.

The term **folic acid** was coined in 1941 by Henry K. Mitchell, who isolated it from leafy spinach. *Folium* is the Latin word for "leaves." It was the ninth B vitamin to be isolated and was given the designation vitamin B_9. The structure of the molecule was defined and synthesized by Robert B. Angier in 1945.[54]

In 1962, Victor Herbert, MD, from the Mount Sinai Hospital and Medical School in New York, placed himself on a folate-deficient diet, confirming vital amine status, and recorded his findings. At one month, the microbiological assay of folate measured lower than the normal findings. In the second month, the number of lobes of the nuclei in the white cells, called neutrophilic polymorphonuclear leukocytes (PMNs), increased; this is characteristic of low levels of both folic acid and vitamin B_{12}. In the third month, folate levels in red blood cells fell and the cells became

---

[54] Herbert, V., "Drugs Effective in Megaloblastic Anemias: Vitamin B_{12} and Folic Acid," In Goodman, L. S., and Gilman, A. (eds.), *The Pharmacological Basis of Therapeutics*, 4th edition, Macmillan, 1971, 1414–1444.

larger and fewer in number, a condition known as megaloblastic anemia (doctor lingo for large young-cell anemia).[55]

Functions of Folic Acid

Folic acid is one of the B vitamins needed to sustain a healthy brain and nervous system. Folic acid is required either directly for neuronal growth or for developing new nerve cell connections or synapses. It is also required to lower homocysteine, thus lowering arterial plaque in blood vessels going to, or within, the brain, providing better blood flow and oxygen.

Folate is the salt of folic acid and the form found in nature. The best sources of folate are dark leafy vegetables, beans, yeast, egg yolk, and liver.

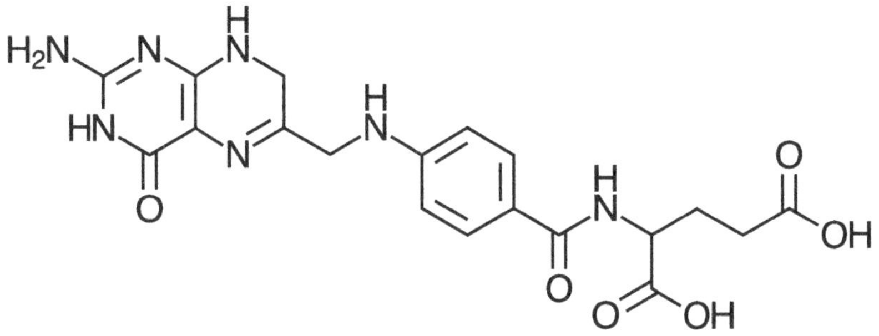

Folate, Dihydrofolate

---

[55] Herbert, V., "Biochemical and Hematological Lesions of Folic Acid Deficiency," *American Journal of Clinical Nutrition*, 1967, *20*(6), 562–569, https://doi.org/10.1093/ajcn/20.6.562.

Folic Acid, Pteroylglutamic Acid

Folic acid is produced in a laboratory. It is heat stable and can be placed into tablets but degrades rapidly in light. Folate found in green leafy vegetables can lose more than 70% of its activity in three days, can be leached out by cooking in water, and is destroyed with heat at temperatures above 105 degrees Fahrenheit. This makes fresh vegetables a better source than cooked vegetables for this vitamin. But fresh means fresh, and every hour since harvesting more folate is lost.

Folate is further transformed to folinic acid. The purpose of this transformation, with the participation of vitamin B_{12}, is to produce methyl groups (-CH_3), to alter molecules, or to turn on or turn off genes.

Folinic Acid, Luecovorin

Folic acid is a common form of this vitamin, but recently a newer, more bioavailable compound has been offered by many purveyors of supplements: Metafolin,[56] which is L-5-methyltetrehydrofolate (L-5-MTHF; the L signifies leftward rotation of polarized light by the molecule and is frequently dropped in many notations and discussions). This is a natural, metabolized form of folate. This is an acceptable form to consume because of its bioavailability, and it readily passes the blood-brain barrier to nurture the brain.

Metafolin (Levomefolate Calcium), 5-MTHF

Cardiovascular Disease

Vitamin B_{12} and folic acid have a close interactive relation metabolically. Both are involved in the transport of methyl groups for the production of DNA, RNA, and the conversion of amino acids. Folate acts as a coenzyme to transform thymidine and purines to products that will be used to construct stands of DNA and RNA. Folate and vitamin B_{12} work together to transform amino acids by moving a **methyl group (-CH3)** from one molecule to another. The most significant amino acid transformation is turning homocysteine into methionine.

Too much homocysteine is a risk factor for vascular disease. Elevated levels of homocysteine promote the fatty buildup in blood vessels that causes heart attacks, strokes, and peripheral vascular disease. The preferred range for homocysteine in the blood is less

---

[56] Metafolin is a registered trademark of Merck KGaA, Darmstadt, Germany.

than 10.0 micromole per liter. Above this level, there is rapid accumulation of arterial plaque that blocks blood flow. In some areas such as the brain, increased homocysteine promotes lipid accumulation that impedes blood flow and reduces oxygen flow to the brain, reducing optimal function and producing brain fog, atrophy, and if obstruction is complete, a stroke. Supplemental folic acid, or folate, can prevent this cascade of events and make you more mentally sharp, improve your memory, and maybe even make you more cooperative.

The conversion of homocysteine to methionine is accomplished by adding a methyl group ($-CH_3$) to homocysteine. Adding additional vitamins to help lower higher-than-normal homocysteine levels, greater than 10.0 ng/ml, usually begins with 400 mcg of folic acid, 500 mcg of vitamin B_{12}, and 250 mg of vitamin B_6. If this is inadequate to lower the homocysteine, 500 mg of betaine and 100 mg of riboflavin daily is added.[57]

Brain and Nervous System Health

When studying vitamins, doctors and nurses learn that folic acid is stored in the liver, with a fair amount in the red blood cells required for their rapid turnover and DNA production. Usually, storage implies that that is where the most folic acid can be found. But just look at this list of tissues and fluid assays:

Tissues and Fluid Assays for Folic Acid	
Tissue	Folic acid level (ng/ml)
Liver	6–12
Serum	5–15
Cerebrospinal fluid	16–21

---

[57] Strain, J. J., et al., "B-Vitamins, Homocysteine Metabolism and CVD," *Proceedings of the Nutrition Society*, 2004, *63*(4), 597–603, https://doi.org/10.1079/pns2004390.

| Brain tissue | 12–26 |
| Red blood cells | >280 |

It appears that the liver has the lowest concentration of folic acid and that other tissues that are more metabolically active may require more or concentrate it more than the liver. Does this high level of folate in the spinal fluid and brain tissue mean it has a higher need and maybe is essential for the growth, maintenance, and preservation of tissue? Knowing that folic acid is needed for proper development of the neural tube to prevent brain malformations and spinal cord malformations such as spina bifida, would it not also follow that folic acid is required for healthy maintenance and function of the brain to prevent atrophy?

The brain is the most metabolically active organ in the body. It needs nutrients, oxygen, and exercise. Contemporary wellness activity and concern is often directed to the cardiovascular system, exercise for the muscles, and calcium for the bones, but what about that soft mass in your head that controls it all? What have you done for your brain today?

Improvement in cognitive function was demonstrated by the FACIT Trial in the Netherlands, using 800 micrograms of folic acid daily. This study followed 818 patients for three years, beginning in 1999 and ending in 2004. The patients selected for the study had elevated homocysteine levels between 13 and 26 micromole per liter (mcmol/L). This group was selected because it was thought that they would benefit the most from folic acid's homocysteine-lowering effect. The dose was not large at 800 micrograms—the RDA in America is 400 mcg. The control group received a placebo.

At the three-year mark, this trial showed that with folic acid, global cognitive function (specifically memory) was significantly better, sensorimotor speed (i.e., reaction times and balance) improved, and the speed of information processing had increased. In the three-year period of this study, those who took folic acid developed the performance of people 4.7 years younger in memory tests.[58] At this small dose, both serum folate levels and erythrocyte folate levels rose, and the homocysteine level fell. The biggest gain was the 4.7 years toward youthful brain function.

Folic acid benefits the brain by two different mechanisms: The first is a direct effect on brain nutrition, taking part in development and repair, and the second is an indirect effect by lowering homocysteine. High homocysteine promotes atrophy of the hippocampus, a portion of the brain involved in the process of memory.[59] From this information, it comes as no surprise that a low folate level is associated with Alzheimer's disease, dementia, and depression.

Dementia, depression, and Alzheimer's are related to a lack of vitamin B_{12} and, to some extent, other B vitamins. The B vitamins work together and support each other's function, as well as working as coenzymes. I am discussing each vitamin individually, but keep in mind that they often work in concert to have their full impact. This is why you will often see the B vitamins prepared with many in the same capsule or tablet, called a B complex. They may be called B-50 or B-100, which means that B-50 contains 50 mg of B_1, 50 mg of B_2, 50 mg of B_3, and so forth. The B-100 complex contains 100 mg of B_1, 100 mg of B_2, 100 mg of B_3, and so forth. Any of the B vitamins can also be bought individually and taken individually, as needed.

Preventing Birth Defects

Folic acid has been shown to be related to neurologic birth defects such as **spina bifida**, a defect in the development of the spinal cord that secondarily causes the bony arches of the lumbar

---

[58] Durga, J., et al., "Effect of 3-Year Folic Acid Supplementation on Cognitive Function in Older Adults in the FACIT Trial: A Randomised, Double Blind, Controlled Trial," *Lancet*, 2007, *369*(9557), 208–216, https://doi.org/10.1016/s0140-6736(07)60109-3.

[59] Den Hiejer, T., et al., "Homocysteine and Brain Atrophy on MRI of Non-Demented Elderly," *Brain*, 2003, *126*, 170–175, https://doi.org/10.1093/brain/awg006.

vertebra to fail to grow and protect the spinal cord from exposure just below the skin. Babies can be born with this defect, visible at birth, or **anencephaly**, which is a markedly defective development or the absence of parts of the brain, either the cerebral or cerebellar hemispheres, and proper bone structure to the skull. **Anencephaly** is not a viable condition. Both these developmental defects occur between the 21st and 27th day from conception. This development is so early in the pregnancy that most women do not even know they are pregnant.

Neural tube defects (NTD) such as spina bifida and anencephaly can be avoided if women take sufficient folic acid at least one month prior to conception and during the first month of pregnancy. The US Public Health Service recommended 400 mcg of folate in the periconceptual period to avoid NTDs. Consequently, since 1998, the FDA has required the fortification of grain so that the average person's diet would include 100 mcg of folic acid per day. The Centers for Disease Control reported that this has reduced the incidence of NTDs by 26%.[60]

Tolarova reported in *Lancet* in 1982 that **cleft lip**, **hair lip**, and **cleft palate** are related to low folic acid and can be prevented by periconceptional supplementation with folic acid. She recommended that women who had delivered children with cleft lips be supplemented with folic acid to avoid second children with the same condition. In her cohort or group, 85 women participated in full supplementation, and this group had only one recurrence, or less than 1%. The control group contained 212 women who did not receive supplements. Fifteen children with cleft lips were born to women in that group—a recurrence of 7.4%. This is more good evidence that folic acid is needed for fetal development.

---

[60] Higdon, J., et al., "Adverse Pregnancy Outcomes," "Folate," Linus Pauling Institute, Oregon State University, last updated December 2023, https://lpi.oregonstate.edu/mic/vitamins/folate#adverse-pregnancy-outcomes.

Low levels of folate are implicated in other complications of pregnancy, such as heart defects, limb malformations, premature delivery, low birth weight, miscarriage, preeclampsia, and placental abruption.[61]

Folic Acid and Cancer

Folic acid, in my opinion, reduces cancer of the breast, colon, pancreas, and prostate. Reviewing the literature is at best confusing, because a pure study of any one of these cancers and folate is hard to find. The most influential external factor is alcohol. Alcohol reduces folate, and less folate permits homocysteine levels to rise. This influence of alcohol and homocysteine is impossible to separate definitively, but looking at studies where these were addressed, alcohol did not help.

Giovannucci and colleagues, in a study involving 45,000 professional men, showed that the risk of colon cancer doubled with two alcoholic drinks per day. Furthermore, they found that men who were homozygous for the C677T MTHFR polymorphism reduced their risk for colon cancer if they took at least 650 mcg of folic acid a day.[62]

Folic acid recently has been implicated in the rise of prostate cancer; many articles can be found on the internet making this association. Trying to understand these articles is difficult at best. What the writers report is that with folic acid, the incidence of prostate cancer is 9%. The incidence, according to the National Cancer Institute, is as high as 35% in men between the ages of 65 and 74.[63] I think that focusing too narrowly on the statistics does not

---

[61] Tolarova, M., "Periconceptual Supplementation with Vitamins and Folic Acid to Prevent Recurrences of Cleft Lip," *Lancet*, 1982, *2*(8291), 217, https://doi.org/10.1016/s0140-6736(82)91063-7.

[62] Giovannucci, E., et al., "Alcohol, Low-Methionine—Low-Folate Diets, and Risk of Colon Cancer in Men," *Journal of the National Cancer Institute*, 1995, *87*(4), 265–273, https://doi.org/10.1093/jnci/87.4.265.

[63] Prostate Cancer Screening (PDQ)—Health Professional Version. Editorial Board, National Cancer Institute, 2024.

give credence to these reports. Additionally, looking at where these reports come from is most interesting. The reports that say folic acid promotes prostate cancer are by and large generated in the United States. Studies performed outside of the United States do not support this finding. In fact, some researchers such as Dr. Simon Collin of the University of Bristol's Department of Social Medicine have reported the opposite; he said that in a study conducted in 2009, he and his team did not find any association between prostate cancer and the commonly studied "folate gene" (MTHFR). If this existed, he said, the variation in enzymes that regulate folate levels could be demonstrated. The laboratory studies do not support the statistics presented. He called the statement that folate increases prostate cancer an "unfounded hypothesis."[64]

The incidence of breast cancer can be reduced with folate, as reported in a 1999 *Journal of the American Medical Association* (JAMA) article. Again, a direct effect of folate in cancer may involve an indirect route of folate's effect on the metabolism of homocysteine. More than two drinks of alcohol a day decreases folate and increases the risk of breast cancer. Taking 600 mcg of folic acid or more a day decreases the risk of breast cancer by about half.[65]

Folic Acid Deficiency

Folic acid is necessary for the production of nucleic acids, DNA, and RNA. These are the essential building blocks of life. All growth requires folic acid, and because of this feature, deficiencies appear where there is the most rapid growth and cell turnover. The systems associated with folic acid deficiencies are the production of red and

---

[64] Collin, S. M., et al., "Association of Folate-Pathway Gene Polymorphisms with the Risk of Prostate Cancer: A Population-Based Nested Case-Controlled Study, Systematic Review, and Meta-Analysis," *Cancer Epidemiology, Biomarkers & Prevention*, 2009, *18*(9), 2528–2539, https://doi.org/10.1158/1055-9965.EPI-09-0223.

[65] *JAMA*, 1999.

white blood cells, gastrointestinal lining cells that control absorption, and fetal spinal cord and brain development in the first few weeks of pregnancy.

Traditional medicine has focused mainly on these three areas because they are the most common problems that occur in medicine. Oncology, the area of medicine involved with the study and treatment of cancer, has developed a fourth major deficiency of folic acid: deficiencies provoked by the use of chemotherapy (methotrexate), which either consumes or blocks the effect of folic acid.

These problems are important and develop when the deficiency is significant. They cannot be ignored. They must be addressed and corrected. Because of their importance, they often capture doctors' and patients' attention, leaving little curiosity to ask the question of what else it does.

Primarily, it corrects the deficiencies that lead to the symptoms, or conditions, of tiredness, irritability, loss of appetite, shortness of breath, psoriasis, brain fog, Alzheimer's, forgetfulness, depression, cleft lip, cleft palate, heart defects, breast cancer, colon cancer, elevated homocysteine levels, and arterial plaque formation. These are not problems that develop suddenly; they are insidious, creeping into our lives slowly and ever so gradually that a change from the norm is not noticed. This is because the stores of folic acid in our body, mainly the liver, can last about three months. Add to this the four months that an average red blood cell lives, and it is more than half a year before changes such as anemia from folate deficiency appear in the blood. Symptoms of anemia may occur anytime in this spectrum and vary in severity so that who knows when it started, but there you are.

The more difficult situation most people find themselves in is not a full deficiency of folic acid, where the body folate level is zero, but in a situation where it is somewhere close to zero and nowhere near the optimal level for all systems to run well. This may mean they will have some days with few problems, but on most days, they will experience tiredness, forgetfulness, and brain fog. It is in this area that most people find themselves. These are the people who benefit the most from supplementing folic acid.

The best description I ran across describing the effects of taking folic acid is the most amusing characterization of a vitamin that I have ever heard: "upon taking folic acid you will first notice that your mind is more alert, the memory is improved, and you will be more cooperative."[66]

According to the National Institutes of Health's Office of Dietary Supplements, the recommendation for folate intake is listed below.[67]

Recommended Dietary Allowance (RDA) for Folate		
Life stage	Age	Intake (mcg/day)
Infant	0–6 months	65
	7–12 months	80
Child	1–3 years	150
	4–8 years	200
	9–13 years	300
Adolescent	14–18 years	400
Adult	19 years and older	400
Pregnant	All ages	600
Breastfeeding	All ages	500

[66] "Folate," Linus Pauling Institute, 2023.
[67] NIH, "Folate," last updated November 1, 2022, https://ods.od.nih.gov/factsheets/Folate-Consumer/.

Folic Acid Sources and Supplements

Food sources of folate are green leafy vegetables, spinach, citrus fruit, asparagus, lentils, and garbanzo beans and fortified foods—that is, folate has been added to increase or to replace what was destroyed by the preparation or to prolong shelf life (e.g., bread). Fortified foods are not my favorite selections for folic acid, as they often do not have the other nutrients normally found with folic acid.

Folic acid supplements can be found in the form of tablets, capsules, powders, and liquid for oral consumption or intravenous injection. Folic acid is available individually or combined with other B vitamins such as in a B-complex formulation, with all the B vitamins, in a multivitamin, or only with one other B vitamin such as a folic acid and vitamin B_{12} combination. Folic acid in a strength of 1 mg or greater requires a doctor's prescription.

Folic acid is a synthetic form of folate used in many supplements. The body does not use folic acid directly; it must be metabolized first to dihydrofolate and then tetrahydrofolate by the intestines to be bioactive and absorbable. Tetrahydrofolate is transformed into either 10-formyltetrahydofolate or folinic acid (5-formyltetrahydrofolate), and then they both can be formed into 5,10-methenyltetradydrofolate. This product, 5,10-methenyltetradydrofolate, is converted to 5,10-methylenetetrahydrofolate, then methyltetrahydrofolate reductase (MTHFR), and finally 5-MTHF. This is a complicated series of chemical names to describe the process that folic acid and folate go through to become the final useful forms the body needs to promote normal DNA synthesis, metabolize homocysteine, preserve nervous system structure and function, maintain the endocrine system, and support digestive health.

A final product that requires no additional steps is methylfolate, a naturally occurring folate designated 5-methyltetrahydrofolate (5-MTHF). Metafolin is a commercially prepared form of 5-MTHF.

Another midway metabolite, folinic acid (5-formyltetrahydrofolate), is also a highly absorbable, bioavailable form of folic acid that I recommend.

Different manufacturers use different names, complicating the selection process when looking for a folic acid supplement. Besides the label saying "folic acid," the package sidebar of "Supplement Facts" may say "folate," "folinic acid," "methylfolate," or "Metafolin." All are acceptable forms of folic acid. Nonprescription dosages are usually limited to 400 to 800 mcg per day. This dosage can be purchased as an individual ingredient or in a multivitamin.

Prescription folic acid tablets come in 0.4 mg, 0.5 mg, 1.0 mg, and 5.0 mg. Compounding pharmacies that prepare tablets or capsules at your doctor's request and made up only for you may go as high as 10–15 mg or more. There are prescription multivitamins that contain larger doses of folic acid, or methylfolate for stubborn cases of homocysteine, or prenatal vitamins for expecting mothers, such as Cerefolin, Foltx, CitraNatal, and NataFort.

Folic Acid Injection, USP, is a sterile solution of sodium folate intended for intravenous (IV), intramuscular (IM), or subcutaneous (SC) injection. It is made by adding sodium hydroxide to folic acid. This forms sodium folate and is often referred to as simply folate. It is a yellow substance that degrades rapidly in light to a brownish color, at which point it has no nutritional benefit. It is resistant to heat below 250 degrees Fahrenheit, but it deteriorates on exposure to light in solution.

Mostly, I give folic acid as part of an IV solution in a drip, or I add it to a Myers's cocktail as an intravenous push, with no ill effects. Given as an intramuscular injection, it tends to sting for a few minutes. I prefer the IV route for folic acid because this way, my patients do not have to experience discomfort.

Leucovorin is a commercial name for folinic acid. It is often used for methorexate "rescue"—that is, where too much methorexate was used in chemotherapy, blocking the transformation of folic acid to folinic acid on its way to the active form of methyl folate, or 5-MTHF. It is also an antidote for methyl alcohol poisoning at 1 mg/kg (maximum 50 mg) IV to reduce the metabolic production of formate.[68] Methyl alcohol causes acidosis, is an inhibitor of mitochondrial function, and causes blindness.

---

[68] Carey, C. F., Lee, H. H., and Woeltje, K. F. (eds.), *The Washington Manual of Medical Therapeutics*, 29th edition, Lippincott-Raven Publishers, 1998, 514.

Vitamin B12

Benefits of Vitamin B_{12}

- Prevents and treats canker sores
- Prevents and treats pernicious anemia
- Reduces depression
- Improves multiple sclerosis
- Reduces the risk of macular degeneration
- Relieves nerve pain, tingling, and numbness
- Slows the progression of Alzheimer's disease
- Reduces ringing in the ears
- Required for the production of DNA and RNA
- Supports immunity
- Treats rosacea
- Reduces heart disease
- Improves postoperative dementia and polyneuropathy
- Provides an energy boost
- Improves the quality of sleep

History of Vitamin B_{12}

The two most common forms of vitamin B_{12} for both oral use and use by injection are cyanocobalamin and methylcobalamin. The term **cobalamin** is applied generically to all the molecular forms of vitamin B_{12}. During the process of developing an understanding of B_{12} deficiencies, other terms have been used to describe B_{12}: **antipernicious anemia factor, Castle's extrinsic factor, and animal protein factor**. These terms developed as sources of B_{12} in clinical practice became effective. The antipernicious anemia factor related to the benefit of feeding patients whole raw beef liver, which contains 1 microgram (mcg) of B_{12} per gram (g) of liver. Castle introduced the idea of intrinsic and extrinsic factors in 1929 and demonstrated it in 1934. Castle's extrinsic factor relates to feeding beef muscle to patients; muscle contains 2 mcg of B_{12} in each 100 g of beef. In the 1940s, animal protein factor was found to be necessary for growth in some animals fed an all-vegetable diet.

Pernicious[69] anemia was the starting point for the discovery of B_{12} deficiency. The first modern medical reference to this disease occurred in 1824 by Combe, who thought it was possibly related to the digestive system. In 1855, Combe and Addison described the symptoms of pernicious anemia. In 1925, Whipple and Robscheit-Robbins were studying dogs that had anemia and that benefited from being fed liver. This observation prompted George Minot and William Murphy, in 1926, to try feeding patients with pernicious anemia raw liver. This corrected the anemia, and the red cells became normal. These experiments began the search for the "antipernicious anemia factor" in liver.

Working in the same field in 1929, W. P. Castle proposed from his observations that two factors are needed to correct pernicious anemia: an **extrinsic factor** in food and an **intrinsic factor** in normal gastric secretions. He isolated the intrinsic factor, a glycoprotein, in 1934. This is produced in the parietal cells of the stomach lining. Vitamin B_{12} was first isolated in 1948 by two separate groups: Rickes and colleagues in the United States and Smith and Parker in England. That same year, West showed that injections of the newly isolated red crystalline substance successfully treated pernicious anemia.[70]

---

[69] "Pernicious, adj. 1. ruinous; highly hurtful, 2. deadly, fatal. 3. evil or wicked"; Bernhart, C. L., and Stein, J. (eds.), *The American College Dictionary*, Random House, 1964.

[70] Herbert, V., "Drugs Effective in Megaloblastic Anemia, Vitamin B_{12} and Folic Acid," In Goodman, L. S., and Gilman, A. (eds.), *The Pharmacological Basis of Therapeutics*, 4th edition, Macmillan, 1971, 1414–1415.

The next year, in 1949, Pierce and his coworkers isolated two forms of vitamin B_{12}: cyanocobalamin, which has a cyanide group, and hydroxocobalamin, which does not. Dorothy Hodgkin, in 1955, identified the molecular structure of vitamin B_{12}, cyanocobalamin and the coenzyme forms, using X-ray crystallography. That same year, vitamin B_{12} was synthesized from bacteria and fungi cultures by Woodward in the United States and by Eschenmoser in Switzerland. Woodward continued to work on vitamin B_{12} until he could synthesize the molecule entirely from chemicals in 1973.

Functions of Vitamin B_{12}

Vitamin B_{12} is important for cell production and maintenance. Primarily, it is involved in the process of making DNA. All cells have DNA; it is the basis of the life code and cell reproduction. Without B_{12}, there would be no cells and no life. B_{12} deficiency is most pronounced in types of cells with rapid growth, turnover, or repair—that is, red blood cells and nervous tissue, as they experience the most growth and repair—but all cells require B_{12} to remain healthy.

B_{12} is also required as a cofactor for two enzymes: methionine synthase, which is required for the conversion of homocysteine to methionine, and L-methylmalonyl-CoA mutase, which is required for a few metabolic conversions, including fat and carbohydrate metabolism.[71]

The most pronounced effects of B_{12} deficiency are neurological symptoms of numbness and tingling in the hands and feet, difficulty walking from damage to the myelin sheaths of nerves, disorientation, dementia, memory loss, loss of smell and taste, breathlessness, and

---

[71] Drake, V.J., "Micronutrients and Cognitive Function," *Linus Pauling Institute Research Newsletter*, Spring/Summer 2011, 12–14,
https://lpi.oregonstate.edu/sites/lpi.oregonstate.edu/files/pdf/newsletters/ss11.pdf.

poor concentration. It also causes anemia in the form of very large red blood cells, called **megaloblastic** (large young-cell) **anemia**. If this anemia is left untreated, additional symptoms such as delusions and hallucinations will develop, and these are not reversible with treatment at this late stage of the disease. Poor repair of the intestinal tract and generalized debility are other symptoms.

The molecule of vitamin B_{12} is the largest of the vitamins. Briefly, it is four corrin rings and a nucleotide holding a cobalt atom, and attached to it is an anionic radical. The radicals are interchangeable, yielding up to six different molecular forms of vitamin B_{12}. The most common and abundant form of B_{12} is **cyanocobalamin**, the crystalline form with a cyanide group attached to the central chelated cobalt atom. The body can take this form of the molecule and, through enzymes and the help of folic acid, metabolize it to **methylcobalamin** (methyl B_{12}), an active form of B_{12}.

The Six Forms of Vitamin B12	
Permissive name	Radicle -R
Cyanocobalamin (vitamin B_{12})	-CN
Hydroxocobalamin (vitamin B_{12a})	-OH
Aquocobalamin (vitamin B_{12b})	$-H_2O$
Nitrocobalamin (vitamin B_{12c})	$-NO_2$
5'-deoxyadenosylcobalamin (coenzyme B_{12})	5'-deoxyadenosyl
Methylcobalamin (methyl B_{12})	$-CH_3$

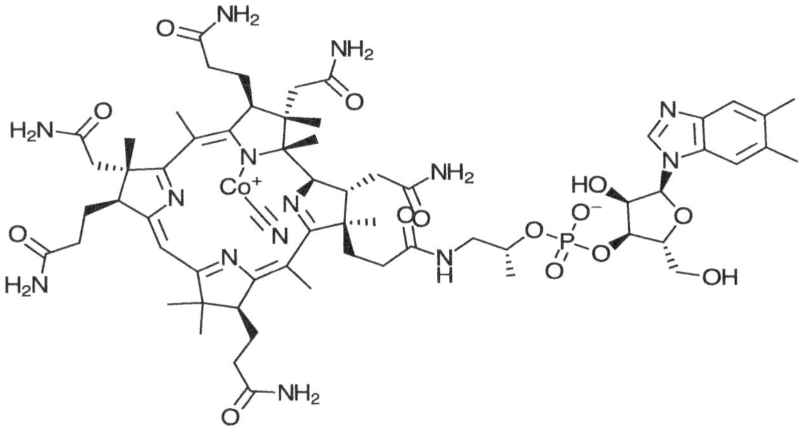

Cyanocobalamin, B_{12}

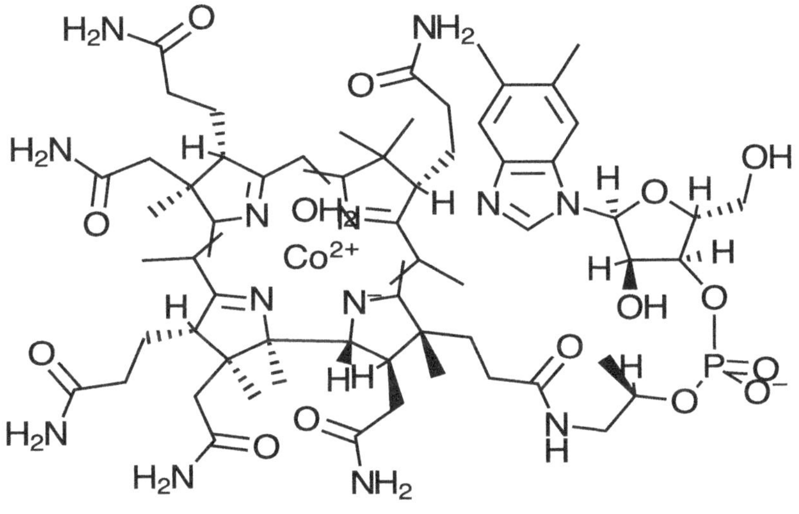

Hydroxocobalamin, B_{12a}

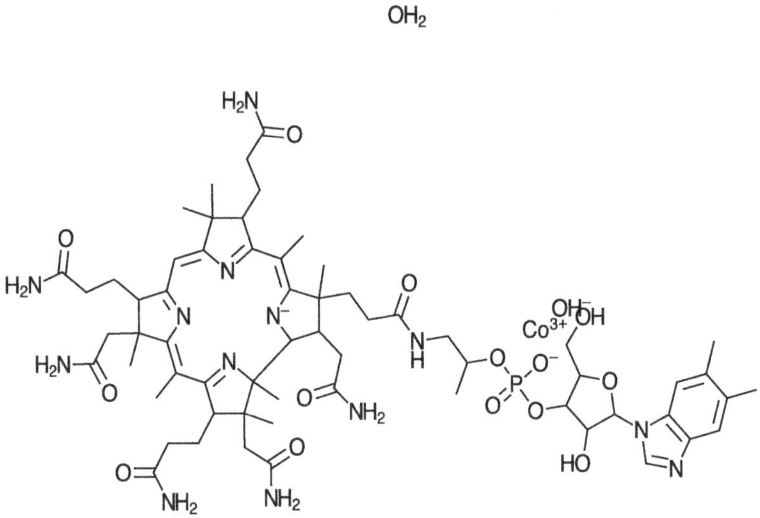

Aquocobalamin, B_{12b}

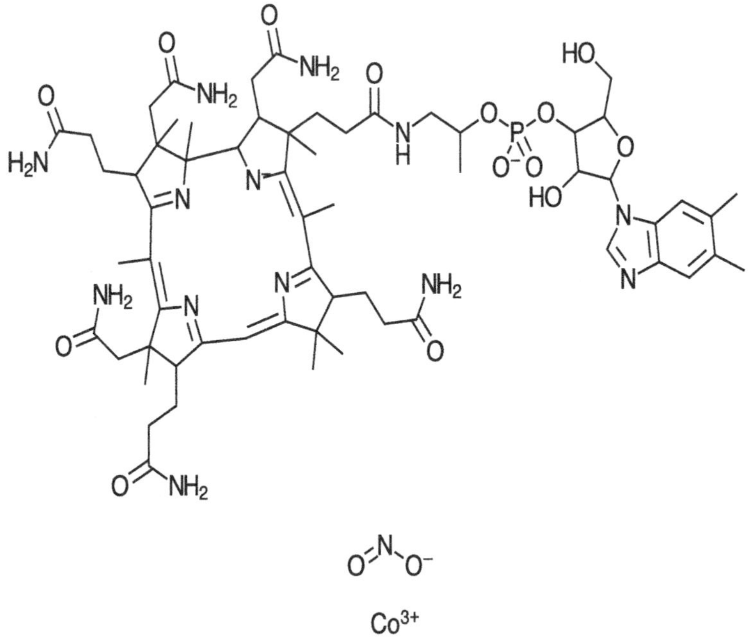

Nitrocobalamin, B_{12c}

5'-Deoxyadenosylcobalamin, Coenzyme B$_{12}$

Methylcobalamin, Methyl B$_{12}$

Vitamin B_{12} affects cell production and maintenance and is required as a cofactor for two enzymes. A B_{12} deficiency can also cause neurological symptoms, megaloblastic anemia, poor repair of the intestinal tract, and generalized debility. Other functions include improved energy levels, a lower risk of macular degeneration, the prevention of canker sores, and improvements in mood.

Improved Energy Levels

Many people claim that taking a Vitamin B_{12} shot or a sublingual spray increases their energy levels, allowing them to tackle difficult tasks. Some science does back this up. Cyanocobalamin is converted to an active form called adenosylcobalamin, one of the six forms of B_{12}, and it interacts with the enzyme methylmalonyl-CoA mutase in the mitochondria to help produce energy.[72] Young cells have more mitochondria than older cells and, as you would expect, more energy. In the mitochondria in the cell is where oxygen and sugar come together with the help of such things as coenzyme Q-10 to produce energy in the way cells can use it.

Reduced Risk of Macular Degeneration

Macular degeneration affects 10% of 70-year-olds and 30% of 80-year-olds. A significant study showed that B_{12} has been proven to treat not only anemia but also vision problems. William G. Christen and his team reported in 2009 that age-related macular degeneration occurred 41% less frequently in people who took vitamin B_6, B_{12}, and folic acid to reduce their homocysteine levels in a 7.5-year randomized, double-blind, placebo-controlled study.[73] More than 5,200 women participated in the study, and the participants were

---

[72] Levine, S., "To B or Not to B: All the Ways Our Body Relies on Folate and B12," *FOCUS, Allergy Research Group Newsletter*, October 2011, 8.

[73] Christen, W. G., et al., "Folic Acid, Pyridoxine, and Cyanocobalamin Combination Treatment and Age-Related Macular Degeneration in Women: The Women's Antioxidant and Folic Acid Cardiovascular Study," *Archives of Internal Medicine*, 2009, *169*(4), 335–341; Christen, W., "B Vitamins Could Lower Risk of Macular Degeneration," *Archives of Internal Medicine*, February 23, 2009.

evenly divided into those who received the vitamin combination and those who received a placebo. In the placebo group, 82 women developed macular degeneration, compared to only 55 in the treatment group.

Usually, the vitamins that are promoted for age-related macular degeneration (AMD) are vitamins A, C, and E, zinc, copper, and lutein. This study sheds new light on the problem in that these are not the only nutrients that preserve vision. Besides being nutrients, the combination of B vitamins lowers the homocysteine level, preventing microvascular clotting and preserving arterial function in the eyeball.

If taking vitamins such as B_{12} will prevent you from developing this type of central vision blindness, this is a significant finding. Moreover, that this article was published in a major American Medical Association publication, *Archives of Internal Medicine*, gives weight to its significance. The next time a doctor argues that there is no proof vitamins work, suggest that they should read their own major professional literature. The reason doctors do not know about these things is that they do not read the available mainline journals. They are looking for the newest drug to impress their patients to show that they are on top of things. Many people are impressed by this, to their own detriment. **Drugs have side effects; vitamins have side benefits.**

Prevention of Canker Sores

Canker sores are not lethal, but they are annoying. In 2009, Dr. Ilia Volkov, a family physician at the Ben-Gurion University, presented a study where 58 random patients were placed in a double-blind, placebo-controlled trial using vitamin B_{12} to prevent canker sores, or recurrent aphthous stomatitis. The study lasted one year, and the crossover point was at six months. Either a placebo or 1,000 mcg of vitamin B_{12} were given at bedtime. The treated group suffered fewer ulcers every month, with no ulcers found in the sixth month. At six months, the treated group became the placebo group and began to develop more ulcers each succeeding month from the time of crossover.[74]

I recommend vitamin B_{12} in any form—lozenges, sublingual drops, capsules, or shots will do the job nicely.

Treatment of Mood Disorders

People who are diagnosed with depression often also have vitamin B_{12} and folic acid deficiencies. Both these vitamins are used to produce neurotransmitters or chemicals that are used for one cell to talk to another. Treatment with B_{12} has been implicated to help mood disorders.

Vitamin B_{12} Sufficiency

Vitamin B_{12} sufficiency is dependent on having enough in the diet, ingesting it, absorbing it, and utilizing it. In utilizing B_{12}, there must be sufficient folic acid, as the two are needed to help each other pass along the methyl group (-CH3) and form methylcobalamin, but renal function is required for the elimination of excess folic acid. If folic acid is not metabolized to tetrahydrofolate, large amounts of asymmetric dimethylarginine accumulate and interfere with the nitric oxide needed for endothelial function (dilatation of arteries to accommodate larger blood flow). Patients in renal failure treated with cyanocobalamin tend to accumulate cyanide and have less of a relaxing factor, similar to nitric oxide. Treating renal patients with methylcobalamin lowers both homocysteine and asymmetric dimethylarginine.[75] In short, when renal failure is present, please seek

---

[74] Volkov, I., et al., "Effectiveness of Vitamin B12 in Treating Recurrent Aphthous Stomatitis: A Randomized, Double-Blind, Placebo-Controlled Trial," *Journal of the American Board of Family Medicine*, 2009, *22*(1), 9–16, https://doi.org/10.3122/jabfm.2009.01.080113.

[75] Spence, J. D., and Stampfer, M. J., "Understanding the Complexity of Homocysteine Lowering with Vitamins: The Potential Role of Subgroup Analyses," *JAMA*, 2011, *306*(23), 2610–2611.

professional guidance in the use of folic acid and vitamin B_{12}. Both methyl folate and methylcobalamin are the better choices.

The Institute of Medicine, through the Food and Nutrition Board, in 1998, revised the dietary reference intakes (RDI) for vitamin B_{12} to be increased for elderly adults above the age of 50. This was done to accommodate the poor absorption with age, and it was advised that this be accomplished by adding B_{12} to cereals and advising the use of oral supplements. The latest RDI[76] is listed below:

Dietary Reference Intakes (RDI) for Vitamin B_{12}		
Life stage	Age	Intake (mcg/day)
Infant	0–6 months	0.4
	7–12 months	0.5
Child	1–3 years	0.9
	4–8 years	1.2
	9–13 years	1.8
Adolescent	14–18 years	2.4
Adult	19 years and older	2.4
Pregnant	All ages	2.6
Breastfeeding	All ages	2.8

---

[76] Institute of Medicine (US) Standing Committee on the Scientific Evaluation of Dietary Reference Intakes and its Panel on Folate, Other B Vitamins, and Choline, *Dietary Reference Intakes for Thiamin, Riboflavin, Niacin, Vitamin B6, Folate, Vitamin B12, Pantothenic Acid, Biotin, and Choline*, National Academies Press, 1998, https://www.ncbi.nlm.nih.gov/books/NBK114310/pdf/Bookshelf_NBK1143 10.pdf.

No upper limit (UL), or maximum level, of daily nutrient intake has been identified for vitamin B_{12}. No cases of toxicity have been reported or linked to any condition or death. The usual laboratory reference range used by BioReference Laboratories for vitamin B_{12} is 211–946 picograms per milliliter (pg/ml). In my practice, I like to see the lower level of B_{12} above 500 pg/ml so that tissue levels are adequate—what I call a more optimal level. Remember that the RDA, and now the RDI, is the level that the Food and Nutritional Board considers just enough not to have any signs of abnormality, or even be close to death. I prefer to have a higher level of B_{12} to enjoy robust health. In my practice, I advise supplements of B_{12} in sublingual, capsule, and injectable forms. Many of my patients have levels that range from 500 to more than 2,000 pg/ml. This is protective, I believe, against early brain atrophy and shrinkage, and it allows people to maintain function for the longest possible time.

The most active forms of B_{12} in humans are **hydroxocobalamin, adenosylcobalamin,** and **methylcobalamin**. All the cobalamins are stable at high temperatures but easily break down in light. Vitamin B_{12} does not need refrigeration. It can be kept at room temperature, but it must be protected from light in a dark-brown bottle or wrapped in aluminum foil.

Throughout most of the discovery of vitamin B_{12} deficiency and treatment, attention was focused on pernicious anemia and the neurological manifestations. Biochemistry defined the structure of the molecule and the metabolic processing of cyanocobalamin to some of its intermediate and active forms. There are six forms of vitamin B_{12}. Some are more active than others, and some are intermediate forms that interact with forms of folic acid to eventually become methylcobalamin. This process of going from cyanocobalamin to methylcobalamin can be skipped by taking the newly available methylcobalamin, but I do not fully recommend it.

Starting with the natural form of cyanocobalamin found in food, this molecule goes through its six forms in an interaction with folic acid, as folic acid passes through various molecular forms to become methyl folate. Besides going through molecular conversion, both vitamins pass along a single carbon methyl (-CH3) group that they then pass on to the DNA and other molecules. The short explanation of this process is that they need each other to become the active forms that exert influence and do the work of vitamins.

In nature, a blend of vitamins is best, and I feel that a blend of the different forms of a vitamin is also good. As we learn more about vitamins, we will find reason to use one form over another. We do not know everything about vitamins and what the intermediate forms do. To cover our bets, both the cyanocobalamin and methylcobalamin forms should be used. After all, most vitamins do not have side effects—they have side benefits.

Vitamin B_{12} Deficiency

The symptoms of vitamin B_{12} deficiency include fatigue, shortness of breath, weight loss, anorexia (diminished appetite), constipation or diarrhea, vague abdominal pain, inflammation with burning of the tongue called glossitis, peripheral neuropathy (nerve pain or numbness), and loss of positional or vibratory sensation in the extremities with muscle weakness and loss of reflexes, like demonstrated with the hammer and knee-jerk test.[77] In people over 60 years of age, neurological symptoms may present before signs of anemia. Poor nerve function leads to falls, and low B_{12} levels accelerate brain atrophy, vertigo, multiple sclerosis, and diabetic neuropathy. Less common symptoms are paranoia (megaloblastic madness), irritability, depression, and yellow-blue color blindness.[78]

---

[77] Hvas, A-M., and Nexo, E., "Diagnosis and Treatment of Vitamin B12 Deficiency: An Update," *Haematologica*, 2006, *91*(11), 1506–1512.
[78] Berkow, R., and Beers, M. H. (eds.), *The Merck Manual*, 17th edition, 1999.

Vitamin B_{12} Deficiency and Neurological Problems

Mild deficiency leads to neurological problems of numbness; tingling in the hands and feet; loss of appetite, taste, and smell; memory loss; poor concentration; poor sleep quality; impotence; spinal cord degeneration; disorientation; and dementia. Although pernicious anemia can develop from severe B_{12} deficiency, a mild to moderate deficiency of the B vitamins leads to neurological problems. B_{12} and folic acid are needed for development of the brain and nervous system. If they are needed for development of the nervous system, it just makes sense that they are also needed for maintenance. The exact mechanism of how B_{12} deficiency affects the neurological system is not known. Your brain grows every day. It makes new connections from one cell to another, called a synapse, as it records a memory, a thought, or an experience.

Cognitive Impairment

Cognitive impairment is expected with normal aging, but it is accelerated in dementia. Shrinkage of the hippocampus, an area of the brain important for memory, was shown to be less when vitamins B_{12}, B_6, and folic acid were added to the diet. Smith and colleagues studied 168 people over the age of 70 for 24 months, documenting the brain size with cranial MRIs at the beginning and at the end of the study. Normal brain atrophy was 8% per year. For those on the vitamins, the loss was decreased by 24%.[79]

Brain Atrophy

Brain atrophy is associated with Alzheimer's disease and progresses as mental function deteriorates. In the Oxford Project to Investigate Memory and Aging (OPTIMA study), a prospective five-year study conducted by Vogiatzoglou and colleagues at the

---

[79] Smith, A. D., et al., "Homocysteine-Lowering by B Vitamins Slows the Rate of Accelerated Brain Atrophy in Mild Cognitive Impairment: A Randomized Controlled Trial," *PLoS One*, 2010, 5(9), e12244, https://doi.org/10.1371/journal.pone.0012244.

University of Oxford on 107 men and women aged 61 to 87, lower vitamin B_{12} levels were associated with more brain volume loss than in those with higher B_{12} levels. The researchers concluded that B_{12} level is a modifiable factor and that by raising it, the rate of brain loss can be reduced.[80]

The OPTIMA study indicated that vitamin B_{12} deficiency is associated with increased atrophy of the hippocampus and the medial temporal lobe in Alzheimer's disease and that lower folate levels are related to hippocampal and amygdala atrophy.[81] I find this information useful from a practical standpoint and recommend to my patients that if they want to preserve good brain health, they need to take the B vitamins. Doctors who give B_{12} shots are often criticized by their colleagues for engaging in a useless process. But from the OPTIMA study, which is only one of many studies, it is apparent that B_{12} supplementation is one of the best things you can do for your brain.

Spinal Cord Degeneration

Severe vitamin B_{12} deficiency, as found in pernicious anemia, is associated with spinal cord degeneration. I find this fact reason enough to use B_{12} in any injury or disease of the nervous system.

Homocysteine

Without going into too much chemistry while we are talking about the brain, I want to refer back to homocysteine. Vitamin B_{12} is required to remove homocysteine from the blood to prevent the vascular disease problems of atherosclerotic plaque formation and poor artery dilation, called endothelia dysfunction. Vitamin B_{12} is required for methylation—that is, to add a methyl group (-CH3) to homocysteine. The new methylated product is called **S-**

---

[80] Vogiatzoglou, A., et al., "Vitamin B12 Status and Rate of Brain Volume Loss in Community-Dwelling Elderly," 2008, *Neurology*, 71(11), 826–832, https://doi.org/10.1212/01.wnl.0000325581.26991.f2.
[81] Ibid., 826.

adenosylmethionine. A deficiency of S-adenosylmethionine is known to be related to white-matter demyelination, another form of brain atrophy.[82] Yet another reason B_{12} is needed for your brain health.

Causes of Vitamin B12 Deficiency

The causes of B_{12} deficiency can include poor ingestion, digestion, and absorption.

Dietary Restrictions

Dietary restrictions, as found with a vegetarian or vegan diets, limits exposure to the B_{12} in red meat. Vitamin B_{12} is found only in animal-sourced foods (ASFs) or fortified foods; it is not made in the plant world.[83]

Gastrointestinal Issues

People with insufficient stomach acid, a condition termed **achlorhydria**, cannot digest meat and liberate the B_{12} from food. The stomach wall may not produce the **intrinsic factor** needed to facilitate absorption. Long-term use of acid-blocking medications (Nexium, Protonix, and Prilosec) decreases the hydrochloric acid (HCl) available for digestion. Pancreatic insufficiency indicates a lack of enzymes needed for digestion to free up the B_{12}. Diseases of the bowel, such as celiac disease, Crohn's disease, and irritable bowel syndrome, and lap banding and small bowel resection (removal of sections of the bowel for injury, disease, or to promote weight loss) limit vitamin absorption. Recently, a rare genetically inherited lack of intrinsic factor called **Imerslund–Gräsbeck** syndrome has been identified.[84] Atrophic gastritis, usually found in the elderly, is a

---

[82] Ibid., 831.
[83] Allen, L. H., "How Common Is Vitamin B-12 Deficiency?" *American Journal of Clinical Nutrition*, 2009, *89*(suppl), 693S–6S, https://doi.org/10.3945/ajcn.2008.26947a.
[84] Hvas and Nexo, "Diagnosis and Treatment of Vitamin B12 Deficiency," 1510.

condition where the stomach produces fewer digestive factors, leading to less absorption of select nutrients.

Rheumatoid Arthritis

There can be rapid utilization of B_{12} in some diseases. For instance, I have noticed that patients with rheumatoid arthritis consume vitamin B_{12} rapidly and have difficulty maintaining B_{12} at optimal levels without frequent injections. At the higher levels of B_{12}, the symptoms of rheumatoid arthritis are reduced.

Gastric Atrophy

On the more practical side, the most common cause of vitamin B_{12} deficiency in America is aging of the stomach lining, called gastric atrophy, leading to low production of the hydrochloric acid needed for the digestion of food. It is estimated that of the adults over the age of 60, 10% to 15% have vitamin B_{12} deficiency.[85]

Prescription Drugs

Another common cause of B_{12} deficiency is the use of prescription drugs that interfere with digestion or absorption or cause interference at the cellular level.

Hormonal contraceptives, either with the combination of **desogestrel** and **ethinyl estradiol (EE)** or **depot medroxyprogesterone acetate (DMPA)**, will lower B_{12} levels 20% and 13%, respectively, versus a normal 3% decline on nonhormonal contraception, as reported by Berenson and Rahman in a study of 703 women at the University of Texas Medical Branch, Galveston.[86]

A group of drugs known as **proton pump inhibitors (PPI)**, used to reduce stomach acid, reduces the amount of acid needed for

---

[85] Drake, "Micronutrients and Cognitive Function."
[86] Brunk, D., "Vitamin B12 Levels Are Diminished in OC Users," *Internal Medicine News*, May 1, 2012, 19.

digestion and the release of B_{12} from food.[87] Examples are omeprazole (Prilosec) and lansoprazole (Prevacid), rabeprazole (AcipHex), pantoprazole (Protonix), and esomeprazole (Nexium). The PPIs are much stronger than the H2-receptor antagonists in controlling stomach acid secretion. Anyone taking these drugs should have their vitamin B_{12} levels checked if they are used for more than two years and monitor for developing neurological problems such as numbness, tingling, gait disturbance, falls, and memory problems.

H2-receptor blockers also reduce the production of stomach acid, but not to the extent of PPIs. H2-blockers were, in 1978, the first drugs used to reduce stomach acid and treat duodenal and stomach ulcers. That first group of drugs included cimetidine (Tagamet), famotidine (Pepcid), nizatidine (Axid), and ranitidine (Zantac). You may be blocking more than acid with these drugs and do yourself more harm than good.

Initially, patients using H2-blockers and proton pump inhibitors were advised to use them for no more than 6 weeks or, for stubborn cases, a maximum of 12 weeks. It was not long before one prescription led to another, then another, and before anyone knew it, years of treatment. Vitamin B_{12} is not the only nutrient that is blocked. All sorts of nutrients pass through the intestinal system undigested and unabsorbed. Could these modern drugs be helping to provoke some of our modern medical problems like Alzheimer's disease, osteoporosis, obesity, hypertension, and diabetes? I believe the evidence is building that many of our major health problems are related to the drugs we take and the quality of the food we eat.

In support of the H2-blockers and PPIs, I do have to say that with their introduction in the '70s, the practice of performing a subtotal gastrectomy or removal of part of the stomach to treat

---

[87] Higdon, J., et al., "Vitamin B12," Linus Pauling Institute, Oregon State University, last updated October 2023, http://lpi.oregonstate.edu/infocenter/vitamins/vitaminB12/.

ulcers came almost to a complete halt. It was a great benefit. But too much of a good thing has gone too far, and it has created its own problems of poor nutrition–provoked conditions.

Metformin (Glucophage) is known to reduce the absorption of vitamin B_{12}, with blood levels reduced up to 30%.[88] Taking it for a prolonged period may cause subtle but slowly progressive neurological numbness that mimics symptoms associated with diabetes. Some portion of the numbness may be inherent to the diabetes, but another portion may be from reduced vitamin B_{12}. Diabetic symptoms of poor nerve function begin when the level of B_{12} is below 460 picograms per milliliter (pg/ml) and not 250 pg/ml, which was the accepted cutoff.[89] Quest Laboratories reports show a normal range of B_{12} as 200–1,100 pg/ml, which is even lower than the textbook. In my opinion, the lowest level should be at least 500 pg/ml, or even higher. In my practice, I like to see my patients in the 1,000 to 2,000 pg/ml range. Fortunately, the poor absorption of B_{12} can be corrected by either increased oral supplementation or injections. Reduced B_{12} blood levels can be corrected with either method.

Nitrous oxide, a common form of anesthesia used by the medical and dental professions, can make B_{12} inactive by oxidizing the molecule. The effect can be subtle or pronounced: sensory loss, peripheral neuropathy, muscle weakness (called myelopathy), or encephalopathy (any abnormal changes in the brain). The most severe case of nitrous oxide toxicity that I treated was in a young man who used this gas recreationally to enhance his orgasms. He reported a very heightened experience by adding nitrous oxide, but the downside was he could neither walk nor stand after his session

---

[88] Andrès, E., Noel, E., and Goichot, B., "Metformin-Associated Vitamin B12 Deficiency," *Archives of Internal Medicine*, 2000, *162*(19), 2251–2252, https://doi.org/10.1001/archinte.162.19.2251-a.
[89] Vinik, A. I., and Strotmeyer, E. S., "Diabetic Neuropathy in Older Adults," In Sinclair, A. J., Morley, J. E., and Vellas, B. (eds.), *Principles & Practice of Geriatric Medicine*, John Wiley & Sons, 2010, 751–767.

of pleasure. His presentation was a combination of leg spasms and weakness so severe that he could not stand up even if he held on to the bed rail. He did recover completely but required hospitalization, injections of cyanocobalamin daily for one month, and physical therapy.

Drugs used to prevent seizures are of great benefit but can lower vitamin B_{12} and folate levels. Dilantin (phenytoin), Mysoline (primidone), and phenobarbital can provoke megaloblastic anemia. The drop in B_{12} and folate may even be responsible for some of the neuropsychiatric side effects attributed to the drugs. It has been observed that while patients are on these drugs, correcting their low vitamin levels often makes the drugs less effective in controlling seizures.[90]

Vitamin B_{12} absorption can also be blocked by alcohol, vitamin B_6, pyridoxine at high levels, and tapeworm infestations.[91]

Diagnosing Vitamin B_{12} Deficiency

Diagnosing B12 deficiency may begin with an assessment of the symptoms of deficiency, such as fatigue, muscle weakness, pins and needles, and gastric changes. More often than not, the doctor will perform a **complete blood count (CBC)** as part of the laboratory component of a history and physical examination. In case of deficiency, the results will indicate anemia—that is, a hemoglobin level lower than 11.7 grams per deciliter (g/dL)—and a mean corpuscular volume (MCV) greater than 100.0 femtoliters (fL). MCV is the average size of the red cells. Looking further, the doctor may do a serum vitamin B_{12} level test. A normal B_{12} level is between 200 and 1,100 picograms per milliliter (pg/ml). A rarely used indirect test for B_{12} deficiency is testing **methylmalonic acid levels** to check whether they are elevated. B_{12} is necessary for the conversion of this

---

[90] Toman, J., "Drugs Effective in Convulsive Disorders," In Goodman, L. S., and Gilman, A., *The Pharmacological Basis of Therapeutics*, 4th edition, Macmillan, 1971.
[91] Langan, R. C., and Zawistoske, K.J., "Update on Vitamin B12 Deficiency," *American Family Physician*, 2011, *83*(12), 1425–1430.

acid to succinate, which is required for carbohydrate and fat metabolism. The utility of this test is to distinguish B_{12} deficiency from folic acid deficiency megaloblastic anemia. Methylmalonic acid levels are normal in pure folic acid anemia.

Some tests have fallen out of favor in recent years because in clinical practice, the results did not affect the selection of treatments. One such test, the **Shilling test**, employed radioactive cobalt, which is part of the molecule of cyanocobalamin. The radioactive cyanocobalamin was given without and with intrinsic factor to try to determine whether the defect was in the insufficient production of intrinsic factor from the stomach lining or poor absorption in the distal small intestine. Fortunately, this test is not currently used and not needed. Usually, the treatment for B_{12} anemia is intramuscular injections of B_{12}, which bypasses both the intrinsic factor in the stomach and the absorption in the small intestine.

Sometimes, a bone marrow examination is performed as well as a microscopic examination of the peripheral blood. This may be necessary when the presentation is not classical. Often, a review of the blood smear may suggest macrocytic anemia, where the red cells are few in number and large in size. The white cells are affected as well; they have a high rate of turnover, as fast as five days. The nuclear material (the nucleus of the cell) is hyper segmented, more than the usual two to three lobes. Today, an examination of the bone marrow is not essential to make the diagnosis of vitamin B_{12} anemia.

Two other tests used to define the cause of B_{12} deficiency, besides poor diet and poor absorption, are the measurements of **intrinsic factor transcobalamin II-B_{12}**, which comes from the gastric (stomach) parietal cells, and **intrinsic factor antibodies**. Intrinsic factor antibodies are characteristic of and unique to pernicious anemia, which in medical terms is called **pathognomonic**: symptoms or findings indicative of this one disease. Pernicious anemia is considered an autoimmune disease because the antibodies are directed at oneself. It has been observed to occur when other autoimmune diseases such as Graves' disease, thyroiditis, and vitiligo are present.

Vitamin B_{12} Deficiency and Folic Acid

Folic acid has a special warning in regard to vitamin B_{12} deficiency. If vitamin B_{12} deficiency is not properly diagnosed and the anemia is thought to be due to a lack of folic acid or if someone begins taking folic acid for fatigue, a serious error could occur. Folic acid will correct the fatigue and anemia of B_{12} deficiency, but it will not correct any of the neurological conditions. If the B_{12} level is too low for too long, the neurological problems will not be corrected even with B_{12} injections. I caution you to see a physician to help with this important treatment selection. This is why you will often see vitamin B_{12} and folic acid in a combination pill to avoid making just this mistake.

Vitamin B_{12} Sources and Forms

Vitamin B_{12} is reported to boost energy and used by many. It was initially used only in intramuscular and intravenous routes, but now, many oral and sublingual forms are commonly found in grocery and convenience stores. Many supplement companies sell B_{12} lozenges, sublingual sprays, sublingual drops, and tablets, which the body converts to adenosyl cobalamin that interacts with methyl malonyl CoA mutase. These two substances are used by the mitochondria to help produce energy.[92] The fastest-acting delivery systems are the lozenges, sprays, and drops applied to the mucus membranes.

---

[92] Levine, "To B or Not to B," 8–9.

Use of Vitamin B_{12} Supplements in Practice

I have used vitamin B_{12} injections in my practice from the very beginning. This was often by patient request. Many said that it increased energy, improved well-being, and helped to combat chronic fatigue. I often obliged because it has no ill effects and no toxicity at the dosages I use, and I was doing something instead of just giving the patient talk therapy.

I am a member of ACAM, the American College for Advancement in Medicine, and all members are listed on the ACAM website. From this website, I began receiving calls from people with problems who needed help with alternative medicine. I would do things for patients that their own doctors would not do—nothing experimental or difficult, but something unique to that person and their problem. It usually required professional knowledge, experience, and the extra time to explain the realities of the problem and what we wish to accomplish. This is how my experience in this field developed. Someone with a medical problem would come in for a consultation and would have heard of a therapy or treatment, and then asked if I would do it for them.

It has happened more than once that I have never heard of the treatment or protocol and have to tell the patient that I will have to study the subject and get back to them. It is common for my patients to give me homework assignments, taking me to new areas I never thought I would be. If I find that the treatment is benign, the substances have a low toxicity, or the treatment has been ignored or overlooked by the pharmaceutical industry, I am willing to work with them.

I ran into one such problem about six years ago: a petite young medical student, 23 years old. She drove about 50 miles to see me and asked me to help her with her **multiple sclerosis (MS)**, which she had been diagnosed with three years earlier, with the diagnosis confirmed with a spinal tap and an MRI. She came in with a protocol she had researched in an effort to avoid future attacks and impairment.

I had treated patients with MS before, but she presented me with a list of vitamins for daily injection that contained no steroids or immune modifiers. The list was simple enough: thiamine, B_{12}, liver extract, and vitamins B_3, D, C, and E. Vitamin B_{12} and thiamine were the major factors in this protocol and required intramuscular (IM) injections. I did not see any danger and said I would provide her with the prescriptions and guidance for the treatment. I asked her if she had ever given herself an injection before, as the protocol required two every day. She had not. I asked her to drop her pants so we could get started. I gave her the first injection into the anterior right thigh and explained how to load the syringe, hold the muscle, use the alcohol and put the needle in, push the plunger, and remove the needle. I did the right thigh; she did the left. She was a quick study, and I wrote the prescriptions.

On this protocol, she did not have any further attacks of MS. Follow-up MRIs showed fewer white spots, and life was good. She interrupted her medical school training to go to Washington, DC, and the NIH to complete her PhD in medicine and then finished her MD program. While she was in Washington, she would take the train twice a year to see me and refill her prescriptions. She never had a relapse for the six years I treated her. I assume she is writing her own prescriptions now and doing just as well.

Vitamin B_{12} Terminology

It is time to talk about "new terms." The old notion that Vitamin B_{12} is a placebo to make people feel good is being chipped away with a better understanding of its function. Recently, I read a commentary in *JAMA* describing metabolic B_{12} deficiency, defining it by the elevation of plasma **methylmalonic acid**.[93] Serum B_{12} may be in the

---

[93] Spence and Stampfer, "Understanding the Complexity of Homocsyteine Lowering with Vitamins."

normal, or euboxic (which means the check mark is in the correct box), range, but the processes it affects may be suboptimal. This, I feel, reflects that the normal ranges for B_{12} may be misstated. I aim for a higher lower limit of 500 picograms per milliliter (pg/ml) and not 200 pg/ml as the "reference range" used by Quest Diagnostics. I feel that a higher lower limit will eliminate the metabolic deficiency.

A side note on how a laboratory comes up with a **reference range**: Usually, 10,000 or more laboratory assays of, say, serum B_{12} are run, a bell curve is produced, the outliers at the extremes are eliminated, and voilà—a reference range for this sample area or neighborhood is produced. The reference range does not reflect the optimal and healthiest range, but, as I say to my patients, it reflects the range found in the neighborhood, and do you want to be like the neighborhood or do you want to be younger and healthier? This neighborhood range difference is more apparent in the measurement of vitamin D variation if the sample neighborhood is Miami, Florida, versus Portland, Oregon. Considering vitamin B_{12}, the neighborhood range will depend on the amount of meat and fortified foods people eat. Remember that a reference range is a reference, not a correct answer. In fact, a value within the bounds of the range may not be optimal. I have seen reference ranges change over time, even in the same neighborhood.

Types of Vitamin B_{12} Supplements

The first known form of vitamin B_{12} to treat deficiency was chicken liver and calves' liver—first in the raw form, then, as it was learned it is heat stable, in the cooked form. In the elderly, it is better absorbed in the supplement form than when the vitamin is bound to food. This may be because of insufficient digestive enzymes in the elderly. Today, it can be given in pill form, powder, lozenges, and sublingual drops.

In the pill preparations, vitamin B_{12} comes in tablets and capsules and as both cyanocobalamin and methylcobalamin. Common dosing is 400 mcg, 500 mcg, 600 mcg, and 800 mcg daily.

Recently, more supplement manufacturers are producing methylcobalamin in the oral capsule form in combination with **Metafolin**, a methylated form of folic acid. The powder is usually cyanocobalamin, whereas the sublingual lozenges and drops are methylcobalamin. The drops under the tongue are fast acting, quickly absorbed, and pleasant tasting. Methylcobalamin is the preferred form for neurologic defects such as brain aging, peripheral neuropathies, Alzheimer's disease, muscular dystrophy, and Parkinson's disease. Cyanocobalamin works well for anemia. Dosage size for methylcobalamin in sublingual lozenges and drops range from 1 mg (1,000 mcg) to 5 mg.

I have found a unique form of B_{12a} in lozenges that contains a combination of 2 mg of B_6 and 800 mcg of calcium folinate: hydroxocobalamin, available in 2,000 mcg doses for sublingual use. Hydroxocobalamin is produced from bacteria. The product is manufactured by Biotics Research in Rosenberg, Texas. The amount of B_6 is insignificant, but the level of folate is a reasonable usual dose. Key Compounding Pharmacy in Kent, Washington State, offers hydroxocobalamin in a nasal spray and in sublingual drops. Both companies have online stores. Life Extension manufactures several B_{12} supplements. Its B12 Elite lozenges contain adenosyl cobalamin and methylcobalamin combined in a 1,000 mcg dose.

Injectable forms of B_{12} are cyanocobalamin, which until recently was cheap and the most commonly available. Methylcobalamin is now also available for both intramuscular and intravenous use but is much more expensive. It is lighter in color, more like a pink color than the red of cyanocobalamin. The intramuscular dose is limited by how much of a bleb or bubble can be comfortably injected into the muscle. In the arm, I usually do not like to inject more than 1.5 ml. In the buttock, 3 ml is the limit. Intravenously, 5 ml can be given with other vitamins and minerals with no ill effects.

A prescription form of B_{12} for delivery by way of a nasal spray is Nascobal (cyanocobalamin, USP). A metered spray of 500 mcg is used in one nostril per week and is not to be administered within one hour before or after eating hot foods or drinking hot liquids. It is expensive and requires a doctor's prescription. Nonprescription sprays for sublingual use, intended to boost energy, are available from Dr. Mercola, from Mercola.com or local vitamin shops.

A synthetic carrier has been developed that replaces intrinsic factor to promote intestinal absorption. This patented molecule is called **Eligen**, and its chemical name is sodium N-(8-[2-hydroxybenzoyl] amino) caprylate (SNAC). It is essentially a small amino acid.[94] This vitamin B_{12} and SNAC complex helps the B_{12} rapidly pass through the lining of the intestines into the blood, without altering the structure or biological activity of the vitamin. It is absorbed 10 times faster than B_{12} alone, and over time, total absorption is twice as high. It is usually found as Eligen B12 as 100 mcg tablets.

---

[94] Singh, B., "Are You Getting Enough Vitamin B12?" *Life Extension*, January 2010, *16*(1), 83–91.

Biotin

Benefits of Biotin

- Helps other B vitamins to convert carbohydrate to energy
- Helps restore brittle nails and hair
- Improves cracking of the corners of the mouth
- Helps correct peripheral neuropathy
- May improve function in patients diagnosed with multiple sclerosis
- Helps heal dermatitis

History of Biotin

Biotin is found in a diet that contains egg yolk, sardines, walnuts, peanuts, cauliflower, bananas, and brewer's yeast. The first indication that a substance was lacking for good nutrition was in 1927, when it was observed that dermatitis and hair loss developed in people who restricted their egg consumption to only raw egg whites. Egg whites contain a protein called **avidin** that binds to biotin and prevents its absorption. This might be found in homemade mayonnaise but not in commercially prepared products. Biotin is also required for the proper growth of yeast. It was first identified in pure form in 1935 and called **vitamin H**. Shortly thereafter, in 1942, the chemical structure was worked out in the laboratory.[95]

---

[95] "Biotin," *Encyclopedia Britannica*, last updated July 2024, https://www.britannica.com/science/biotin.

Functions of Biotin

Biotin is one of the eight water-soluble B vitamins. It is a critical nutrient for the production of energy, embryonic growth, repair of peripheral neuropathy, and repair of mucous membranes, and it prevents cradle cap.

Biotin, $C_{10}H_{15}N_2O_3S$

As a water-soluble vitamin, it is not subject to storage in the body and must often be replenished. The question arises whether biotin is a vitamin. Remember, the definition of a vitamin is that without it, life will end. For this vitamin, it is difficult to make the call. Much of the literature puts the daily amount necessary for life at a measly 50 mcg. It is almost impossible to avoid, as it is found in so many common foods (eggs, nuts, fish, and vegetables) and produced by bacteria in the gut. It is almost impossible to reach a state where one ingests no biotin. To test the rule that a lack of this vitamin produces death is near impossible.

Biotin and Multiple Sclerosis (MS)

Biotin is being investigated for use in the treatment of MS. Biotin is a cofactor for acetyl-CoA carboxylase, an enzyme needed for the production of myelin synthesis. Myelin is a complex of lipoprotein layers that act as a protective sheath for the axons of nerve cells, protecting them and speeding up the transmission of electrical impulses. MS is a condition where the myelin sheath deteriorates, followed by the deterioration of the axon and death to the nerve cell in either the brain or spinal cord. This leads to loss of normal nerve function and permanent impairment.

Treating early MS patients with 100–300 mg of biotin has shown improvement in function with little downside. Patients with MS are typically treated with prednisone, but biotin would be a candidate for a therapeutic trial with little risk. It is cheap and has no known toxic effects.[96]

A note of caution when using high-dose biotin: It will not harm the patient, but it is known to interfere with the results of some laboratory tests—testosterone, DHEA-sulfate, progesterone, estradiol, thyroid function, 25-hydroxyvitamin D_3, and vitamin B_{12}. The solution is to stop the biotin several days before laboratory blood testing.[97]

---

[96] Cree, B. A. C, et al., "Safety and Efficacy of MD1003 (High-Dose Biotin) in Patients with Progressive Multiple Sclerosis (SPI2): A Randomized, Double-Blind, Placebo-Controlled, Phase 3 Trial," *Lancet Neurology*, 2020, *19*(12), 988–997, https://doi.org/10.1016/s1474-4422(20)30347-1.
[97] Gaby, A. R., "Biotin and Multiple Sclerosis," *Townsend Letter*, October 2021, 10–12.

Biotin Deficiency

The National Academy of Science suggests an adequate intake (AI) of biotin as outlined below.[98]

Adequate Intake of Biotin		
Life stage	Age	Daily intake (mcg)
Infant	0–6 months	5
	7–12 months	6
Child	1–3 years	8
	4–8 years	12
	9–13 years	20
Adolescent	14–18 years	25
Adult or pregnant	19+ years	30

There is no recommended daily allowance (RDA) for biotin, as no reputable studies consistently show hair loss, brittle nails, or dermatitis. Likewise, there is no tolerable upper intake level (UL), as there no consistent reports of ill effects or toxicities.

Laboratory values for biotin range from 133 to 329 picomoles per liter (pmol/L) in serum and 18 to 127 millimoles per 24 hours

---

[98] Institute of Medicine (US) Standing Committee on the Scientific Evaluation of Dietary Reference Intakes and its Panel on Folate, Other B Vitamins, and Choline, *Dietary Reference Intakes for Thiamin, Riboflavin, Niacin, Vitamin B6, Folate, Vitamin B12, Pantothenic Acid, Biotin, and Choline*, National Academies Press, 1998, https://www.ncbi.nlm.nih.gov/books/NBK114310/pdf/Bookshelf_NBK1143 10.pdf.

(mmol/24h) excretion in urine. Deficiency is better noted in the urine or with the development of symptoms: dermatitis, hair and nail changes, and peripheral neuropathy.[99] Pregnancy and breastfeeding consumes biotin, as does the use of antiseizure medication. If symptoms occur, higher doses of biotin may be needed.

Many commercial products promote biotin for hair loss, but this refers to thinning hair or small patches of hair loss. It will not correct genetic male-pattern baldness, horseshoe baldness, or a receding hairline. Likewise, female-pattern baldness, which usually presents as global thinning, will not be affected. What it will do is be of some help from hair loss from chemotherapy, autoimmune diseases such as lupus, COVID-19, stress, hormonal imbalance, and thyroid conditions. The usual dose of biotin is 8–16 mg daily.

In addition to biotin for hair loss, especially in hair loss from COVID-19, I have found that the addition of **saw palmetto**, an herb, speeds up the return to normal for the hair follicles. Remember, hair growth is slow, 0.3 to 0.4 mm per day or six inches per year. I recommend 320 mg of saw palmetto once or twice a day. It usually is found mixed with nettle root, Pygeum bark, and pumpkin oil.

Brittle nails are not a one-nutrient problem. They may need biotin plus gelatin, which is one of the building blocks of collagen. Gelatin can be bought in capsules or liquid. Remember, your body cannot make collagen without vitamin C. Hypothyroidism is another cause for slow-growing, thin, and brittle nails.

Biotin Supplements

Biotin, or B_7, comes in tablets, capsules, soft gels, powders, injectables, and liquids for sublingual application. It is also added to shampoo and conditioner. Many purveyors of biotin list the tablet

---

[99] Ibid.

or capsule size in micrograms instead of the expected milligram size. You will see 5,000 mcg, which translates to 5 mg, or 10,000 mcg, which translates to 10 mg. 1,000 mcg = 1 mg. I guess the bigger number implies that you get more, but in reality, the amounts are the same.

Biotin is available from Life Extension, Pure, Nature's Bounty, Now, Jarrow, and Solgar.

Vitamin C

Benefits of Vitamin C

- Prevents scurvy
- Reduces the incidence of flu
- Reduces bladder cancer
- Increases the rate of wound healing, including after surgery
- Strengthens connective tissue (skin, tendons, and blood vessels)
- Reduces the incidence of tuberculosis and most infectious diseases
- Improves peptic ulcer disease
- Reduces hyperthyroidism
- Optimizes pregnancy and lactation
- Necessary for the function of drug metabolizing enzymes
- Reduces the symptoms of herpes simplex
- Reduces the symptoms of allergies
- Reduces the risk of cataracts
- Reduces gallbladder and kidney stones by a third
- Prevents liver spots on the skin
- Facilitates iron absorption
- Associated with uric acid metabolism and used to treat gout
- Reduces C-reactive protein (CRP) and hypertension
- Reduces or eliminates toxicity
- Prevents reflex sympathetic dystrophy

History of Vitamin C

Vitamin C is the most significant vitamin for humanity. Of all the vitamins, its story is the longest and most convoluted, and it is the most controversial, praised, vilified, suppressed, and exalted of any substance isolated by humanity. Its possession, or lack of it, has altered the history of humanity more than any substance on a national or personal level, without people even knowing it. The effects of vitamin C were known long before anyone understood what it is. To make the link between diet and good health is easy, but to define what good health is and what diet is needed to achieve it is puzzling. A fortified city under siege can be starved to death if no outside source of vitamin C can be found, as the human body cannot manufacture it, unlike most animals. Yet some men, such as Captain Cook, were observant of nutritional needs. Although Cook had never heard of Vitamin C, he knew where to find it and how to store it, ration it, and benefit from it.

As evidenced by the mention of the seafarer Captain James Cook, the story of vitamin C is also the story of scurvy. A total lack of vitamin C causes scurvy. This relationship between a nutrient and a disease is the main point of this book. Vitamin C and scurvy is the classic example often presented to make the argument, but others abound. Some connections are straightforward and easy to see, like thiamine (B_1) and beriberi or calcium and strong bones.

Scurvy

Scurvy has been reported for thousands of years. The condition was most pronounced when armies or fortified towns under siege were cut off from their supplies of fresh fruits and vegetables. However, although the disease was known, it was poorly understood. The period between stopping vitamin C intake to the presentation of the disease was variable, and no single factor was attributed to its cause. A poison, in contrast, has a much more direct, positive relationship to an effect. Taking arsenic or drinking bad water provokes abdominal pain, sickness, and even death. A disease of deficiency, such as scurvy, is caused by not ingesting something, so an absence of action causes the disease. The thought process to arrive at the cause is thus a bit more complicated.

Scurvy initially presents as soft spongy gums; loose teeth; teeth falling out; exuberated growth of skin around hair follicles; corkscrew-shaped hairs; bruising easily; fatigue; ruptured capillaries, tendons, and ligaments; and then lung and kidney troubles before death. The disease became problematic and isolated on long sea voyages during the Age of Exploration. Vasco da Gama, in 1498, on his trip from Lisbon to Calicut, India, lost 60% of his crew to scurvy. The body's stores of vitamin C are so limited and the effects of scurvy so devastating that it is a wonder that so many took to the seas for long voyages.

The first mention of the treatment of scurvy that I found was by Jacques Cartier, who discovered the St. Lawrence River. Twenty-five of his men died of scurvy on this trip. While they stayed the winter in Quebec, an Indian advised him to make a brew of the leaves and bark of the arbor vitae tree as treatment. This quickly brought them back to health.

The British admiral George Anson had a similar experience with scurvy in late 1740 to June 1741 during a journey to the Island of Fernandez that lasted more than six months. He started the voyage with six ships and 961 men. When he arrived, he had only 335 remaining crewmembers, with more than half dying from scurvy. A Scottish physician in the Royal Navy, **Dr. James Lind**, knew of Admiral Anson's tragedy and had a similar experience on the *Salisbury* in 1747. Lind's journey lasted 10 weeks, and 80 men from a crew of 350 developed scurvy. He took the opportunity to conduct trial therapies in hopes of developing a treatment for this condition.

Lind selected 12 men who had already developed scurvy and created six treatment groups of two men each. The trial treatments were as follows:

1. Cider, one quart per day
2. Elixir vitriol (copper sulfate), 25 drops taken three times per day
3. Vinegar, two spoonfuls three times per day
4. Garlic and mustard seed, three times per day
5. One lemon and two oranges to be eaten each day
6. No treatment for the last two men, who served as control subjects

The citrus fruit group responded so well that in six days, one returned to full duty and the other was assigned as nurse to the other five groups.[100]

Dr. Lind went on to publish his findings in 1753 as ***A Treatise of the Scurvy***. In this paper, he set forth his idea that scurvy was a disease of deficiency and detailed his proposed treatment of citrus fruit. Little by little the cause of scurvy was being approached, but the substance we know as vitamin C was far from discovery. Lind and others continued to work with the citrus fruits of lemons, limes, and oranges, but with little success. To save space on ships during long voyages, they tried to make a condensed syrup called rob. The juice of oranges, lemons, and limes was boiled down for easier storage and transport, but the heating process destroyed the vitamin to low levels, and what remained was oxidized to where none, or insignificant amounts, remained.

Lind began to doubt his own theory on antiscorbutic treatments, as the results after the first experiment were poor and not reproducible. The process of making rob and then storing it took him away from the original ascorbic acid. It was known that scurvy could get better after being on shore and eating fresh fruits and

---

[100] Lind, J., *A Treatise of the Scurvy*, 1753.

vegetables, but to pack enough perishables on board a ship for long voyages without them rotting was next to impossible. He experimented with dehydrating both oranges and lime juice. He made rob, but he did not know that these physical changes, such as heating the liquid, also changed the molecule to an oxidized form that made it useless to prevent scurvy.[101]

Captain James Cook sailed the Pacific Ocean, often away from land more than six months at a time. He had a practice of ordering his men to gather fresh fruits and vegetables any time they landed on an island. This was something other captains did not do because the fruits and vegetables were new and strange to them. Cook was aware of the experiments of Dr. Lind but found that rob was of little value in preventing scurvy. He tried carrot marmalade; carrots contain no Vitamin C. At the time there was a meal called dehydrated soup, starting with less water, but Cook produced better results with the soup when he added the local wild vegetables. His method of island hopping, in conjunction with his use of cabbage in the form of sauerkraut, was so successful that on his second voyage to the Pacific, he lost no one due to scurvy. Cabbage contains about 30 mg of vitamin C per 100 g of cabbage. On Cook's ships, the daily ration of sauerkraut was about 150 g.

Captain Cook made good observations and applied practical solutions for the prevention of scurvy, but still no molecule or exact substance was identified. Cook was recognized for his scientific contributions and awarded the Copley Medal and made a fellow of the Royal Society of London.

It was not until the early 20th century that vitamin C was finally isolated. In 1928, Albert Szent-Gyorgyi, while working on a chemical biological oxidation process, discovered a new substance he called hexuronic acid. It was isolated from both cabbages and adrenal glands. As a reducing agent or antioxidant, it protected apples and

---

[101] Badger, G., *The Explorers of the Pacific*, 2nd edition, Kangaroo Press, 1996.

bananas from oxidizing, or going brown. In 1932, the American investigators Waugh and King showed that the substance Szent-Gyorgyi had isolated was vitamin C, a compound they isolated from lemon juice, and that it had a significant antiscorbutic effect. Szent-Gyorgyi, with the help of English chemist W. M. Haworth, determined its structural formula. Hexuronic acid prevented scurvy—it was the antiscorbutic substance. Szent-Gyorgyi changed the name hexuronic acid to ascorbic acid.[102]

Notable Contributions to the Study of Vitamin C

The study of vitamin C has been marked by several researchers who made valuable contributions to the fields of nutrition, medicine, and biochemistry. Frederick R. Klenner, MD, and Linus Pauling, PhD, deserve an honorable mention for their contributions.

Frederick R. Klenner, MD

A discussion of vitamin C would be incomplete without mentioning Frederick R. Klenner, MD. He was a pioneer in the medical uses of vitamin C, practicing in Reidsville, North Carolina. He first came to attention in 1948, when he began to treat polio patients with intravenous vitamin C. He would treat them in the acute infective febrile stage and early convalescence of the disease, which helped the body to fight off the infection and prevented the subsequent motor paralysis.

From 1943 to 1947, he successfully treated 41 patients with viral pneumonia. He published an article about his work in the *Journal of Southern Medicine and Surgery* titled "Virus Pneumonia and Its Treatment with Vitamin C." This four-year period gave him a good

---

[102] Ibid.

understanding of dosages, frequency, and mode of treatment for the polio epidemic of 1948.

Dr. Klenner's use of vitamin C was mainstream medicine at the time. During the polio epidemic of 1948–1949, he treated 60 polio patients and cured every one of them. This fact alone should command any doctor or patient to pay attention to this therapy. Dr. Klenner presented a summary of his work on polio at the annual session of the American Medical Association on June 10, 1949, in Atlantic City, New Jersey.[103]

In 2021, Martin Zucker, an author who has written extensively on alternative medicine over the last 40 years, wrote about an interview he conducted with Dr. Klenner in June 1978. Zucker published this article in the *Townsend Letter* because he thought the information was valid and relevant to doctors of integrative medicine.

Dr. Klenner was a general practitioner specializing in diseases of the chest, and as a general practitioner, he delivered more than 400 babies. The interview with Zucker centered on his use of vitamin C in 322 pregnant women. Dr. Klenner gave the women 4 g of oral vitamin C per day in the first trimester, 6 g per day in the second trimester, and 10 g per day in the third trimester. The vitamin C had the effect of reducing labor, which is defined as starting with the first contraction and ending with the delivery of the baby, from an average of 24 hours to 3 or 4 hours, and never more than 6 hours. Reducing the length of labor translates into less pain.

In addition, the perineum was more flexible and returned to its normal form after delivery. The women reported fewer stretchmarks, and in many cases, none were evident. Hemorrhaging in the mother or infant was nonexistent. There was not a single

---

[103] Braun, P. A. D., "Klenner and Vitamin Therapy," *Nutritional and Preventative Medicine—Chronic Illness Care*, 2012; Saul, A. W., "Hidden in Plain Sight: The Pioneering Work of Frederick Robert Klenner, MD," *Journal of Orthomolecular Medicine*, 2007, *22*(1), 31–38.

miscarriage in any of the 322 pregnancies. In this series of pregnancies, the Fultz quadruplets were born; one weighed 3 pounds and the rest were 2 pounders. None needed special attention or resuscitation, and all were alive and well at the time Zucker wrote his article in 2021. No deformities were reported. Following delivery, Dr. Klenner had the babies on 50 mg of vitamin C daily up to the age of six months, increasing it to 500 mg daily and then 1 g daily at one year, and adding 1 g for each year of life up to 10 g at age 10. He kept it at 10 g daily thereafter.[104]

Dr. Klenner wrote a book, published in 1959 in collaboration with Fred H. Bartz, titled *The Key to Good Health, Vitamin C: Don't Lose This Key for It Might Lock or Unlock Your Life!* He explained his introduction to scurvy through treating patients and described how he learned to use vitamin C. At the end of the book, which is only 99 pages long, he referred to the work of other doctors. One reference, out of many, jumps off of the page. It was written by Dr. P. Berkenau in 1940. I cannot improve upon what he said, so I will print it as it appears in the book. The information is just as relevant today as it was in 1940.

ALL SENILE PATIENTS LACK VITAMIN C

A senile patient is forgetful, confused, his speech rambles. He repeats a question that has just been answered. Memory is so poor the individual does not recognize members of his own family.

Dr. P. Berkenau made a study of "senile dementia" patients at the Warneford Hospital, Oxford, England in 1940. He found all of his patients short of C. No exceptions. "A deficit of 1,500 mgs, may be regarded as pathological (disease causing)." The deficit of these patients varied from 2,400 to 3,000 mgs.

---

[104] Zucker, M., "Vitamin C Pioneer Frederick R. Klenner, MD: An Historic Interview," Orthomolecular Medicine News Service, *Townsend Letter*, June 2021, 65.

Plaques appeared in the brain of senile patients identical to those found in alcoholics. This indicates a poisonous origin. Hence senile patients and those approaching old age need substantial quantities of vitamin C to protect their brain from damage and to fight infection.

P. Berkenau, Journal of Mental Science, vol. 86, page 675, 1940.[105]

In this short reference to his article, he was telling us a clue to a major medical problem today. My father would often say that if you cannot read between the lines, you do not deserve the answer. Take this information and protect yourself.

This brings us to the question that goes with every vitamin and mineral: How much is the right amount? Dr. Klenner said, "I am now satisfied that **no two people are precisely alike in their need for C.**" He further noted that everyone would have to find their own minimum and maximum dosage. Some things can be handled with as little as 30 mg per day; other conditions will require 10 g per day. Klenner favored the higher doses in his treatments, and reported that other users of vitamin C, such as doctors who used it in cancer treatments, indicated that a patient with cancer may be in need of at least 4,550 mg of vitamin C daily.[106] In fact, he felt it might take 4,000–5,000 mg of vitamin C to satisfy the daily need of someone experiencing the burden of cancer. In support of his use of higher doses, Dr. Klenner claimed that vitamin C causes no pathologic changes, has no toxic effect, and does not cause allergic reactions.

In his book, Dr. Klenner reported that he used vitamin C to treat hypercholesterolemia, hypertension, water loss from burn injury, atherosclerosis, glaucoma, the common cold, hepatitis, polio, and most viral diseases. He reported that the method he used to discover

---

[105] Klenner, F. R., and Bartz, F. H., *The Key to Good Health, Vitamin C: Don't Lose This Key for It Might Lock or Unlock Your Life!* Graphic Arts Research Foundation, 1971, 68.
[106] Ibid., 42.

a patient's need for vitamin C was to measure the excess that appeared in the urine. When the vitamin is found in the urine, it means that the body's requirements have been met. Initially, he used Benedict's solution to detect vitamin C in the urine, but later he developed the silver nitrate test on urine to test for vitamin C.

Today, there are several commercially made tests to test for ascorbic acid. These tests come in the form of a dipstick that can be dipped into the urine. The color change of the stick is then compared to the color chart on the container. If no ascorbic acid is found in the urine, it means that the current dosage of vitamin C is insufficient for the needs of the condition.

Klenner believed people cannot produce vitamin C because we lost the gene to produce the enzyme **l-gulonolactone oxidase**. This enzyme facilitates the transformation of glucose to ascorbic acid. We share this genetic deficiency with two other mammals: monkeys and guinea pigs. This means our only source of ascorbic acid is our diet.[107]

Linus Pauling, PhD

A major investigator in the understanding and application of vitamin C was Linus Pauling, PhD, a scientist who worked in diverse fields and who was recognized as one of the two greatest scientists of the 20th century. To advance the theory and application of inorganic chemistry, he wrote textbooks, including ***General Chemistry***. He was one of the founders of molecular biology, coined the term **orthomolecular chemistry** (which means the right molecule or proper molecule), demonstrated the chemical structure of sickle cell disease, and promoted the use of vitamin C for the treatment of the common cold and cancer. In 1994, he gave his last

---

[107] Smith, L. H. (ed.), "Clinical Guide to the Use of Vitamin C: The Clinical Experiences of Frederick R. Klenner, MD, Abbreviated, Summarized, and Annotated," 2004.

interview with Tony Edwards of the BBC's *Q.E.D.*[108] and Patrick Holford at the Power of Prevention Conference.

Dr. Pauling recommended vitamin C for the treatment of arterial plaques in coronary artery disease, strokes, and peripheral vascular disease. He promoted the concept that plaque formation of atherosclerosis was caused by **lipoprotein A** and not just by **low-density lipoprotein (LDL)**. Pauling said that more than 20 milligrams per deciliter (mg/dL) of **lipoprotein A** in the blood initiates the deposition of plaque on the arterial wall. He claimed that a particular amino acid, **lysine**, in the wall of the artery attracts lipoprotein A. He proposed that this nontoxic amino acid could be given to increase the concentration of lysine in the blood, attracting and attaching to lipoprotein A for elimination by the body before lipoprotein A attaches to the arterial wall, initiating the plaque.

Lysine is an essential amino acid that is obtained from the diet, which means the body cannot manufacture it. A person must obtain it from their food. The most abundant source of lysine is meat, but this nontoxic substance can be obtained in supplement form, as 500 mg tablets or capsules. He proposed that everyone should be taking vitamin C two or three times a day. To this should be added lysine. He recommended at least 2,000 mg of lysine a day in divided doses.[109]

Vitamin C and lysine is a much gentler treatment for hypercholesterolemia than niacin and less damaging than statin drugs that will deplete your enzyme Co-Q-10, reducing your energy level and producing muscle pain that might not go away even when the statin drug is discontinued.

---

[108] The Latin abbreviation for *quod erat demonstrandum*—"which was to be demonstrated," or confidently saying in plain English, "I just logically proved my argument."

[109] Edwards, T., and Holford, P., "The Last Interview," Institute for Optimum Nutrition, 1994, https://towerlaboratories.com/Pauling_Last_Published_Interview.html.

Functions of Vitamin C

This vitamin has mystical powers to ward off the common cold and the flu, alter the course of cancer, send fear through oncologists, and drive a stake thought the heart of Big Pharma. This is such a controversial substance that a simple internet search about vitamin C will return no less than 1.5 million articles, and the list grows daily. There has been so much praise, so many good recommendations, so much written about the benefits, the healing powers, the good health, the longevity, the restoration of youth, and well-being that articles written to expose or discredit it carry little weight. Oncologists claim that it harms cancer protocols and interferes with their treatment. Needless to say, considering the damage to the poor cancer patient from the chemo, the alleged production of kidney stones, and the interference with the good intentions of medical care, it is unimaginable that we are talking of the same molecule.

A molecule, something so small and yet so important to human life. Something men have literally sailed the seas for and because of. Possession of it gives one human strength and vitality. Without it, you die. Vitamin C, also known as ascorbic acid, is essential to people and their health and lives.

Most species, except for people, monkeys, and guinea pigs, can produce ascorbic acid from glucose. There is a cascade of chemical reactions that start from glucose and ends as ascorbic acid.

Glucose → l-Gulonolactone Oxidase → Ascorbic Acid

Glucose is converted to glucuronic acid, which is converted to **gulonic acid**, which is converted to **gulonolactone**. In humans, guinea pigs, and monkeys, the final step of the conversion to ascorbic acid, which requires the enzyme **gulonolactone oxidase**, has been lost.[110] Burns, in 1959, reported that this inability to convert gulonolactone to ascorbic acid is because of a gene-controlled enzyme "deficiency."[111] The gene to convert glucose to ascorbic acid is present in humans, as was found in the Human Genome Project, but the ability to activate that gene to produce the enzyme gulonolactone oxidase, has been lost.[112]

Ascorbic acid is not an end product but a molecule that is converted to metabolites such as **dehydroascorbate** or **urinary oxalate**; unconverted ascorbic acid is excreted.[113] If the serum concentration is less than 2 milligrams per deciliter (mg/dL), little is excreted by the kidneys, and it is retained to be converted to dehydroascorbic acid and back to ascorbic acid again through reversible oxidation-reduction functions. No molecule stays in any one form for long. The hydrogen atom, which is the proton donor, disassociates from the rest of the molecule, leaving the ascorbate anion.

Ascorbic Acid   **Ascorbate**

The molecule on the left is ascorbic acid; the molecule on the right is the ascorbate anion without its hydrogen that becomes negatively charged when exposed to oxygen. At this location another atom may be added to make a salt, such as sodium ascorbate,

---

[110] Goodman and Gillman, *Pharmacological Basis of Therapeutics*, 4th edition, 1971, 1668.
[111] Ibid.
[112] Milne, R. D., *PC Liposomal Encapsulation Technology*, Life's Foundation Books, 2004, 78.
[113] Ibid.

calcium ascorbate, or potassium ascorbate. These preparations may be easier on the stomach than the ascorbic acid form.

This ascorbate anion has an extra electron, giving it a negative charge of -1. This ascorbate form can be transformed with the help of iron or copper, oxygen, and hydrogen to produce hydrogen peroxide. It is through this mechanism of producing hydrogen peroxide that vitamin C promotes its antibacterial, antiviral, and anticancer effect.

To be precise, vitamin C is found in citrus fruit, but this is not citric acid. The chemical formula for ascorbic acid is $C_6H_8O_6$; for citric acid, $C_6H_8O_7 \cdot H_2O$; and for glucose, $C_6H_{12}O_6$.

Prevention of Scurvy

The primary benefit of taking vitamin C is the prevention of scurvy. It has the ability to maintain cell adhesion by the formation of the glue, or ground substance, that keeps cells together. It is not only the glue—within it can be found small fibrils of collagen that give it strength. In deficiency states, these collagen bundles disappear and the glue becomes watery. When a person has scurvy, the tendons and ligaments lose strength and rupture, blood vessels hemorrhage, and the framework of organs cannot support itself. The vitamin C molecule does not become incorporated in collagen but somehow facilitates the binding of proline and lysine to from fibers. This weakness appears in bones at the epidiaphyseal growth plates. Tooth sockets weaken, and teeth fall out.

The prevention of scurvy is simple. It requires only 30 to 60 mg of ascorbic acid a day. Surprisingly, scurvy still exists today in people who do not eat fresh fruit and vegetables. As recently as 2008 *American Medical News* carried a story of scurvy occurring in people who have diets with little or no vitamin C. A 57-year-old man complained of shortness of breath and bruising from the thigh to the ankle. He was divorced and toothless, and it was discovered that he ate only processed food and no fresh fruit or vegetables. A child examined at Columbia University Medical Center developed scurvy because he limited his diet to ice cream and crackers. The disease is often found in people who live alone, the elderly, and children with behavior problems.

The Centers for Disease Control (CDC) reported that from 1979 to 2005, 57 people died from scurvy in the United States. The National Health and Nutrition Examination Survey estimated that 14% of men and 10% of women have vitamin C deficiency.[114]

Osteoporosis

According to Dr. Marian Hannan of Harvard Medical School's Institute for Aging Research in Boston, the results of the 15- to 17-year follow-up to the Framingham Osteoporosis Study, which involved 5,209 men and women, indicated that taking vitamin C reduced hip fractures by 44%.[115] The lowest-intake group averaged 97 mg per day and the highest-intake group took an average of 305 mg per day.

Wound Healing

When it comes to wound healing, it is not vitamin C alone that is helpful but a blend of ingredients that together rebuilds ligaments, connective tissue, skin, and new scar tissue. In my practice, I recommend nutrient support to promote quicker and more complete healing. A good initial blend of supplements is

- 500–1,000 mg of vitamin C three to four times a day;
- 500–1,000 mg of quercetin a day;

---

[114] Elliott, V. S., "Scurvy Rare, but Cases Still Are Popping Up," *American Medical News,* September 22/29, 2008, 26.
[115] Sahni, S., "Vitamin C Intake Tied to Lower Hip Fracture Risk," *Internal Medicine News,* October 1, 2008.

- 20–50 mg of zinc glycinate, zinc citrate, or zinc picolinate per day;
- 500 mg of lysine once or twice a day;
- a B complex; and
- 5,000 units of vitamin D per day.

Good healing begins with good ingredients. The body needs food for both fuel and building blocks. Vitamins and minerals give the process that extra ingredient to facilitate good construction. These are not the only nutrients needed for repair, but they should be considered a basic essential.

In 1972, Irwin Stone described some of the attributes of ascorbic acid in fighting bacterial infections:

1. It is bactericidal or bacteriostatic and will kill or prevent the growth of pathogenic organisms.
2. It detoxifies and renders harmless the bacterial toxins and poisons.
3. It controls and maintains phagocytosis.
4. It is harmless and nontoxic and can be administered in the large doses needed to accomplish the above effects without danger to the patient.[116]

The mechanism of bacterial death is similar to that for viruses. Ascorbate and oxygen catalyzed by copper or iron produces hydrogen peroxide to inactivate the organisms. It performs this at concentrations as low as 1 mg/dL, as was shown by Boissevin and Spillane in 1937.

Vitamin C deactivates the toxins of diphtheria, tetanus, staphylococcus, and dysentery. It is, by and large, harmless in high doses. I often give 25 to 50 g intravenously over the course of one or two hours in my office. Vitamin C is a natural antihistamine by two mechanisms: It prevents the release of histamine from the mast

---

[116] Stone, I., *The Healing Factor: Vitamin C Against Disease*, Grosset and Dunlap, 1972.

cells and increases the detoxification of histamine. Histamine can be lowered in the blood, and a lower blood level translates to fewer symptoms. Two grams of oral vitamin C daily will lower blood histamine 38% in one week.[117]

The Semmelweis Reflex

Vitamin C is effective with antibiotics for the treatment of infections, especially sepsis. **Sepsis** is the body's reaction to a severe infection, characterized by the production of an outpouring of cytokines, or chemicals of inflammation, that is so damaging that it can bring about death. The four characteristics of sepsis, according to the **Sepsis Alliance**, are **TIME**: time, infection, mental decline, and extreme illness. Even if treated, a good proportion of patients with sepsis die. Most patients will experience shortness of breath, a rapid pulse, low blood pressure, fever, and mental confusion. The infection can progress rapidly from sepsis to severe sepsis and to septic shock.

Dr. Paul Marik is an intensive care physician who works at Sentara Norfolk General Hospital in Virginia. He began to treat sepsis patients with intravenous vitamin C, corticosteroids, and thiamine and produced significant results.

An observational study conducted in 2016 and published in *Chest*, a medical journal, revealed the information before the numbers were massaged.[118] **Observational analysis** means that the findings are raw data, which allows the reader to draw their own conclusion. The study involved examining 47 sepsis patients before

---

[117] Johnston, C., et al., "Antihistamine Effect of Supplemental Ascorbic Acid and Neutrophil Chemotaxis," *Journal of the American College of Nutrition*, 1992, *11*, 172–176.
[118] Marik, P. E., et al., "Hydrocortisone, Vitamin C and Thiamine for the Treatment of Severe Sepsis and Septic Shock: A Retrospective Before–After Study," *Chest*, 2017, *151*(6), 1229–1238, https://doi.org/10.1016/j.chest.2016.11.036.

the protocol was started and the first 47 patients immediately after the protocol was started. In the untreated group, 19 patients died, whereas in the treated group 4 patients died. To be included in the study, patients were required to have sepsis. It did not matter what other conditions they had. The goal was to gather observational data. The results look like a simple win protocol.

The protocol followed in the study, or the Marik protocol, involved intravenous (IV) administration of the following:[119]

- 1.5 g of vitamin C every 6 hours for four days or until discharge from the ICU
- 50 mg of hydrocortisone every 6 hours for seven days or until discharge from the ICU, tapering on the third day
- 200 mg of thiamine every 12 hours for four days or until discharge from the ICU

The study has been criticized—the sample was too small, it was not a parallel study of the two groups at the same time, the patients were not properly selected . . . There is no shortage of criticism, as in any endeavor. But is this really criticism, or is it professional jealousy? There is no doubt that professional jealousy is at the root of many scientific or medical debates. Both fields are highly competitive, and the stakes are high. Personal reputation and peer recognition are at stake.

Paul Marik, MD, proposed and placed in action a therapy that is simple, easy to implement, and effective. He characterizes the criticism that he receives as the **Semmelweis reflex**. Dr. Ignaz Semmelweis was a Hungarian physician at the University of Vienna in 1847, when he implemented antiseptics and handwashing prior to obstetrical procedures, significantly reducing puerperal fever, a form of sepsis that develops after gynecologic procedures and childbirth.

---

[119] Rezaie, S., "The Marik Protocol: Have We Found a 'Cure' for Severe Sepsis and Septic Shock?" REBEL EM blog, April 7, 2017, https://rebelem.com/the-marik-protocol-have-we-found-a-cure-for-severe-sepsis-and-septic-shock/.

It saved many lives. It was cheap and effective. Semmelweis was not thanked for his contribution but was denied departmental promotions by his superiors and suffered professional jealousy.

Dr. Marik's protocol, often referred to as the **HAT protocol** for the combination of hydrocortisone, ascorbic acid, and thiamine, is cheap, easy to implement, and effective. It was brought to attention not through medical journals, even though it was published in *Chest*, but by the airing of the report on **National Public Radio (NPR)**. The medical community was unable to suppress the information with its method of peer review and criticized the discovery as "science by press release."

Common Cold and Respiratory Illnesses

In a systematic review of eight studies, where the daily intake was 500 mg to 2,000 mg per day, Harri Hemila, MD, PhD, reported that vitamin C supplementation reduced the incidence of the common cold by 45% to 91% and the incidence of pneumonia by 80% to 100%.[120]

The combination of vitamin C and zinc has a synergistic effect on components of the immune system, lymphocyte proliferation, chemotaxis, natural killer cell activities, hypersensitivity, growth, and wound healing. Vitamin C prevents damage from oxidation to lipids, proteins, and DNA, in addition to having a regenerating effect on other antioxidants such as glutathione and vitamin E, to their active forms. Moreover, cytochrome P-450 and drug-metabolizing enzymes are supported by vitamin C. Inflammatory mediators

---

[120] Hemilä, H., "Vitamin C Supplementation and Respiratory Infections: A Systematic Review," *Military Medicine*, 2004, *169*(11), 920–925, https://doi.org/10.7205/milmed.169.11.920.

benefit from vitamin C, boosting cytokines IL-1, IL-6, tumor necrosis factor-alpha, leukotrienes, and prostaglandins.[121]

The intracellular concentrations of vitamin C in neutrophils decrease with age, as does neutrophil function. The oral administration of vitamin C to the elderly increases both the concentration of vitamin C and the function of neutrophils to reduce the duration of respiratory tract infections such as sinusitis, bronchitis, and pneumonia and skin infections such as the herpes simplex virus.[122]

Allergy Symptoms

Ascorbic acid can reduce the effects of allergies, but it is not the only substance that is effective in this regard. Often, I advise someone who has trouble with allergies to take not only vitamin C but to simultaneously take **quercetin** and **bromelain**. Quercetin stabilizes the mast cell membrane, inhibiting the release of the histamine, and bromelain reduces the proinflammatory prostaglandins and increases the anti-inflammatory prostaglandins.[123]

Gastric Cancer

Gastric cancer is more prevalent in people with a low consumption of vitamin C, as well as low vitamin E and beta-carotene intake. This is believed to be amplified when there is a

---

[121] Wintergerst, E. S., Maggini, S., and Hornig, D. H., "Immune-Enhancing Role of Vitamin C and Zinc and Effect on Clinical Conditions," *Annals of Nutrition and Metabolism*, 2006, 50(2), 85–94, https://doi.org/10.1159/000090495.
[122] Ibid.
[123] Haggag, E. G., et al., "The Effect of a Herbal Water-Extract on Histamine Release from Mast Cells and on Allergic Asthma," *Journal of Herbal Pharmacotherapy*, 2003, 3(4), 41–54; Taussig, S. J., "The Mechanism of the Physiological Action of Bromelain," *Medical Hypotheses*, 1980, 6(1), 99–104, https://doi.org/10.1016/0306-9877(80)90038-9.

gastric infection of **Helicobacter pylori** that also consumes these nutrients. Without eradicating the infection but supplementing with these vitamins, the incidence of gastric cancer decreases.[124]

Herpes Simplex

Herpes simplex infections treated with just 200 mg of vitamin C showed a 57% reduction in the duration of symptoms—4.2 days versus 9.7 days in those treated with a placebo.[125] The usual level of vitamin C for prophylaxis of Herpes simplex is 500–3,000 mg daily and up to 10,000 mg in divided doses for five to ten days for an acute flare-up, provided there is good bowel tolerance.

Rectal and Familial Polyposis

Ascorbic acid, given orally, was used by DeCosse and his group in Milwaukee in 1975, as he reported in *Surgery*, to reduce rectal and familial polyposis.[126] A measurable reduction in both the size and number of adenomatous polyps was reported to occur in a time frame of four to six months.

Viability of Pregnancy

A decrease in threatened, spontaneous, and habitual abortion was reported by Javert and Stander in a paper they authored in 1942 while at the Department of Obstetrics and Gynecology, Cornell University Medical College and the New York Hospital.[127] They

---

[124] Kim, H. J., et al., "Effect of Nutrient Intake and Helicobacter pylori Infection on Gastric Cancer in Korea: A Case-Control Study, *Nutrition and Cancer*, 2005, *52*(2), 138–146, https://doi.org/10.1207/s15327914nc5202_4.
[125] Gaby, A. R., "Natural Remedies for Herpes simplex," *Alternative Medicine Review*, 2006, *11*(2), 93–101, 96.
[126] DeCosse, J. J., et al., "Effect of Ascorbic Acid on Rectal Polyps of Patients with Familial Polyposis," *Surgery*, 1975, *78*(5), 608–612.
[127] Javert, C. T., and Stander, H. J., "Plasma Vitamin C and Prothrombin Concentration in Pregnancy in Threatened, Spontaneous, and Habitual

measured blood levels of vitamin C and vitamin K, demonstrating one or both of these vitamins to be low with these conditions. Besides abortion, their symptoms usually included easy bruising, bloody nose, bleeding gums, and vaginal bleeding—that is, the nature of a threatened abortion. It was rare to see abortions where the vitamin C level and the prothrombin time, or the time it takes for plasma to clot, were normal. Prothrombin is a functional measure of vitamin K. An incidental finding was that infants with cerebral hemorrhage had depressed blood levels of vitamin C.[128] Levels in umbilical cord blood were found to be higher than those in maternal blood in abortion states, showing the need to protect and benefit the fetus. Diet and income did not have a relation to abortion like vitamin C level did. The same applied then as applies today: Many believe that they eat a balanced diet, but knowledgeable awareness is often found lacking when measuring blood levels.

Heart Attack Recovery

Recovery from a heart attack is quicker and more pronounced when vitamins C and E are present. During a heart attack, the local tissue surrounding the muscle that was the so-called ground zero of the attack also becomes deficient in oxygen, but to a lesser extent than the muscle itself. This marginal area becomes a zone of **hibernating tissue**, which is not dead but is under oxidative stress, producing toxic products of oxidation. As blood flow to the area returns, this milieu of cellular waste washes downstream and causes more damage, which is termed **ischemia of reperfusion**.[129] This

---

Abortion," *Surgery, Gynecology, and Obstetrics*, 1943, *47*(3), 436–437, https://doi.org/10.1016/S0002-9378(15)30772-9.
[128] Ibid.
[129] Saitoh, Y., and Miwa, N., "Cytoprotection of Vascular Endotheliocytes by Phosphorylated Ascorbate through Suppression of Oxidative Stress that Is Generated Immediately after Post-Anoxic Reoxygenation or with Alkylhydroperoxides," *Journal of Cellular Biochemistry*, 2004, *93*(4), 653–663, https://doi.org/10.1002/jcb.20245.

blood contains oxidized material, cellular metabolic products that are in a greater concentration than usual, to upset the normal functioning of the muscle fibers in terms of electrical excitability, contraction, and aerobic respiration. This produces effects ranging from symptoms of angina or chest pain, weak muscular contractions that manifest as heart failure, low blood pressure, and shock, to electrical disturbances of rate or rhythm, felt as palpitations or skipped beats, to the worst: no sign of life. Less free radical damage is produced if an antioxidant like vitamin C is present.

In a large study of post–heart attack patients, the Multicenter Pilot Myocardial Infarction and VITamins (MIVIT) Trial, participants were given 1,200 mg of vitamin C and 600 units of vitamin E daily for one month. This protocol was found to reduce combined new heart attacks, the death rate, and severe complications by 20%.[130]

Patients with a heart rhythm known as atrial fibrillation produce products of oxidative stress that damage the mitochondrial DNA. The **mitochondria** are small organelles in cells that produce energy. If these are damaged, the cell has less energy to function with, and in this case, the cell muscle is weaker and less efficient.

Elimination of Toxicity

Vitamin C has the ability to neutralize poisons and return denatured tissue to normal. This was one of the early observations when ascorbic acid was used in a clinical setting. Infusions of vitamin C have the ability to neutralize venom from snake bites and spider bites. Dr. Klenner reported in his book the story of a dog being bitten by a large rattlesnake.[131] This was for sure a death sentence for

---

[130] Jaxa-Chamiec, T., et al., "Antioxidant Effects of Combined Vitamins C and E in Acute Myocardial Infarction. The Randomized, Double-Blind, Placebo Controlled, Multicenter Pilot Myocardial Infarction and VITamins (MIVIT) Trial," *Kardiologia Polska*, 2005, *62*(4), 344–350.
[131] Klenner and Bartz, *The Key to Good Health*.

the dog. Not having any antivenom or similar products, Dr. Klenner treated the dog with IV vitamin C. This treatment returned the dog to health with no delirious effects from the snake venom.

This is a great attribute for vitamin C. Detoxing has often been reported for heavy metals and organic compounds. The most difficult to explain has been the detoxing of organic compounds, but now an explanation has been presented by Thomas E Levy, MD, JD. In a book he wrote, he provided an explanation of the detoxing mechanism. All toxins denature the normal molecules by oxidation: by removing two electrons, initially destabilizing the electrical charge of the molecule, and in turn, the denatured molecule becomes the disease. The toxin has the ability to affect the host, causing the malfunction of an enzyme or altering the structure of a protein. What you see is the effect of the toxin on the previously normal tissues. If the toxin can gain two electrons, it would not be a toxic molecule. And if the host molecule could gain two electrons, returning the molecule to a normal balanced charge, there would be no disease.[132]

This is certainly an innocuous procedure, with no ill effects, and certainly worthy of a trial treatment in any doctor's office or emergency room following an insect or animal bite. A physician starting with only the information of a bite should start with Ascor (vitamin C for IV administration), 10 g in 250 ml of lactated Ringer's solution over 15 to 30 minutes. For a person 150 pounds and above, the physician should give 20 to 25 g of Ascor in 500 ml of lactated Ringer's solution over 30 minutes to one hour. Should rabies be possible in relation to an animal bite, this would be an excellent course of action. Dr. Klenner said that "vitamin C is deadly to all types of viruses and their toxins." Vitamin C has been successful in reversing the toxic effect of everything that it has been tried on.

---

[132] Levy, T., *Vitamin C, Infectious Diseases, and Toxins: Curing the Incurable*, Xlibris 2002.

Many harmless treatments are used to detox organic toxins, all of which function by adding an electron pair and which are often referred to as **electron donors**. They are hydrogen peroxide (H_2O_2), ozone therapy (O_3), and, of course, vitamin C. The process of reversing oxidation, or giving back the electrons, is called **reduction**. This permits the molecules to return to their normal chemical and metabolic functions.

If any sizable amount of repair of oxidized tissue is undertaken, especially with hemodynamic changes, it is advisable to add magnesium chloride ($MgCl_2$) to prevent arrhythmias.

Neurosurgical Benefits of Vitamin C

Dr. Klenner reported in his book that vitamin C has a diuretic effect and a dehydrating effect on the brain.[133] This is apparent with the infusion of vitamin C at levels above 20–25 g. People receiving vitamin C intravenously at 50 g may complain about headaches and general fatigue. At this concentration, it may take anywhere from 12 to 24 hours to recover. Because of this effect, I generally limit my dose to 25 g per treatment, my reasoning being that any treatment should not make you ill if I am trying to make you better.

This effect is brought about by an intravenous solution of vitamin C being higher in osmolality than the local tissues. To equilibrate the tissues and fluid, water is taken from the tissues into the blood for elimination by the kidneys. There is no better example of this than with my patient, Genevieve. We called her Gene. Gene was 48 years old when we met, and at that time she had had a glioma brain tumor for eight years. Initially, when the seizures presented, she had a CT scan and an MRI of the head, followed by a brain biopsy to confirm the tumor. The biopsy left her with such increased seizures and headaches that she refused further treatment. She had been badgered by her surgeons and oncologist for years to have

---

[133] Klenner and Bartz, *The Key to Good Health*.

surgery to remove the mass, but she had a bad gut feeling and refused to have the surgery. She then found me and asked if there was anything I could do that would help her. I started her initially on Myers's cocktail, and then vitamin C alone, starting at 2.5 g and increasing it to 5 g, 7.5 g, 12 g, and finally delivering 15 g intravenously in 500 ml of lactated Ringer's solution. This concentration of vitamin C had a favorable effect on her for a few days after the treatment. Headaches and seizures were greatly reduced.

The inflammation around the tumor also provoked cerebral edema or swelling of the brain. The higher osmolality of the vitamin C infusion pulled water from the brain, reducing the swelling, reducing the headache, and reducing the frequency of the seizures. Besides these benefits, the immune system was better able to slow the expansion of the tumor and keep it localized.

Gene was treated weekly for nearly two years at my office with reasonable success—fewer seizures and headaches—in keeping with her wishes to avoid surgery, if possible. This was not a cure for her brain cancer; it was a treatment to slow tumor growth and reduce the symptoms. Increasing sleepiness, a crescendo of seizures, and headaches brought her and her family to change course, opting for surgery. She was so disappointed with the treatment she received from the prestigious New York hospitals that she followed up on a prior consultation she had made at Massachusetts General Hospital to have the surgery there if she deteriorated.

On arrival to the hospital, she had an MRI. The findings were enough to prompt the doctors to move her surgery forward two days. Everyone was expecting the worst. She underwent surgery with a large horseshoe-shaped scalp incision, an equally large bone flap, and, finally, extraction of the tumor, which was pretty much walled off by the immune system, fortified by vitamin C. Surprisingly, her postoperative recovery in the hospital was only five days. She was scheduled to have two weeks in rehab, but she refused, as she felt so well that she insisted on returning home and resuming her vitamin C drips. Again, she was driven by her gut feelings. On seeing her in my office, it was hard to comprehend that a week before she had brain surgery, and not just a biopsy hole but with half of the brain exposed.

The Effects of Vitamin C on Cancer

This is a brief description of the landmark paper that Big Pharma fears the most: "Supplemental Ascorbate in the Supportive Treatment of Cancer: Prolongation of Survival Times in Terminal Human Cancer."[134] In November 1971, in Glasgow, Drs. Ewan Cameron and Linus Pauling began a trial involving cancer patients. To be included in the trial, at least two independent clinicians must have determined that continuing with any conventional form of treatment would offer no further benefit. Participants were divided into two groups. The control group comprised 1,000 patients who met the above criteria; the treatment group comprised 100 patients who were matched for age, sex, type of cancer, and stage compared to the control group. The treatment group was started on 10 g of intravenous ascorbic acid daily; after the first week, the vitamin C was given orally. Those in the treatment group reported better well-being and lived longer than those in the control group. Their quality of life was better, and a few even went on to return to work. Sixteen people in the treatment group outlived all the patients in the control group, and some were still alive and healthy seven years later.[135]

Vitamin C can improve the quality and longevity of life of someone with cancer. It can provide an extension to life; it is a betterment to the quality of life. Dr. Linus Pauling considered this

---

[134] Cameron, E., and Pauling, L., *Proceedings of the National Academy of Sciences of the United States of America*, 1976, *73*(10), 3685–3689, https://doi.org/10.1073/pnas.73.10.3685. The full unedited report is in the Appendix.
[135] Newbold, H. L., *Vitamin C against Cancer*, Stein & Day, 1979, 339–354.

study and its results and determined that the taking of vitamin C could prolong life by as much as 16 years. Even healthy people can increase their longevity, as did Dr. Pauling. He lived until the age of 93, and he did not start taking high doses of vitamin C until he was in his 70s.

Cataracts and Macular Degeneration

New information is coming to light as a byproduct of eye surgery. A common surgery today is for the removal of cataracts. **Cataracts** are a hardening and a cloudiness of the lens of the eye that limits clear vision. They occur in some older individuals and are thought to develop from ultraviolet light, chemical exposure, seed oils, and even microwave frequencies. The proteins of the lens develop cross-structural binding causing the lens to lose flexibility and reducing the passage of light.

The current treatment for cataracts is to remove the hard cloudy lens and replace it with a plastic lens, restoring vision, often without the need for corrective glasses. The procedure requires an incision at the border of the cornea and sclera, or white of the eye. The fluid in the anterior chamber, the area between the cornea and the lens, leaks out and is lost during the procedure. After the cataract is removed, a plastic lens is inserted, and the incision is sutured closed. The ciliary body, which is located at the border of the cornea and sclera, replenishes the fluid in the anterior chamber, and through normal flow, the fluid passes to the vitreous humor in the center of the eye. The new fluid increases the pressure in the eyeball to help maintain its spherical shape.

This procedure is now commonly performed, which has presented an opportunity to gather information from many patients that was not possible before. Micro quantities of fluid from the anterior chamber have been collected from many patients and analyzed to find out what factors cause cataract formation. One of the substances that was measured was the amount of vitamin C in the aqueous humor of the anterior chamber. The concentration of vitamin C was on average 39 times more concentrated in the anterior chamber than in the blood. Vitamin C in the anterior chamber was 2.04 millimoles per liter (mmol/L) versus 0.052 mmol/L in the blood.[136] Remember, these are people with cataracts. Concentrations of vitamin C in the anterior chamber were stratified, showing an inverse relation between vitamin C and patients with the worst cataracts. The lower the amount of vitamin C in the anterior chamber, the worse the cataracts were. They were very hard and very opaque. A greater amount of vitamin C in the anterior chamber permitted the lens to remain flexible and retain greater clarity.

The eye is an active extension of the brain, and it requires much energy and oxygen to process light images into nerve impulses all day long. It processes close to 20 images per second all day long. The vitamin C in the anterior chamber in a healthy person ranges from 20 to 70 times the concentration that is found in the blood. Vision can be preserved by taking extra vitamin C. I suggest taking 2,000 mg of vitamin C two or three times a day, or what you can tolerate. There are commercial eye vitamins, such as PreserVision, but I think that the 250 mg of vitamin C in the formula is much too low. If you take this or Ocuvite, with 150 mg of vitamin C, take additional vitamin C.

The benefit of vitamin C is well known to my patients with cataracts and macular degeneration who have received vitamin C infusions. Ophthalmologists have commented to my patients that they see an improvement in their eyes, saying that they do not know what they are doing but to keep doing it. Certainly, these mainstream physicians cannot admit that vitamin C is critical for eye health and risk professional isolation by advising nutrients over drugs.

---

[136] Huang, W., et al., "Extracellular Glutathione Peroxidase and Ascorbic Acid in Aqueous Humor and Serum of Patients Operated on for Cataract," *Clinica Chimica Acta*, 1997, *261*(2), 117–130, https://doi.org/10.1016/S0009-8981(97)06520-0.

Another independent study found that the ciliary body in the eye concentrates ascorbic acid more than any other organ in the body. The concentration of ascorbic acid in the eye is anywhere from 18 to 71 times higher than that found in the blood.[137] These measurements of vitamin C in the eye constitute the first objective information that the health of the eye is correlated with nutrients, specifically vitamin C, and patients can take a proactive position in preserving vision by taking additional ascorbic acid.

Other substances found to be beneficial to the eye in preventing cataracts are **glutathione**, an antioxidant; **N-acetyl cystine (NAC)**; and **alpha-lipoic acid (ALA)**.[138] NAC and ALA contribute to glutathione levels. High levels of glutathione are found in normal lenses, with progressively decreasing levels with the worsening of cataract development. To prevent cataracts, 500 mg of glutathione may be taken orally daily, although the intravenous form is more effective. You can also take 600 mg of NAC or 300 mg ALA once or twice a day.

Vitamin C Deficiency

Scurvy

Scurvy is a disease of deficiency. The presentation begins with weakness, restlessness, and rapid exhaustion. Additionally, ascorbic acid is necessary for the construction of collagen, connective tissue, bones, and teeth. It is required for the formation of intercellular cement, called ground substance—the glue that keeps cells together. Without it, structural integrity is lost and the cohesion between the

---

[137] Taylor, A., et al., "Vitamin C in Human and Guinea Pig Aqueous, Lens and Plasma in Relation to Intake," *Current Eye Research*, 1997, *16*(9), 857–864, https://doi.org/10.1076/ceyr.16.9.857.5039.
[138] Huang, W., et al., "Extracellular Glutathione Peroxidase and Ascorbic Acid."

cells of the tendons, ligaments, and blood vessels weaken and lose support. The disease goes on to produce broken blood vessels in, for example, the whites of the eyes, called subconjunctival hemorrhages. The joints swell because of both the accumulation of intracellular fluid and bleeding into the joint and surrounding joint tissue. The gums become swollen and soft, and the teeth fall out. The skin of someone with scurvy has the most characteristic and unique appearance in that the hair follicles become more pronounced, and the surrounding skin becomes red and may bleed.

Scurvy is easily confused with arthritis, bleeding diseases, and the gum disease called gingivitis. The associated laboratory tests for these diseases are normal with suspected scurvy. The normal serum level of ascorbic acid is 1 to 2 milligrams per deciliter (mg/dL). The lower limit of normal is about 0.5 mg/dL, with less than 0.15 mg/dL associated with the disease itself.

So how much vitamin C should one take? And how did anyone come to that number in the first place? The recommended dietary allowance (RDA) of vitamin C is 60 mg per day.

A Note on Recommended Vitamin Intake

The new term for recommended dietary allowance (RDA) introduced by the US Food and Drug Administration (FDA) is **daily values (DV)**. In medicine, changing the name of something that has been around for many years gives it a semblance of progress and innovation. In effect, RDA and DV are the same thing. The name change was made to relate the recommended intake to the average serving size. But the quantity of food that makes up a serving size adds further confusion. Generally, a serving size is a cup, or four ounces. This is handy for liquids, but for solids such as berries or chunks of meat, the weight measure of four ounces is a serving.

Dr. Lind, the Scottish physician who conducted the original trials of treating scurvy in sailors, found that one lemon and two oranges cured scurvy. That was the starting point. In fact, it was found that as little as one lime or one orange per day cured or prevented scurvy. This was the therapy for a long time, even before the molecule of vitamin C was defined. Citrus fruits were noted to have antiscorbutic effects. Many years later, after the molecule of vitamin C was defined and could be measured, the amount of vitamin C in an orange was measured and found to be about 60 mg. From this rough observation of disease prevention, one orange worth of vitamin C prevents scurvy. Therefore, 60 mg of vitamin C is the recommended dietary allowance of vitamin C to prevent scurvy.

It is by examples like this one that RDA, or DV, values have been assigned to vitamins and minerals. Other examples include a lack of thiamine (vitamin B_1) causing beriberi and a lack of iodine causing cretinism in children or an enlarged thyroid, or goiter, in young adults. Little by little the connection between lack of nutrients and disease began to coalesce. As the ability to measure substances improved over time, more extensive experiments began to yield more accurate lower limits of the daily recommended amounts. Dr. Linus Pauling, who recommended that vitamin C be taken for the prevention and treatment of the common cold and flu, reported that 10 mg of vitamin C is all that is needed to prevent scurvy in most humans.

Finding the lowest amount of vitamin C to prevent scurvy did much to establish the concept of nutrition-based diseases. This opened a new area in medicine—that a lack of something could cause a disease. This was very much contrary to the concept of the germ theory of Louis Pasture, which held that coming into contact with bacteria caused a disease. These are two very diametrically opposed ideas that fit together well.

RDA and DV are good starting points. We now know from the study of vitamins and minerals at what point a lack of them promotes disease and what amounts are sufficient to treat and cure diseases.

Sadly, I must report that most vitamins had a "lower than" value that promoted disease and a "higher than" value that cured diseases. But some, such as vitamin D, had an assigned value for the RDA. Search as you may, and I have done that for some, it is impossible to find the science behind the number.

The next thought concerns whether there is a point where too much is harmful. Is there a toxic level? Remembering that most of these substances come from food, how much is too much? There is a movement today to regulate, under the international Codex agreement, the sale of vitamins and minerals. People eat food by the pounds. Can this be harmful? When isolated from beef, can vitamin B_{12} be toxic? Interestingly, most vitamins do not have side effects but do have side benefits. As eaten, most are not toxic. Only when given intravenously, and then only in massive amounts, do vitamins begin to act as a drug and may present toxic effects. The argument can be made for water—it is generally safe, can be taken even in large amounts with no harm, but then too much of a good thing can be overdone, and even orally, one can induce water intoxication. Too much water dilutes the salts of the body and upsets the compartmental composition of water and minerals such as sodium, potassium, magnesium, and chloride. This interferes with muscle contraction and may provoke seizures. Death is possible.

All substances have a toxic level that should not be exceeded. Generally, these are not as low as the literature would like you to believe. Every year in the fall, there is a health scare or warning that through the medical literature published in a reputable medical journal, misstated conclusions or observations, or a meta-analysis is picked up by a radio or television news department and reported in a sound bite or a teaser for a short report for the six o'clock or eleven o'clock news. This makes "good copy" and has shock value. This is not good information.

My favorite is the **meta-analysis**. This is a fancy term for a book report or article report. In this analysis, there was no firsthand research, no firsthand trials, and no original work. What the reviewer did was gather 10 to 20 reports that support their view or hypothesis. Pretty much, the reviewer's bias was paid by someone who has an interest in promoting or stopping someone from using a product. Few, or usually no, reports are included in the reviews that support the opposite conclusion. This meta-analysis is presented to the public as a factual report. It is factual, but not all encompassing and not representative of the available information.

But wait, there is more. There is the **meta-meta-analysis**. It would be silly if it was not so harmful. This is a report where someone does a book report from a group of book reports and produces evidence to support their opinion. The term meta-meta-analysis sounds like very sophisticated science. This is usually published without peer review or shame; it is crunched down into a teaser for a sound bite for TV or radio or plastered in the headlines of some newspaper to attract readers. Misinformation or incomplete facts are sent into the public domain, with most listeners or readers left in confusion. This is tabloid science at its best.

Causes of Vitamin C Deficiency

There are two sides to the equation: the need for and loss of vitamin C. Most of this chapter is about the need for vitamin C and how much is required. I want to point out the areas of loss, of which there are three: metabolic needs, bowel loss, and loss from the kidneys. A person's metabolic needs change with the activities and requirements related to states of body repair and fighting disease. Bowel loss results from rapid transit time or reaching the limit of bowel absorption. The bowel has a limit to how much vitamin C it can absorb, and if more is presented, it will pass right through, taking extra stool with it. This is called **bowel tolerance**, which also refers to the maximum dose of vitamin C a person can take and absorb. Bowel tolerance changes with the needs of the body. When you have a cold or infection, your need will increase, and because of this need, absorption is increased and bowel tolerance will increase.

The third form of loss is from the kidneys. The kidneys have a threshold for ascorbic acid, known as the **renal threshold**: If the concentration of vitamin C in the blood is less than 1.3 mg per 100 ml, no vitamin C will appear in the urine.[139] It can at least hold that minimal concentration in the blood. If the blood concentration can reach 5 mg per 100 ml from supplements or eating fresh fruit and vegetables, there will be more to service the immune system and structures of the body. The vitamin C will be metabolically consumed, and it will be eliminated by the kidneys until the blood concentration falls below 1.3 mg per 100 ml. This threshold is the concentration of vitamin C that the kidneys can maintain. From this point, the further reduction of vitamin C will be from metabolic consumption and not kidney loss.

Chronic Scurvy

I am introducing you to a new name for chronic problems that I believe have a common cause: **chronic scurvy**. These problems are all related. I feel that these modern chronic conditions are due to insufficient vitamin C. The standard American diet, also known as the SAD diet, does not include enough fresh fruit and vegetables, leaving it devoid of essential vitamins and minerals. Modern processing and cooking destroy vitamins. For example, cooking vegetables to 105 degrees Fahrenheit will degrade vitamin C and folic acid. Long distribution routes and sorting times increases the field-to-table time, leading to more depletion of vitamin C in the food.

The medical conditions that I place in the category of chronic scurvy are all modern-day problems that keep getting worse. The

---

[139] Faulkner, J. M., and Taylor, F. H. L., "Observations on the Renal Threshold for Ascorbic Acid in Man," *Journal of Clinical Investigation*, 1938, *17*(1), 69–75, https://doi.org/10.1172%2FJCI100929.

frequency with which they are occurring is increasing. Let us start with a short list: osteoarthritis, osteoporosis, and torn ligaments and tendons of the knees, hips, shoulders, and back. The structure of the body is falling apart. Years ago, did you ever hear of so many structural problems of the eye that you hear about today? Blood vessels bleeding in the back of the eye, torn retinas, detached retinas, and cataract development. Sagging skin, crepey skin, premature aging of the skin, striae or stretch marks from pregnancy or from rapid weight gain, posterior thigh cellulite, and poor wound healing. Leaky gut syndrome, metastatic lesions, diminishing life expectancy, spontaneous abortion, and the explosion of Alzheimer's disease may all be related.

Vitamin C deficiency may be the cause. Acute scurvy, as you will remember, causes hemorrhagic or bleeding gums, loose teeth that may fall out, hemorrhaging into the skin at the base of hair follicles, anemia, lassitude, weakness, irritability, muscle and joint pains, snapped tendons, bleeding of the conjunctiva of the eye, and swelling in the lower extremities.

The factor that ties all these conditions together is collagen. Every one of these conditions is related to poor maintenance of structure, often described by the effects of poor structure or function. Medical professionals will describe what they see before them or what is under the microscope. Looking deeper into the molecular level of these structures, deeper than the eye can see, may be the answer. Each student of vitamin C, from Dr. Lund to Dr. Cameron, Dr. Campbell, and Dr. Pauling, contributed to the understanding and the healing power of vitamin C. Dr. Klenner, I feel, is the most overlooked and forgotten contributor to the broad use of vitamin C. In *The Key to Good Health*, he reported many conditions that depend on vitamin C to support the underlying conditions of chronic scurvy.

A good example is coronary disease. Attention has been paid to arterial plaque, the narrowing of the artery, and the development of a thrombus or blood clot to fully obstruct the flow of blood. As these pioneers of medical research have shown or suggested, it is injury to the internal structure of the collagen within the muscular layer of the arterial wall, not the surface of the lining of the artery. Cholesterol plaque is expressed from the injured cell itself and not from the diet or produced in the liver.[140] Correct the damaged collagen structure and the body will remove the plaque. This theory has been proven by the experiments and autopsies performed on guinea pigs by Dr. Pauling and Dr. Matthias Rath.[141]

Vitamin C Deficiency and Collagen

Collagen is a protein that gives us structure, strength, and flexibility. It is referred to as a **glycosaminoglycan**, a form of polymer made up of units of glycine, lysine, and proline that requires ascorbic acid—that is, vitamin C—for its assembly. If there is insufficient vitamin C, no collagen will be made or repaired. No repair means aging of the structures. Collagen is a protein; it comprises 25% to 35% of all the protein in the body. That is a significant amount of structure that requires vitamin C. This is tissue of the skin, ligaments, tendons, the protein of bones, eyeballs, the valves of the heart, and blood vessels. Another form of collagen is **ground substance**, which is more like a glue made of the same glycosaminoglycan and twisted fibrils of stranded collagen but folded differently. The physical folding of the protein gives it different physical characteristics. They both require vitamin C for construction and repair. Ground substance and stranded collagen are the same thing. Ground substance is the collagen that holds cells together. This lack of glue can lead to leaky gut syndrome and increased permeability in capillaries leading to pulmonary edema or swelling of the legs.

---

[140] Linus Pauling, PhD, in an interview with Harold L. Newbold, in *Vitamin C Against Cancer*, 1979, 22.
[141] Rath, M., *The Heart*, MR Publishing, 2001.

Has your doctor talked to you about your collagen lately? The only doctors who discuss it are dermatologists. They are primarily interested in selling their latest concoctions of collagen pills and creams. Reviewing some formulations, I found that they contain little or no ascorbic acid. So how will the collagen be assembled in your body? It will not. A typical formula is 20 g of collagen and 90 mg of vitamin C, or all collagen and no vitamin C. This will not produce any significant results. It is more important to overdo the vitamin C than the collagen. The basic formula for collagen is vitamin C plus lysine and proline. These two amino acids are the basic building blocks of collagen. They require vitamin C for assembly. Vitamin C is required for the assembly of collagen—it is not incorporated into the structure. To build collagen, grams, not milligrams, of vitamin C are needed daily. I have never heard a cardiologist, general surgeon, orthopedic surgeon, obstetrician, gastroenterologist, or plastic surgeon discuss the need for proper nutrition to support collagen. Eye doctors have vitamins for the eye, but the amount of vitamin C is so low that the effect is meaningless.

Collagen is also needed to prevent metastases. Remember, ground substance is collagen; it is the glue that holds cells together. A tumor mass that has sufficient glue will hold the mass together. It will keep it localized. Not enough glue, and cells will easily disassociate from the primary mass and drift off, seeding new tumors or metastases.

Leaky gut syndrome is yet another intestinal problem where there is not enough glue to hold the cells of the intestines together, permitting the undigested contents of the intestines to enter the body by passing between the cells that are not tightly held together by ground substance.

Another structure that relies heavily on ground substance is the blood-brain barrier. This is made up of the capillary endothelium, the astrocytic sheath, and ground substance that present protection for the brain from water-soluble substances. Loss of ground substance leaves the brain vulnerable to many toxic chemicals and organisms. Could this be a mechanism for Parkinson's disease, autism, Alzheimer's disease, and other neurological issues?

Treating Chronic Scurvy

Treating chronic scurvy requires much more vitamin C than treating acute scurvy does. Acute scurvy can be treated with as little as 30–60 mg of vitamin C per day. That is the amount that can be found in one orange or lime. For chronic scurvy, daily consumption must be at least 4 g, 6 g, or 8 g a day, or if you think in milligrams, that would be 4,000 mg, 6,000 mg, or 8,000 mg per day. For the best results, let us say you want to take 6,000 mg per day, start with 2,000 mg three times a day—2,000 mg in the morning with food, 2,000 mg with lunch or supper, and another 2,000 mg at bedtime. It is better to spread the total amount over the day than to take it all at once. Taking it once a day will cause a high serum peak concentration, but that will be washed out in four to six hours. Taking multiple doses will create a better-sustained medium level over a longer period, achieving better results. Also, it would be better to take 2,000 mg every two to three hours, boosting the daily total to 8,000 mg, 10,000 mg, or even 12,000 mg per day. For most people, 6,000 mg would be ideal.

Ascorbic acid is the best form of vitamin C, and it is the cheapest. As it is an acid, it may be too acidic for some people. If the acid form causes too much irritation, the salts of vitamin C can be used instead: **sodium ascorbate** and **calcium ascorbate (Ester-C)**. All three forms are absorbed in the stomach. They are taken in as their presented forms. Another popular form is **liposomal-encapsulated vitamin C**. This is ascorbic acid with an attached fatty acid. This is passed on into the intestines, where it is assumed that maybe half the dosage is digested, and the remainder is absorbed. It may not be as effective as ascorbic acid or sodium or calcium ascorbate.

My patient, Ann Marie, was in her 50s. She experienced surgical menopause in her 30s from a hysterectomy and oophorectomy (removal of the uterus and ovaries) and was suffering from mild gastritis and dry eyes to the point that her eyeballs would ache at the end of the day. To build up her immunity and treat her joint pain, I suggested that she take powered calcium ascorbate, as she was experiencing irritation from ascorbic acid capsules. I recommended one teaspoon two to three times a day. She misunderstood me and took one tablespoon of the ascorbate. She reported that the gastritis and dry eye pain resolved immediately. She was overjoyed. That was good to know, and no harm was done, but I admonished her to take a one-teaspoon dose in the future for maintenance. She had been on vitamin A for the dry eyes and stomach irritation, but this was just the boost that she needed. In the world of alternative medicine, combinations of vitamins and minerals are often needed to get the desired effect.

Measuring Vitamin C Levels

The best evaluation for the adequacy of vitamin C is to measure it in the urine. If someone has enough vitamin C in the body, excess amounts will appear in the urine. How much vitamin C appears in the urine is inversely related to the body's demand for vitamin C. For example, if the usual need for the vitamin is 2,000 mg daily but significantly increases to 4,000–6,000 mg when a major infection is encountered, the needs will not be met by giving 2,000 mg or less. It is difficult to measure cellular demand. The method used here is that you are measuring the difference between the known quantity being ingested and the extra or unutilized vitamin in the urine, which represents the current demand of the body. If no vitamin C is found in the urine, the body's needs are not being met and there is a deficit.

A quick test for vitamin C in the urine can be purchased from the **Riordan Clinic Nutrient Store**. They have **VitaCheck-C Strips** that can give results in 30 seconds. They give a quantitative as well as qualitative results. For those of you into the do-it-yourself experience, below is a method that is simple and easy to do at home.

Four solutions are needed to test the amount of vitamin C in urine:

1. An **indicator solution** that turns from clear to dark blue when a balance is reached between the sample concentration and the oxidizing agent. This is cornstarch, one teaspoon dissolved in one cup of water. The best way to prepare it is to add the cornstarch and water to a small jar with a lid and shake the starch and water for a few minutes. Some starch will dissolve in the water; the remainder will settle on the bottom. When you are ready to use the solution, gently shake the jar enough to make the fluid on top is slightly cloudy. You will use the cloudy solution, not the residue on the bottom of the jar, for testing.
2. A **standard solution of vitamin C**. Make this in a one-liter (1,000 ml) plastic or glass bottle. Add 1 g of vitamin C to the water. The easiest method is to open a 1,000 mg (1 g) capsule of vitamin C, add it to the water in the bottle, and mix it. This standard solution concentration will be 1 mg of vitamin C per 1 ml of water.
3. An **oxidizing agent**, either a tincture of iodine or 2% Lugol's solution. Lugol's solution can be found in most vitamin shops, usually sold in a dropper bottle.
4. **Urine** from the patient to be tested.

The necessary tools are small test tubes, from 5 ml to 10 ml size, and either 3 ml syringes or droppers that have volumes marked on the side (e.g., 0.25 ml, 0.5 ml, 0.75 ml, or 1.0 ml).

Set up a minimum of three test tubes, each filled with 2 ml of the indicator solution. Add 2 ml of water to the first test tube, 2 ml of the urine to be tested to the second, and 2 ml of the standard solution of vitamin C to the third.

Now, the testing begins. Add one drop of Lugol's solution to the first test tube that contains the water. It should immediately go from a cloudy solution to a deep blue purple. This indicates that no vitamin C is in the water. To the second test tube, add the Lugol's solution one drop at a time, mixing it after each drop. The deep blue purple should remain after mixing, indicating that the ascorbic acid has been neutralized. Test the third test tube that contains the standard solution of vitamin C with drops of Lugol's solution until it turns a deep blue purple, indicating the end point.

Now, make a chart indicating the number of drops needed to find the end points.

Vitamin C Content by Lugol's Solution		
Sample	Number of drops	Vitamin C content (mg)
No vitamin C	1	0
Urine	3	1
Standard solution of Vitamin C	6	2

From the data in the chart, the urine vitamin C concentration can be calculated. Two milliliters of a standard solution was placed in the test tube. That was 2 ml × 1 mg/ml = 2 mg. The ratio of the drops of Lugol's solution in the urine to the standard solution is 3:6 drops, or 3/6 × 2 mg = 1 mg of vitamin C in the urine.

The takeaway from this test is that if you have no vitamin C in the urine, you do not have enough vitamin C in your body. You have a vitamin C deficit. Having a deficit will lead to diseases of chronic scurvy. To avoid the issues of chronic scurvy, you will need additional vitamin C in your diet to reach blood concentrations of 3–5 mg/ml or more of vitamin C. This requirement can be fulfilled only with the frequent dosing of vitamin C. The best way to maintain an elevated level of vitamin C in the blood is to take smaller frequent doses rather than one or two large doses per day. It is better to take 1,000 mg or 2,000 mg of vitamin C every two to three hours than 4,000 mg or 5,000 mg once a day.

Vitamin C Supplements

Ascorbic acid, a mild acid, is the primary form of vitamin C. Chemically, this is a six-carbon molecule backbone that is referred to as the ascorbate. It is negatively charged and has a positive hydrogen atom that defines it as an acid by being a proton donor. All other forms are salts, where the hydrogen proton is substituted with minerals. Examples of mineral ascorbates are sodium ascorbate, calcium ascorbate, magnesium ascorbate, potassium ascorbate, molybdenum ascorbate, zinc ascorbate, and chromium ascorbate. Without getting too technical, it is the six-carbon ascorbate that is the working portion of the molecule by being the donor of an electron pair, thus making it an antioxidant. This ascorbate can be from either the ascorbic acid or the form of one of the salts, such as sodium ascorbate.

The advantage of using a salt is that it is not too irritating to the stomach lining. In small doses, it is helpful to use magnesium, potassium, or calcium ascorbate if the desire is to increase these minerals as well. However, when the ascorbate dose becomes too large, the minerals may be too concentrated and may produce problems of their own. These include the salts of sodium ascorbate provoking congestive heart failure in patients with heart failure, potassium ascorbate placing renal patients in potassium toxicity, and too much calcium in patients with osteoporosis interfering with the vascular system. Too much calcium in the wrong place is an **index of aging**: calcified heel spurs, calcific tendonitis of the shoulder, deposits in the plaques of arteries, calcium spicules in breast tissue, and stones in the kidney, gallbladder, and semicircular canals in the ear that assist balance.

Calcium ascorbate is known by other names, such as buffered vitamin C and Ester-C. It has no advantage over ascorbic acid, especially when multigram doses of 2–6 g per day are taken. The brand Ester-C is, according to the package insert, a proprietary blend of calcium ascorbate and small amounts of vitamin C metabolites, dehydroascorbic acid (oxidized ascorbic acid), calcium threonate, xylonate, and lyxonate. Besides fillers to bulk up the tablet, citrus bioflavonoids are added: acerola, rutin, and hesperidin complex.[142]

All these forms of vitamin C come in capsule, tablet, chewable, and liquid form. They are available in dosages as low as 50 mg, as well as 60 mg, 100 mg, 200 mg, 250 mg, 500 mg, and up to 1,000 mg per unit. Vitamin C is formulated alone as ascorbic acid crystals, compounded with sugars to fill out the capsule or tablet, or mixed with other vitamins in a multivitamin preparation.

Often, you will see small amounts, such as 3 mg, in an herbal extract as an ingredient. This certainly is not a therapeutic dose, nor is it intended to be. In this situation, the vitamin C is listed on the label and is an ingredient, but its purpose is to act as a preservative to protect the other substances from oxidation. Another example of low-dose vitamin C for its antioxidant preservative effect is in snacks, candy, and prepared foods. Many recipes for home canning of jellies and jams also call for a teaspoon of ascorbic acid crystals as a preservative to maintain freshness and color. When ascorbic acid is used as a preservative, the label lists it in either milligrams or %

---

[142] Linus Pauling Institute Micronutrient Information Center, "Supplemental Forms," n.d., https://lpi.oregonstate.edu/mic/vitamins/vitamin-C/supplemental-forms.

RDA. Do the math—it is not intended to be a measure of nutrition but as public relations to those who do not know better.

Oral forms of vitamin C usually do not come in the liquid form, as this often requires refrigeration after opening to reduce oxidation. It can be found, but the shelf life is short. In its pure form vitamin C is a white crystal, and it turns brown when oxidized. This is the case with most organic compounds. Regardless of the expiration date on the bottle, if the tablets become light brown or discolored, discard them, as they are oxidized and will offer little to no benefit. They will not be harmful, only worthless. Chewable tablets usually are colored orange and have orange flavoring added to suggest the fruit of origin. These too become stale and discolored with exposure to the air, usually in a spotted pattern; when this occurs, toss them out.

Three quality factors to consider when buying ascorbic acid is to look for the l-ascorbic acid, not the d-ascorbic acid or the mixture of the l- and d- isomers. Do not buy the ascorbic acid derived from corn. And do not buy ascorbic acid from China for the reasons of contamination.

Topical forms of vitamin C have recently appeared in many skin care products. Vitamin C is usually blended with other vitamins, hormones, essential amino acids, and oils or creams that act in concert for healthier skin and to give it an inner radiance or glow. Vitamin C is almost never applied as the only nutrient and never in high concentrations. This form is intended to nurture the skin from the outside in by providing nutrients directly to the collagen and structure of the skin. It is not intended to boost internal blood levels or to treat scurvy. The new term for this type of application is called **nutraceuticals**—a word that implies a synergy of nutrients or foods and pharmaceuticals or medicine. Makeup is no longer for covering up defects or blemishes. Applying nutrients to the skin is really a rejuvenation by applying food the skin needs for growth and health.

The cells hold water better and are fuller, softer, and color is restored. The result: Wrinkles are not as deep and pronounced.

Ascorbyl palmitate is a fat-soluble form of vitamin C. The long-chain fatty acid and ascorbic acid are joined together by removing a molecule of water to form a product known as an ester. This **vitamin C ester** is formed to make a molecule that is soluble in both water and oil, and it should not be confused with **Ester-C**, a water-soluble calcium ascorbate. Ascorbyl palmitate has characteristics of a polar molecule in the ascorbic portion of the molecule and nonpolar features in the palmitate portion. The palmitate side of the molecule can be stored in cell membranes and can penetrate the skin in topical forms. It is often used in skin care products and as a preservative in food, medication, and supplements that tend to oxidize readily.

Ascorbyl palmitate is the only form of vitamin C that can be stored in the lipid cell membrane. All other forms of vitamin C are water soluble and excreted by the kidneys. The oral form of ascorbyl palmitate usually is in capsule form and taken with meals, but only at 500 mg to 1,000 mg per day. It is not taken in higher doses like the water-soluble form.

C complex formulas are a combination of vitamin C and bioflavonoids. This is another group of compounds from citrus fruit (lemons and oranges) and plums. The bioflavonoid rutin is derived from buckwheat. It helps in the synthesis of connective tissue and promotes the function of the clotting factors. **Corsitin** from turmeric is another bioflavonoid.

At this point, I must mention **intravenous vitamin C**. This is not a common method of vitamin C delivery, but it is becoming more popular. Ascorbic acid is supplied in liquid form as **Ascor L 500**, in concentrations of 200 mg/ml and 500 mg/ml in 50 ml vials for dilution in the intravenous fluids of dextrose, normal saline, and lactated Ringer's solution. In the liquid form it oxidizes easily, has a short shelf life, and must be refrigerated. I administer this intravenously in the office as part of the Myers's cocktail, diluted in lactated Ringer's solution, or as part of a chelation formula.

Vitamin C is diluted in other fluids and introduced directly into the vein, and generally no major injury occurs and no harm is done. It may feel cold near the injection site if large quantities of vitamin C are immediately taken from the refrigerator and used. The area near the IV may also hurt if it is run in too swiftly. It should never be injected into a muscle or subcutaneous tissue. If you do this, it will burn. And I do not say this casually. I have had intravenous vitamin C myself, and if the needle becomes dislodged or is inserted improperly, it smarts. Do not hesitate to pull that needle out quickly. Small doses do not injure the skin or underlying tissue, but if you experience any pain, you are doing the infusion wrong.

Vitamin C is found in oranges and other citrus fruits; however, the commercial forms and industrial quantities are derived from corn. This is the cheapest source of vitamin C and the most commonly available on the market. Another source of vitamin C (**Ascor L NC** 500 mg/ml) is derived from red beets and is carried by most compounding pharmacies. The red beet vitamin C is slightly more expensive than the corn vitamin C, but I find no difference between them that warrants the added expense and trouble to obtain the less common beet form.

Intravenous versus Oral Supplementation

Intravenous vitamin C is the same molecule as the oral form. Interestingly, the method of delivery is important in achieving the optimal blood and intracellular tissue levels. Vitamin C that is ingested is limited by the ability of the gut to absorb the molecule. The rate and quantity of bowel absorption is limited. In fact, if more vitamin C than the gut can absorb is swallowed, the remainder will pass in the stool. It does not cause diarrhea, but it does cause a loose stool. If this occurs, the remedy is to take a smaller dose. This is why multiple small doses of 500 mg four times a day will yield higher absorption than 2,000 mg once a day. The absorption is more even, and more is absorbed over the day.

Intravenously, doses as large as 50–100 g (50,000–100,000 mg) can be given over one or two hours. The blood concentration can be as high as 400 to 450 milligrams per deciliter (mg/dL). The conventional range in the plasma is 0.2–2.0 mg/dL. At these higher quantities, this is no longer a vitamin, or vital amine; instead, it begins to function as a drug. This brings to light another designation of vitamin C used by some nutritionists: **C1** is used to designate doses less than 100 mg and **C2** doses of more than 100 mg, whether given orally or intravenously.[143] As a drug, it produces large quantities of hydrogen peroxide that the body uses to fight infection and cancer.

These high levels of vitamin C in the plasma fall to normal levels after four to six hours by vitamin C being excreted in the urine. The normal renal threshold level has been reported in various studies as ranging from 1.3 mg/dL to 2.2 mg/dL of blood concentration. It is above this value that the kidney cannot maintain larger concentrations of ascorbic acid in the blood, and it is passed in the urine. In the use of mega doses of vitamin C, much of the ascorbate is passed by the kidneys into the urine. Contrary to modern medical legend and much admonishment by urologists, I have not seen any kidney stones caused by vitamin C. And my practice includes infusing high doses rapidly, such as 50 g in 30 to 45 minutes.

High doses of vitamin C make the blood hypertonic, or very concentrated compared to the amount of water in the blood. Consequently, when an infusion of vitamin C greater than 3 g is performed, the patient usually notes increased thirst as the body tries to dilute the blood to its normal concentration. Having had this myself, I can confirm that this is when water has never tasted so good!

---

[143] Crayhon, R., *Nutrition Made Simple: A Comprehensive Guide to the Latest Findings in Optimal Nutrition*, M. Evans and Company, 1994.

When the ascorbate is over the renal threshold, it is rapidly excreted in the urine. This process of drinking water and urinating goes on for the next two or three hours, until the concentration of the blood normalizes.

The hypertonic effect of vitamin C has a beneficial medical effect in that it can reduce brain swelling from head trauma or brain surgery. Peripheral edema in the lungs and extremities can also be reduced and removed with 10,000 mg to 25,000 mg of intravenous vitamin C. Before the ascorbate is excreted, it donates an electron pair to other molecules in the body, giving it the added function of an antioxidant.

Optimal Daily Dosing of Vitamin C

Daily dosing can be conservative:[144]

Conservative Daily Dosing for Vitamin C		
Life stage	Age	Intake (mg/day)
Infant	0–1 year	30
Child	1–10 years	60
	11–18 years	250
Adult	19–40 years	500
	40 years and older	1,000

---

[144] National Academy of Science, *Recommended Dietary Allowances*, 1989.

Or daily dosing can conform to Dr. Klenner's guidelines:

Dr. Klenner's Daily Dosing for Vitamin C		
Life stage	Age	Intake (mg/day)
Infant	0–1 year	50
Child	1–10 years	1,000 for each year of life*
	11–18 years	10,000
Adult	19 years and older	10,000

Note. *In other words, a one-year-old receives 1,000 mg (1 g) a day, a two-year-old 2,000 mg (2 g) a day, and so on.

When young adults and adults have infections, especially a cold, flu, bronchitis, and pneumonia, they should take the daily dose three or four times a day. A young adult with a cold and developing bronchitis should take 500 mg four times a day. An adult over 40 years old may take 1,000 mg four times a day, providing bowel tolerance allows this. Surprisingly, during an illness absorption is good, as the need for vitamin C is great. The body uses vitamin C to fight infection at the cellular level by producing hydrogen peroxide and supporting lymphocyte formation.

To treat wounds after surgery or injury, a steady intake of vitamin C is suggested at 500 mg four times a day, at minimum. Absorption is better when the dose is split than when taking 2,000 mg once a day.[145]

---

[145] Pauling, L., *Vitamin C and the Common Cold and the Flu*, W H Freeman and Company, 1976, 99.

Assessing Your Vitamin C Levels

How do you know if you are getting enough vitamin C? In the hospital or doctor's office, this question is easy to answer. Do a blood test and measure the blood level. A normal blood level is 1.5 to 2.0 milligrams per deciliter (mg/dL). But what if you are at home and a trip to the office is a big hassle? What is a convenient way to get a good ballpark estimate? Fortunately, there is **VitaChek-C**,[146] a reagent strip to test the urine for the presence of vitamin C. Vitamin C is always excreted into the urine and reflects the concentrations in the blood quite accurately. This is a good at-home urine test that is cheap and easy to perform. It empowers you to take control of a small portion of your nutritional needs, removing the need for needle sticks and having to go to the doctor or laboratory to answer the question "Am I taking enough vitamin C?"

---

[146] Distributed by Longevity Plus, www.longevityplus.com.

Vitamin D

Benefits of Vitamin D

- Lowers blood pressure
- Helps the pancreas produce insulin
- Has an anti-inflammatory effect and inhibits autoimmune diseases
- Stimulates the growth of dendritic cells, which have vitamin D receptors
- Promotes the transportation of calcium into bone
- Stimulates cells to prevent cancer
- Lifts depression and improves mood
- Prevents the flu
- Helps fight chronic bronchitis
- Prevents childhood cough and runny nose
- Improves memory in the elderly
- Reduces seizure rates
- Reduces brain tumor growth
- Treats hypoparathyroidism
- Increases tolerance to pain
- Makes pain medications more effective
- Protects against macular degeneration
- Relieves the pain of diabetic neuropathy
- Reduces risk of breast cancer
- Prevents migraine headaches
- Reduces menstrual cramps
- Promotes REM sleep

Functions of Vitamin D

Vitamin D is a fat-soluble vitamin that helps transport calcium and phosphorous into the bones. Adequate vitamin D prevents rickets in children, osteomalacia (a form of bone softening) in adults, and osteopenia and osteoporosis in seniors. All these conditions are characterized by insufficient calcium in the bones, which leads to abnormal bone formation or bones that easily break or fracture. Vitamin D can be obtained in the diet from fish, cod liver oil, egg yolk, and supplemented foods such as fortified milk and orange juice—or the body can make it from sunlight shining on the skin.

The body makes vitamin D by the action of sunlight on cholesterol in the skin.

Cholesterol

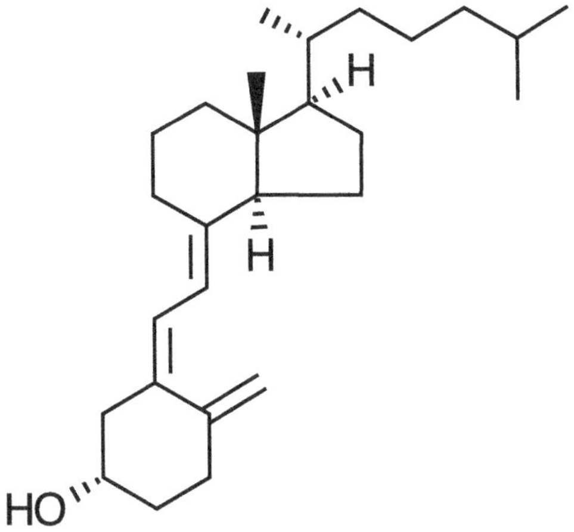

Cholecalciferol, D$_3$

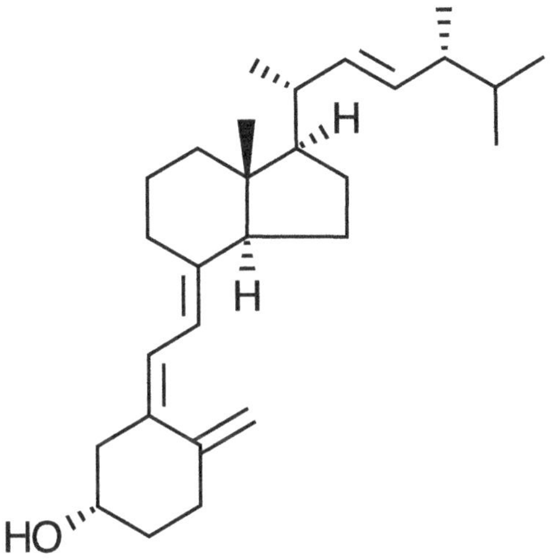

Ergocalciferol, D$_2$

Sunlight is necessary for the energy to make this transformation. In the chemical structure of cholesterol above, an arrow points to the bond that is broken with the energy of sunlight, transforming cholesterol into **vitamin D$_3$, or cholecalciferol**. It is estimated that for people living in New York City, the body does not make any vitamin D$_3$ from November to March because of insufficient exposure to the sun. Therefore, to maintain proper levels of this vitamin, it is necessary to eat foods that are a good source of vitamin D or to take supplements.

Vitamin D and Exposure to Sunlight

Dr. David S. Grimes and his colleagues at the Blackburn Royal Infirmary in England demonstrated a consistent relationship between the amount of sunlight exposure and heart attacks.[147] It helps to live at a latitude where sunlight is more abundant, but that affords no guarantee of adequate vitamin D levels. For the body to produce vitamin D, sunlight must reach and penetrate the skin to reach the cholesterol below the surface to transform it into vitamin D. The sunlight must have **ultraviolet B (UVB)** light to impart the right amount of energy to make the photochemical conversion of cholesterol to vitamin D_3. UVB light is produced in the ultraviolet spectrum in the range of 280–320 nanometers (nm).

UVB levels are affected by the season, specifically by how high in the sky the sun is at a particular time of the year. The amount of absorption of UVB by the ozone layer also varies by time of year and time of day. The sun must be at least 45 degrees above the horizon for significant amounts of UVB to penetrate through the atmosphere. These rays will not arrive in sufficient amounts if the sun is not high enough in the sky, like in the winter months. At a lower angle, the rays pass through too much air that absorbs much of this wavelength of light.

Putting on sunblock to avoid tanning and burning also blocks UVB rays. Secondhand advice from health promoters has made many people avoid the sun altogether. Sitting in a room behind a glass window is not helpful, and neither is sitting in a car with the

---

[147] Grimes, D. S., Hindle, E., and Dyer, T., "Sunlight, Cholesterol, and Coronary Heart Disease," *QJM*, 1996, *89*(8), 579–589, https://doi.org/10.1093/qjmed/89.8.579.

windows up. UVB does not penetrate glass, and though you feel warm from the infrared light, you do not reap the health benefits of the sunlight. Our modern life of tall buildings with the streets in the canyons below, climate-controlled houses and office spaces, and late-night activities, which all appear to be advancements to civilization, have not worked to our benefit. In fact, our lifestyle advances have been ruining our health.

A vacation that includes exposure to sunlight, fresh air, and physical activity makes you feel energized. You have increased vigor. Your body feels better because your vitamin D level goes up. Inflammation is reduced. Your joints work better and present no problems when you get up out of a chair or walk. Your attitude is improved, not only because of the change of venue and exposure to new surroundings but also because vitamin D has **receptors** in the brain. This benefit of sunlight for attitude and depression is easy to comprehend because most people have experienced it—after a series of rainy, dreary days, it is easy to get depressed. On the first sunny day, everyone is happier.

It has been found that the brain has vitamin D receptors that must be stimulated for the nervous tissue to develop to full maturity and functionality. In early childhood development, these receptors must be stimulated for proper brain development. If the brain is not stimulated, some of those cells will die and never develop.

Is There Such a Thing as Too Much Sunlight?

In recent years, warnings about exposure to sunlight have proliferated. These warnings are generally based on good intentions but on little evidence of direct harm and consideration of the type of sunlight someone is being exposed to. Let us talk about some of the fears the medical community is communicating to the general public. Most of the warnings are painted with a broad brush and include little information about beneficial light. The medical community is promoting the use of sunblock, cover-up cream, and UV-blocking sunglasses and planting the fear of skin cancer, the damaging and aging of the skin, and the ultimate fear of developing the deadly skin cancer of melanoma.

In the New York area, the wintertime sun does not get high enough in the sky to penetrate the atmosphere and deliver a full punch of UV light. Much of it is absorbed in the longer path through the atmosphere as it travels tangentially instead of along the shortest route to the earth's surface—that is, perpendicularly downward from above. Summer exposure is more intense, as the light comes from above between the hours of 11:00 a.m. and 3:00 p.m. Remember that high noon in the summer when daylight savings time is in effect is 1:00 p.m. or thereabout, not noon (12:00 p.m.). The scattered light is more effective when it is bounced off water and sand from the lateral spaces and from above. This high-noon light can be very intense, as anyone who frequents the Jersey Shore can attest. In fact, the light can be so intense that it feels like light skin is being seared and cooked.

High-intensity light may feel uncomfortable, burn the upper layer of skin, and cause physical damage to the layers of cells in both the epidermis and dermis. The outermost layer, called the corneous layer, is already dead, and this debris acts as a blocker of light and a physical barrier that affords some physical cushion to the viable tissue below.

In the summer, the light during the day can be divided into strong, damaging light when the sun is high in the sky and less intense light when the sun is lower in the sky, from 8:00 a.m. to 11:00 a.m., and again from 3:00 p.m. to 6:00 p.m. Before 8:00 a.m. and after 6:00 p.m., the rays of the sun are softer. Even though more of the energy of the UV light is absorbed by the air, it still has significant energy to produce vitamin D from cholesterol and promote tanning by stimulating the melanocytes.

Sunburn

I prefer to stay out of the sun when it reaches high-noon intensity. I have fair skin and often burned as a young man from being out in the intense sun. After several sunburns that needed to be treated with aspirin and cool baths for relief, I learned to avoid the intense sun. Sunburn is inflammation of the skin, and the warm to hot temperature is from dilated blood vessels and the increased metabolism of repair. Once the skin has been damaged, it takes two days for the repair process and the effect of the damage to reach its peak. The second day is the worst after a burn.

I experimented with several treatments for sunburn and found that anesthetics such as benzocaine lotions or sprays only sensitized the skin even more. Remember, the skin is red, warm, swollen, painful, and does not work well at retaining heat or cooling. I found that the best treatment for sunburn is to take two 325 mg aspirins three or four times a day and to submerge the arms, legs, and body in a cool, but not cold, bath. Ibuprofen can also be used, and the application of cool, wet towels.

A cool bath may be a tooth-chattering experience because the blood vessels of the skin are dilated, sending blood to the skin for repair. Most of this blood circulating to the skin will lower the core temperature and make you feel cold. The object of the cool bath is not to make you cold but to cool the skin. Water is the active agent. It will lower the temperature of the skin, cooling it. This cooling will help get it back to its normal metabolic rate. After 10 to 15 minutes, you will notice that you transferred much of the heat to the water, and it will be much warmer than when you started. The best part of this treatment is that after the skin is cooled, it will not be as sensitive. If you touch your skin, you will find that the sting of the burn is gone. If some areas are sensitive, stay in the water another 5 or 10 minutes.

When you get out of the bath, you can air-dry or lightly pat yourself dry with a towel before putting your clothes on again. You should be pain free for four to six hours, but then the burning pain will return. Repeat the entire process for relief. This is the best treatment I know of, besides prevention.

If the treatment of aspirin and cool soaks sounds like it takes too much time and effort, it does. I advise prevention. First, stay out of the intense sun at high noon. Get off the beach or get below deck and cover up from 11:00 a.m. to 3:00 p.m. You know how much exposure your skin can take. And take vitamins that prevent burning. To promote tanning and prevent burning, I use 400 mg to 500 mg daily of pantethine (vitamin B_5). Pantethine promotes the production of **melanin**, the product of tanning, and reduces burning. Start taking it two weeks before the anticipated sun exposure to avoid the pain and skin damage.

The Right Amount of Sun Exposure

The most effective sunlight is the less direct sunlight. Take advice from Goldilocks: not too much, not too little—it must be just right. The sun at high noon is too burning, too searing, and too damaging. The sunrays that come from almost overhead with little absorption from the atmosphere are too strong and put too much energy into the skin, damaging the tissue with light, heat, and dehydration. Tanning the skin and producing vitamin D requires just enough energy to stimulate the melanocytes to make pigment and to act on the bonds of cholesterol to break them open to transform it into vitamin D.

It is far better to expose yourself to a slightly indirect light, one that is not as intense, for one hour than to a highly intense light that, on balance, will do more damage than good. Remember, most biochemical reactions occur over time. They occur at lower temperatures than are used in the laboratory. In the laboratory, the chemist uses high temperatures produced by a Bunsen burner, a hot plate, or even a flame and in extreme environmental conditions such as a vacuum or at high pressure. The body performs all its chemical reactions at 98.6 degrees Fahrenheit.

From this normal temperature of 98.6 degrees Fahrenheit up to about 102 or 103 degrees, the body uses higher temperatures to fight off bacterial or viral infections. In the first 24 to 48 hours, even a broken bone will provoke a temperature of 101 degrees. Beyond 103 to 106 degrees, the temperature becomes destructive and has deleterious effects on the body. The system was not meant to function at that temperature. Heat speeds up the rate of the chemical reactions to where they are occurring too fast, consuming too much fuel, or in the parlance of chemists, too much substrate. This goes on to a point where this chemical process we call life is spent and consumed. And when this process stops, there is no life.

In the laboratory, an old rule of thumb was that in the life-viable range of temperature for plants and animals, from above freezing to body temperature, the rate of the chemical reactions double for every increase of 10 degrees Fahrenheit. So at this rate of exposure to heat and UVB radiation, it is easy to damage the skin. Follow nature and take it slow when tanning and building up your vitamin D level. The melanocytes will take days to manufacture pigment. You cannot do it overnight. Small doses of sunlight are better, but if you are short on time, use a sunblock cream or an umbrella to reduce exposure.

Sunblock or sunscreen lotion is intended to block ultraviolet radiation and inhibit damage to the skin by filtering the sunlight. This is the desired effect, but too much blocking will also inhibit the production of vitamin D. This is where good judgment is required to get just the right effect. The process of tanning, with the increase of melanin in the skin, is nature's own sunblock. The more tanned you become, the more the ultraviolet rays are blocked and the less vitamin D is produced. This correlates with the finding that darker-skinned people have lower levels of vitamin D_3. This is one of the mechanisms that prevents vitamin D toxicity. The other mechanism that guards against toxicity is that vitamin D is not a final product but only a step in the cascade, or process, of cholesterol being transformed into vitamin D and then 1,25-dihydroxycholecalciferol and so on, until it is metabolized and eliminated from the body.

Too Much Sunlight Causes Skin Cancer—Or Does It?

Before answering this question directly, I will supply you with some interesting numbers that I found in my research. Most advisors on health issues say to stay out of the sun to avoid skin cancer. If that is the case, how is one expected to produce vitamin D if its formation is related to exposure to sunlight? This is a question that can be more easily answered after you have some knowledge about the yin and yang of sunlight. We are looking for the Goldilocks medium. Not too much, not too little, but just right.

First, some facts about skin cancer. There are three basic skin cancers that account for 98% of all cancers: **melanoma skin cancer**, **squamous cell cancer**, and **basal cell cancer**. The melanoma is the most lethal and difficult to treat, followed by the squamous cell cancer and then the basal cell.

It is interesting that melanoma receives the most attention when it comes to avoiding sunlight but in fact it occurs mostly where the sun shines the least. The most sun-exposed areas of the body are the face, neck, ears, and back of the hands. These areas comprise about 6.5% of the body surface. The least exposed areas are the soles of the feet, pubic region, armpits, groin, and scalp, if it is covered with hair. The site count was developed in an attempt to place a number on the frequency of a skin cancer in exposed compared to nonexposed skin. If sun exposure has a direct effect on the development of skin cancer, the ratio would be one to one (1:1). As an example, if the sun-exposed areas had 100 cancers and the nonexposed areas had only one cancer, the ratio would be 100:1. This would be a strong argument that this cancer is influenced by exposure to the sun. This is the case only with squamous cell cancer of the skin.

The development of basal cell cancer is much less influenced by sunlight. For every basal cell cancer found in the nonexposed areas, 7.2 are found in the sun-exposed areas. The argument here is much weaker than for squamous cell cancer. In looking at the ratio for melanoma, the site count falls to 4.2. Melanoma has little relation to sun exposure, and the findings remain unchanged in a population that, geographically, experiences more hours of sunlight per lifetime. Tripling the hours of sunlight increased the risk of squamous cell skin cancer by 23, basal cell cancer increased by 3.2, and nil for melanoma. Melanoma is the cancer least affected by ultraviolet light, and squamous cell cancer is the most affected. The strongest relation to the development of melanoma, according to Allen Christophers in Australia, is temperature of the skin and the ambient temperatures as they relate to latitude.[148]

Unfortunately, any skin that receives sunlight will make sunlight suspect in the development of cancer. Too much sunlight will promote early aging and a condition called **actinic keratoses**, also called **senile keratoses**, characterized by a small area of reddish scaling that may become elevated, with a grayish top. This is often seen in people who work outdoors, such as sailors and farmers. This is not cancer, but premature aging caused by wind, extreme temperature, and sunlight.

Use your best judgment for sun exposure. Do not seek sun exposure during the most intense time of the day, do not overdo it, and most important of all, if you see you are starting to turn pink, cover up. Use sunblock, put on loose clothing that protects you, and head for the shade.

---

[148] Christophers, A. J., "Melanoma Is Not Caused by Sunlight," *Mutation Research*, 1998, *422*(1), 113–117, https://doi.org/10.1016/S0027-5107(98)00182-1.

Other Functions of Vitamin D

Vitamin D is no longer thought to affect only bones. Many normal soft tissue systems and chemical processes require sufficient Vitamin D to function properly. Vitamin D has also been found to have anti-inflammatory effects that involve autoimmune diseases. It affects the secretion of insulin by the pancreas and the sensitivity of cells to insulin, and through the renin enzyme, it affects blood pressure. This vitamin also stimulates cell differentiation, which means it has some effect on the maturation of cells and in the prevention of cancer. Vitamin D fulfills several other functions, including reducing pain and inflammation, improving sleep, and maintaining cardiovascular health.

Multiple Sclerosis

Multiple sclerosis (MS) has always been a mystery in terms of its cause and treatment. Recently, a relationship was established between MS flareups and the amount of sunlight a person is exposed to. Years ago, it was demonstrated, and written about in many medical textbooks, that the disease is more prevalent in the northern and southern latitudes, away from the equator, and less prevalent in the tropics. It was thought that this may be related to light exposure, and since then, more evidence supporting this theory has been reported. The frequency and number of flareups is closely related to the amount of exposure the patient has to sunlight throughout the year. In winter, when sun exposure decreases and the hours of darkness increase, MS flareups occur more frequently; flareups decrease in summer, when there are more hours of light from a higher angle.

Not surprisingly, vitamin D levels vary with exposure to sunlight. In the winter months, I have found very few vitamin D levels above 30 nanograms per milliliter (ng/ml) in people who are taking no supplements. In the late summer and early fall, if someone participated in outside activities in sunlight, and this is beginning to not be the norm in American life, their serum blood level is above 60 ng/ml.

Another interesting phenomenon I have noticed is in attitude and outlook. Sunlight has the ability to drag you out of the doldrums. For example, if you take an airplane ride, whether you are on a business trip or on vacation, on an overcast day and fly above the clouds, it improves your mood. Even with the stress of flying, checking in, and going through security, coming down below the clouds is a unique experience. Your friends and family members may be happy to see you, but that trip to the sunny side of the clouds has left you a little bit more buoyant and optimistic. Even though your day may have been long and demanding, that extra bit of sunshine made the day easier to get through.

Dysmenorrhea or Painful Menstruation

Dysmenorrhea, or painful menstruation, often referred to as a painful period, is influenced by vitamin D. In a double-blind, placebo-controlled study reported in the *Archives of Internal Medicine*, a single dose of vitamin D was used to reduce pain and discomfort in women aged 18 to 40. No one in the group treated with vitamin D asked for pain relief with nonsteroidal anti-inflammatory drugs (NSAIDs), but 40% of the untreated group did request them. Vitamin D acts by decreasing prostaglandin synthesis and increasing inactivation of the prostaglandins present in the uterus.[149]

---

[149] Lasco, A., Catalano, A., and Benvenga, S., "Improvement of Primary Dysmenorrhea Caused by a Single Oral Dose of vitamin D: Results of a Randomized, Double-Blind, Placebo-Controlled Study," *Archives of Internal Medicine*, 2012, *172*(4), 366–367, https://doi.org/10.1001/archinternmed.2011.715.

Sleep

Vitamin D has a significant influence on sleep and the quality of sleep, according to Gominak and Stumpf.[150] They argued, in an article published in *Medical Hypotheses* in 2012, that there are vitamin D receptors in the hypothalamus and brainstem, areas that initiate and maintain sleep. They did research over two years on 1,500 patients with various sleep disorders such as poor REM sleep, obstructive sleep apnea, insomnia, and headache on awakening. When these patients took vitamin D_3 to achieve a blood level of between 60 nanograms per milliliter (ng/ml) and 80 ng/ml, they experienced restful sleep. They went on to clarify that too little or too much vitamin D_3 was not beneficial. Supplementation with **vitamin D_2, ergocalciferol**, which is the plant form of vitamin D, did not give normal sleep in most individuals studied.

Inflammation

Vitamin D has beneficial effects on reducing inflammation. Inflammation is the healing process that the body initiates to recover from an injury, such as a sprain from a mechanical injury or an infection caused by bacteria or a virus. The clinical characteristics of inflammation are that the area is **red, hot, swollen,** and **sore** and **does not work well**. This includes, for example, swelling in a joint, lung congestion in pneumonia, fever, or local warmth that is apparent. Difficulty in using a sprained or broken joint is troublesome, just as difficulty breathing is apparent if someone has pneumonia or bronchitis.

Vitamin D reduces inflammation, and as the blood level increases, inflammation is reduced. Inflammation is a bit like the immune system gone wild. A bit too much activity in the repair process and things just do not work well. It is in the early stage that

---

[150] Gominak, S.C., and Stumpf, W.E., "The World Epidemic of Sleep Disorders Is Linked to Vitamin D Deficiency," *Medical Hypotheses*, 2012, *79*(2), 132–135, https://doi.org/10.1016/j.mehy.2012.03.031.

things become a bit confused because the body is trying to do two things at once. First, it is trying to remove the toxic or noxious substances from the local tissues, such as blood that may have leaked from the blood vessels due to a traumatic injury or bacteria that may have entered the body. Second, it is trying to repair the broken blood vessels or rebuild tissue that was destroyed by an infection.

Recently, it was found that the process of inflammation requires two types of **macrophages** called **M1** and **M2**. A macrophage is a type of white blood cell that removes dead cells, encloses and kills microorganisms, and stimulates the function of other cells in the immune system. The M1 macrophage is found in the early stages of inflammation. It disassembles the structures of and attacks the foreign organisms or substances. The M2 macrophage is involved with repair and cleaning up the debris. Most of the time, both macrophages are present in the field of injury at the same time, in varying amounts.[151]

In combating cancer, the body develops a boundary of inflammation, a border of white blood cells (lymphocytes, monocytes, and natural killer cells) and antibodies that surrounds the tumor to try to limit its growth. In fact, there is a destructive force to inflammation that does damage to both the invading cells and the body's own normal tissue. This process involves oxidation of the cancer cells and other modulators that, in turn, develop swelling from the increased water the body puts into the area to dilute the ongoing injury. In the big picture, this is interpreted as swelling, or edema. On a chest X-ray of a cancer, this increased water, called an infiltrate, is visible. It is this infiltrate that is visible, not the tumors per se.

The more swelling, the more the local tissues have gone wild, and not much repair is performed until the swelling is reduced. Vitamin D helps reduce some of the wildness of the original injury

---

[151] Yunna, C., et al., "Marcrophage M1/M2 Polarization," *European Journal of Pharmacology*, 2020, *877*, https://doi.org/10.1016/j.ejphar.2020.173090.

and gets the repair process started. It helps suppress some of the proinflammatory messenger chemicals that aggravate the wildness. Some of these messenger chemicals are called **cytokines** and are the substances that cells use to communicate to each other.

Under the influence of vitamin D, the cleanup and repair process is much more orderly and effective. In the winter months, there is much less seasonal stimulus—that is, less sunlight and less vitamin D produced. This is why colds are more common in the winter months. Infections are more difficult to fight when your resistance is down. I have measured **vitamin D$_3$**, the **25-hydroxy** form, in my own patients, and it is often less than 30 ng/ml in those who do not take supplements or experience adequate exposure to sunlight.

Cardiovascular Health

Reducing inflammation is all the buzz lately, and neurology and cardiology are certainly pulled into the discussion when it comes to vitamin D. The plaque areas of blood vessels that make up the obstructions to blood flow are active areas of inflammation with the infiltration of white cells, cholesterol, and triglycerides, as these substances try to repair breaks in the arterial walls. These plaques represent **exuberant repair** to the vessel wall, causing first partial obstruction and then full obstruction, leading to a full heart attack or stroke.

In the development of the plaques as they mature, calcium becomes part of the matrix, making what was a rubbery, flexible repair patch into a hard, nonflexible material on the inner lining of the arterial wall. At this point, movement of the blood vessel, such as bending and flexing of the artery, as the heart contracts and relaxes with each heartbeat may cause a bend that pulls the plaque away from the blood vessel wall. This rupture, or separation of the plaque from the wall, causes immediate repair activity to the area from cytokines and extrinsic clotting factors, released from the vessel wall, to promote platelets and intrinsic clotting factors in the blood to develop a clot at that location. A blood clot develops that is so large that little or no blood at all will pass beyond that point. And there you have a heart attack or stroke.

Cancer

Many cancers are affected by vitamin D. Vitamin D reduces the risk of breast cancer, pancreatic cancer, colon cancer, kidney cancer, brain tumors, and prostate cancer. Many cells have vitamin D receptors that are acted on by the most active form of **vitamin D, 1,25-dihydroxycholecalciferol**. This permits vitamin D to induce changes of development, such as differentiation or inhibition proliferation, invasiveness, blood vessel growth into the tumor, and the ability to metastasize. Vitamin D is just not a vitamin; it is a hormone. This molecule, or the group of molecules called vitamin D, can influence growth and structure, making it more than a nutrient. It controls development. It guides the health of the body.

This has not been well noted in the recent past, as the daily recommended allowance has been too low—200 units for children, 400 units for adults, and 600 units per day for the elderly. I have promoted 5,000 units to elevate the blood level to above 60 ng/ml. This is a quantity found in the summer months in someone in good health and with a respectable level of exposure to sunlight.

Solar radiation has been noticed to reduce the incidence of such cancers as breast, colon, rectal, uterine, ovarian, prostate, esophageal, stomach, pancreatic, lung, and kidney cancer and non-Hodgkin's lymphoma and multiple myeloma. Dark skin, because of the increased melanin, blocks ultraviolet rays, producing less vitamin D.[152]

---

[152] Giovannucci, E., "The Epidemiology of Vitamin D and Cancer Incidence and Mortality: A Review (United States)," *Cancer Causes & Control*, 2005, *16*(2), 83–95, https://doi.org/10.1007/s10552-004-1661-4.

Vitamin D Levels

The National Institutes of Health recommends that adults take about 400 units of vitamin D a day to prevent deficiencies. This is the DRA, or daily recommended allowance. Where this number came from—that a dose of 400 units of vitamin D is necessary to maintain health—is almost impossible to know. Some researchers have suggested that this was an assigned value that was not based on experimental data but on an urge to fill a box in a government table.

Measuring Vitamin D Production

Attempts to determine how much vitamin D the body produces have yielded ranges for different exposures. Exposure to the sun in the summer for 15 to 20 minutes while wearing a T-shirt and shorts produces about 2,000 to 4,000 units of vitamin D. This is a lot more than the 400 units recommended by the National Institutes of Health. A newer unit of measure for the production of Vitamin D is the **minimal erythemal dose**. That is the amount of UVB sunlight needed to produce a slight pinkness to the skin. In an adult, to produce one unit of erythema requires about 20,000 units of Vitamin D_3 produced from sunlight.[153]

If a person stays in the sunlight for a good portion of the day, sunbathing, working in a field, or fishing, they do not experience vitamin D toxicity, as the body metabolizes vitamin D to other end products. In fact, despite all the sun exposure some people experience, they do not experience toxicity. To give lip service to the toxicity of Vitamin D is very easy, but to document the fact is very difficult, if not nearly impossible.

I have been measuring 25-hydroxy vitamin D (D_3) levels in my patients for the last 20-plus years, and the highest value I have found

---

[153] National Institutes of Health, NIH.gov, https://ods.od.nih.gov.

is 98 ng/ml. This was a measurement taken on September 15, after my patient, who worked for the county parks department as a groundskeeper for most of the summer and then vacationed at the Jersey Shore and basked in the sun while on vacation, returned to have his annual medical survey. I have to say his skin was dark from all the tanning he did, but he showed no signs of any toxicity.

Measuring Vitamin D Levels

Testing vitamin D levels is simple and easy. Collection is with a standard serum separator tube (SST), no special refrigeration or freezing of the specimen is necessary, and the results are usually returned in less than a week.

The laboratory usually provides a reference range of what it thinks is normal, based on reviewing many tests and applying statistical analysis to produce a bell curve. I disagree with the method and interpretation of the data. This reference range is what is found in the neighborhood and does not indicate health or the optimal range for health. Initially, a value above 30 ng/ml was considered good, and this was a good starting point for doctors like me to become familiar with assessing lab values. We could use these numbers as a guide in monitoring our patients. More recently, I view numbers above 60 as more compatible with beneficial levels of vitamin D. Higher levels are helpful with problems of depression, anti-inflammatory effects, COVID, and respiratory symptoms.

Because vitamin D levels rise and fall with the seasons, assessing the adequacy of vitamin D levels is a bit more complicated than a simple good or bad reading. It is this undulating behavior of vitamin D values that has made it so difficult to understand its value in relation to the conditions it affects. In 1981, R. Edgar Hope-Sampson coined the term **seasonal stimulus** to describe the effect of variations in vitamin D levels on such diseases as the flu. He noted that the flu has a "season of infliction." A vast number of cases of the flu occur after the winter solstice and abate almost completely by the summer solstice.

Dr. Hope-Sampson was the British physician who recognized the relationship between shingles and its latency from chicken pox. He was a good observer, and after noting the relationship between these two diseases, he was occupied with the seasonal stimulus and influenza epidemics. He not only noted the relationship between flu and the seasons but also noticed that in the tropics, where there is little variation in seasons, there is no seasonal clustering of flu. Unlike major flu epidemics in the temperate climates, flu epidemics occur during the winter months, January, February, and March in the Northern Hemisphere and July, August, and September in the Southern Hemisphere.[154] However, although Dr. Hope-Sampson hypothesized a relationship between solar radiation and flu infections, he did not make the link with vitamin D.

Optimal Vitamin D Levels

So how much is too much? Every substance has an optimal level where everything is in balance. The best estimate is that 40,000 units per day should not be taken for a prolonged period. At these doses, calcium may begin to shift from the bones and kidneys to the blood, producing abnormal deposits in areas such as arteries and joints.

The best advice is to total up all the sources of vitamin D—eggs, fish, fortified milk, and fortified orange juice—and add between 1,000 and 5,000 units of supplemental vitamin D per day. The usual form of vitamin D is listed as vitamin D_3 (cholecalciferol, activated 7-dehydrocholesterol). Bear in mind that 400 units = 10 mg of vitamin D. Sources of vitamin D include the following:

- Egg yolk—25 units

---

[154] Cannell, J. J., et al., "Epidemic Influenza and Vitamin D," *Epidemiology & Infection*, 2006, *134*(6),1129–1140, https://doi.org/10.1017/s0950268806007175.

- Sardines—3 ounces contain 231 units
- Cow's milk—8 ounces contain 100 units
- Fortified cereal—50 units
- Sunlight—20 minutes produces 4,000 units

Vitamin D Supplements

Vitamin D, 25-hydroxy, also called **cholecalciferol** and **activated 7-dehydro-cholesterol**, is referred to as **vitamin D_3**. This is produced when people are exposed to sunlight and is found in egg yolk and fish oils. This is the preferred form, the form used in most supplements, and the form I recommend. Vitamin D_3 is the major circulating form and measured as the storage form of vitamin D. When purchasing vitamin D, look for the designation D_3.

Supplements come in capsules and tablets of 400 units (IU), 800 IU, 1,000 IU, and 5,000 IU. There is a prescription form that is 50,000 units, designed to be taken once a week. A liquid form of D_3 is available in doses of 1,000 units per milliliter (IU/ml), 2,000 IU/ml, and 5,000 IU/ml. Children and teenagers may use 1,000 units per 25 pounds of weight.

Vitamin D_2 is produced from yeast that has been irradiated and is called **ergocalciferol** or **ergosterol**. The body must metabolize it to 25-hydroxyvitamin D and 1,25-dihydroxyvitamin D. It comes in tablets and capsules of 25,000 IU and 50,000 IU and in a liquid form of 8,000 IU/ml. This form is often prescribed by doctors and is carried on hospital and insurance formulary preferred lists because it is cheaper. Remember that most studies were performed on the D_3 form. Vitamin D_2 is sold under the brand names of **Calciferol** and **Drisdol**, and as generic vitamin D without referencing that it is the D_2 form.

Vitamin E

Benefits of Vitamin E

- Helps leg pains from poor circulation
- Reduces heart damage from bypass surgery
- Reduces the severity of sickle cell anemia
- Reduces the severity and progression of Parkinson's disease
- Improves control of seizures
- Reduces the risk of cancer of the lung, prostate, cervix, breast, mouth, and pharynx
- Prevents or delays cataract formation
- Prevents abnormal blood clotting and embolism
- Reduces cellular aging by maintaining cell wall membranes
- Protects against Alzheimer's disease
- Reduces scarring from burns and cuts
- Increases muscle power
- Enhances testicular health
- Prevents spontaneous abortions
- Prevents infant hemolytic anemia
- Strong antioxidant
- Effective antithrombin agent
- Best defense against heart attacks and strokes

What Is Vitamin E?

Throughout this chapter, the definition of vitamin E will be the blend of the eight molecules found in nature that work together to function as an antioxidant with the ability to lower cholesterol and triglycerides, permit normal development of the gonads, provide neurological protection, function as a natural anticlotting agent in the blood, and reduce or inhibit tumor growth. There are two basic groups called **tocopherols** and **tocotrienols**, each with four members with the same side chains but different placements and numbers of methyl groups on the double ring, or **chromanol ring**. This is our working definition of vitamin E in the world of alternative medicine. In contrast, traditional medical doctors use the definition of the Food and Drug Administration (FDA) of vitamin E as **alpha-tocopherol**. They do not consider the other seven molecules that are found in nature. Alpha-tocopherol can be refined, but it is often manufactured in a laboratory. It is lighter in color than the natural eight-molecule forms, and it does not function the same or have the same health benefits.

I start this chapter with this definition because it is crucial to the understanding of vitamin E. Many people know vitamin E is beneficial to their health because they have experienced its effects. Many studies have been performed and reported in the *Journal of the American Medical Association* (*JAMA*) and the *New England Journal of Medicine* that show no benefits of vitamin E or that even claim it is detrimental to health. More often than not, the studies with poor outcomes have used alpha-tocopherol as vitamin E, as defined by the FDA, rather than Mother Nature's definition of a blend of eight molecules as found in hazelnuts, almonds, sunflowers, the annatto plant, and whole grains.

Tocopherols

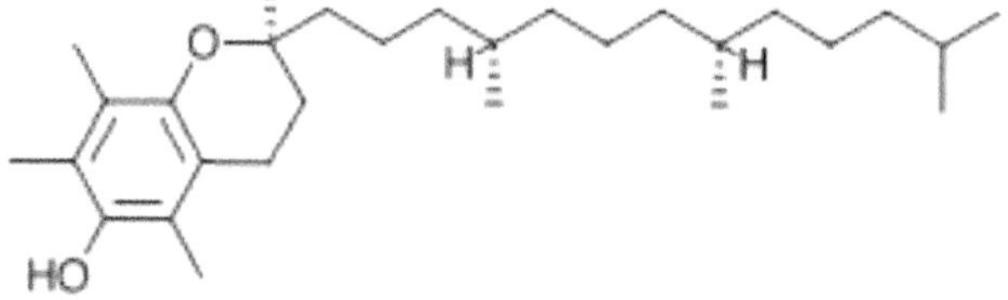

Alpha-Tocopherol

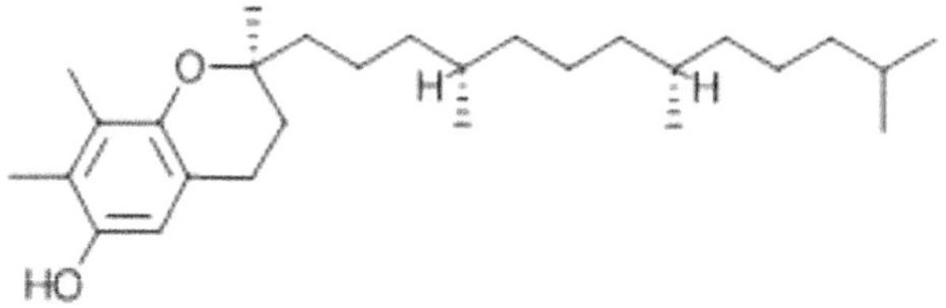

Gamma-Tocopherol

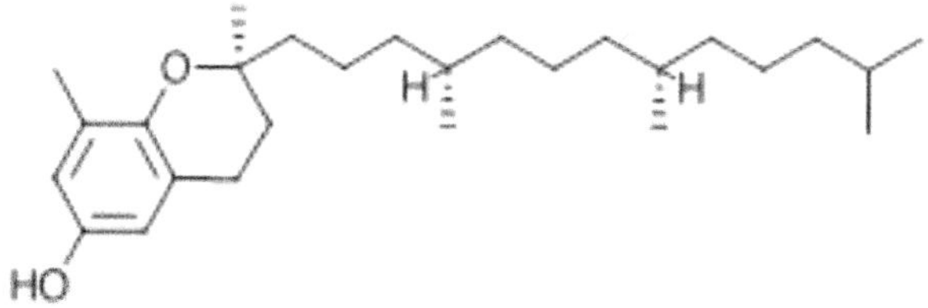

Delta-Tocopherol

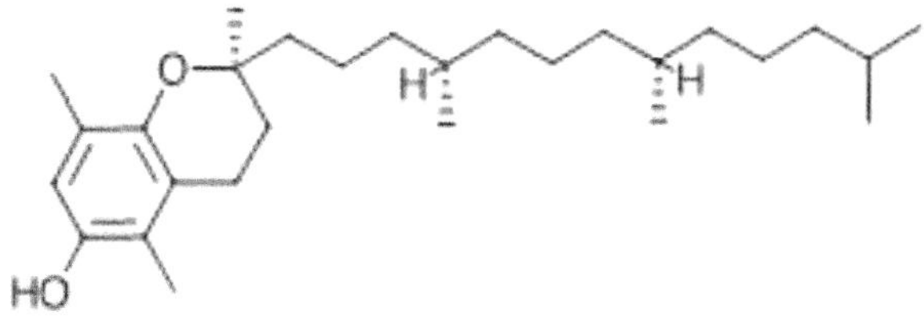

Beta-Tocopherol

Tocotrienols

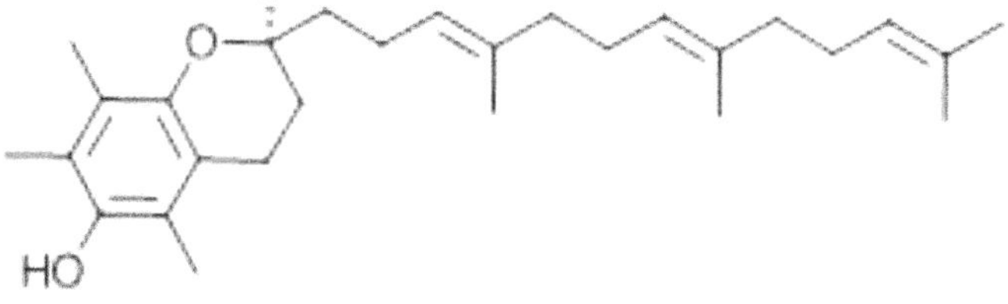

Alpha-Tocotrienol

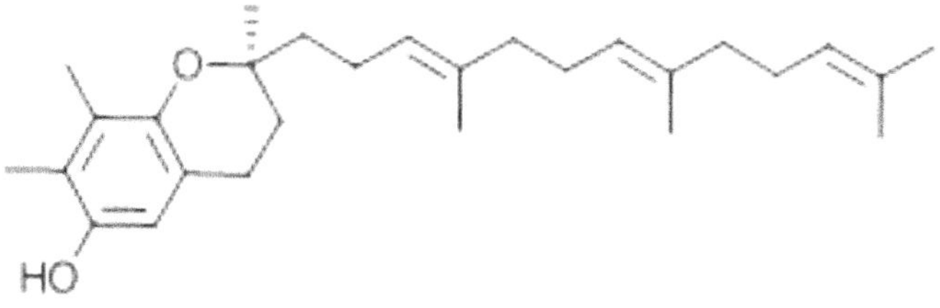

Gamma-Tocotrienol

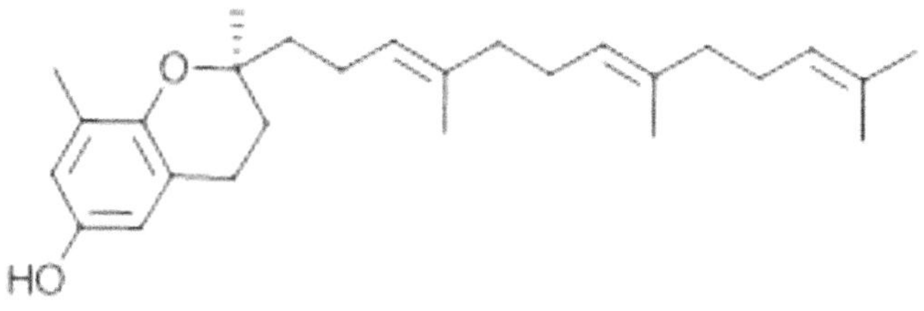

Delta-Tocotrienol

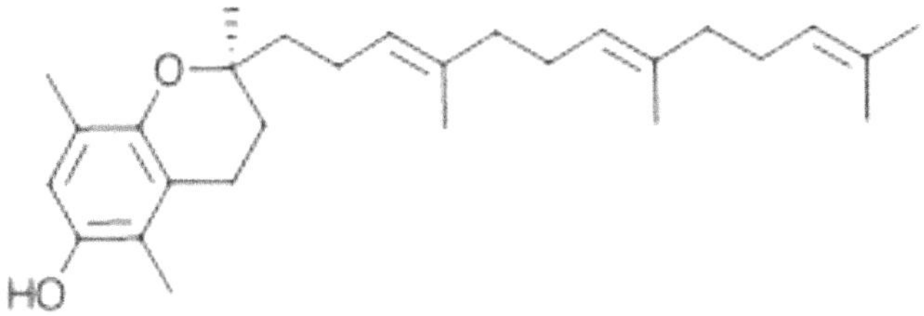

Beta-Tocotrienol

In this book, I use the definition of vitamin E as a blend of the eight molecules: two groups with the tails of tocopherol or tocotrienol and each with four different chroman rings, or heads and side chains designated **alpha, beta, gamma,** and **delta**, to define vitamin E.

The different molecules produced by nature are called **vitamers**. They all have unique functions and molecular weights, the latter because of the number of methyl groups on the chroman head or the amount of hydrogen on the tails because of double or saturated bonding. Alpha-tocopherol is the largest and heaviest of the group, and delta-tocotrienol is the smallest and lightest.

The synthetic alpha-tocopherol is made up of eight different molecules called **isomers**. It is the same number of atoms, and therefore the same molecular weight, but joined in different arrangements. Only one of the arranged structures is found in nature and similar to natural alpha-tocopherol. The other seven are not found in nature and have not been found to be beneficial to humans. From a practical perspective, if you ingest a 400-unit gel cap of synthetic vitamin E, only 50 units of the gel cap will give you any benefits. The other 350 units will have no effect.

Most of the early studies using vitamin E used the natural form of eight molecules with good results. Unfortunately, after it was discovered how to cheaply synthesize alpha-tocopherol in 1938, studies were performed with the one molecule form, and their findings often indicated less, or no, beneficial effects.

I advise you when reading other source material on vitamin E to ask the question "Which vitamin E are they talking about?"

History of Vitamin E

Vitamin E was first recognized in 1922 by Evans and Bishop, who noticed its ability to sustain a pregnancy in rats.[155] These female animals had no problem ovulating and conceiving, but during the pregnancy the fetus would sometimes die and be reabsorbed into

---

[155] Cohn, V. H., "Fat-Soluble Vitamins," In Goodman, L. S., and Gilman, A. (eds.), *The Pharmacological Basis of Therapeutics*, 4th edition, Macmillan, 1971, 1694.

the mother. Treating these rats with vitamin E prevented this from occurring. Similarly, degenerative changes were observed in the testes of male rats. Giving this group of vitamin E restored the testes to normal. Because of these beneficial effects on the rat reproductive system, vitamin E was described as the anti-sterility vitamin. The first human application of alpha-tocopherol was suggested in *The Lancet* in 1931 by Danish veterinarian Philip Vogt-Möller for the problem of habitual abortion.[156]

Evans, who first used vitamin E in 1922 in his rat experiments, went on to isolate it from wheat germ oil in 1936. Two years later, in 1938, Fernholtz identified the molecule's chemical structure, which is similar to the structure of the **Q enzymes**. Many people are familiar with the antioxidant and energy enhancer known as **coenzyme Q10**. It has never been proven that there is any overlapping function, but they help similar problems. That same year, in 1938, vitamin E in the form of alpha-tocopherol was synthesized.

Synthesis of Alpha-Tocopherol

The confusion began in 1938. The availability of a cheap form of chemically produced alpha-tocopherol, commonly called vitamin E, meant many experiments could easily be performed with an abundant supply of the vitamin. But are experiments performed with only one molecule of vitamin E the same as those performed with the natural eight molecules? I suggest that they are not the same.

Opponents to my view say that the most common form of vitamin E found in the blood is alpha-tocopherol, with a little of the gamma and delta and even less of the beta. The reasoning is that if there is little found in the blood, it is not needed or is not important. I respond with the argument that most vitamin E is found in the

---

[156] "Treatment of Habitual Abortion with Wheat-Germ Oil (Vitamin E)," *Lancet*, 1931, https://doi.org/10.1016/S0140-6736(00)47093-5.

liver and fat and less in the blood, which is the alpha form. Gamma and delta are taken up rapidly and are either in the tissues, repairing cell wall membranes, or are being metabolized. Furthermore, studies that have been performed with the alpha-tocopherol only have not shown much of a benefit. Studies performed with the eight-molecule blend of tocopherols and tocotrienols have shown more favorable results.

In the 1940s, two brothers, Drs. Wilfred and Evan Shute, started treating their patients with cardiovascular disease with vitamin E. They reported slowing down and even in some cases reversing atherosclerosis. This concept of lowering the **low-density lipoprotein (LDL)** was picked up in 1992 by Ishwarlal Jialal, MD, and Scott Grundy, PhD, at the University of Texas Southwestern Medical Center, where they initiated studies to measure the effect of vitamin E. In their study, they gave volunteers 800 units of alpha-tocopherol daily and measured the effect. They found that LDL oxidation was reduced by half.[157] The cholesterol level did not change. It is oxidized LDL that is thought to promote the formation of the fatty deposits in the arteries—that is, the formation of atherosclerosis.

Vitamin E is a fat-soluble antioxidant, and vitamin C is a water-soluble antioxidant. It is thought that after vitamin E donates its electrons, its function as an antioxidant does not end entirely. Vitamin C can donate its electron pair to vitamin E, rejuvenating vitamin E and restoring its antioxidant ability. This may explain why small amounts of vitamin E are required in the diet. The molecule can be recycled many times.

The eight molecules of vitamin E are best explained by showing the molecular structure. The left ring of the two ring structures on the left of the diagram determines whether this is an alpha, beta,

---

[157] Jialal, I., and Grundy, S., "Effect of Dietary Supplementation of Alpha-Tocopherol on the Oxidative Modification of Low Density Lipoprotein," *Journal of Lipid Research*, 1992, 33, 899–906.

gamma, or delta molecule by which atom, or group of atoms, occupy the R positions. In alpha-tocopherol, all the R positions are occupied by a methyl (-CH$_3$) group. In delta-tocopherol, only the R$_3$ position is occupied by a methyl (-CH$_3$) group, while R$_1$ and R$_2$ are occupied by a hydrogen (-H) atom. In beta-tocopherol, R$_1$ and R$_3$ each have a methyl (-CH$_3$) group, and R$_2$ has a hydrogen (-H) atom. In gamma-tocopherol, R$_2$ and R$_3$ have a methyl (-CH$_3$) group each, while R$_1$ is occupied by a hydrogen (H) atom

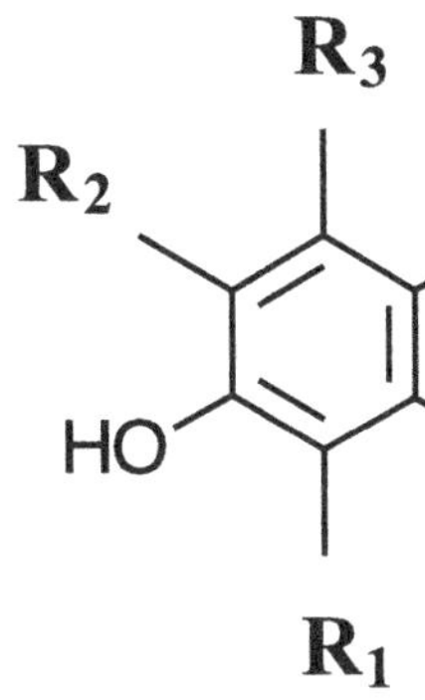

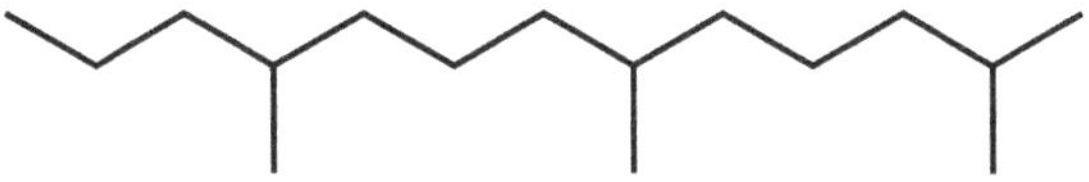

The tail of the molecule is made up of a 13-carbon chain with three methyl side chains. The side chains of the tocopherols are completely saturated.

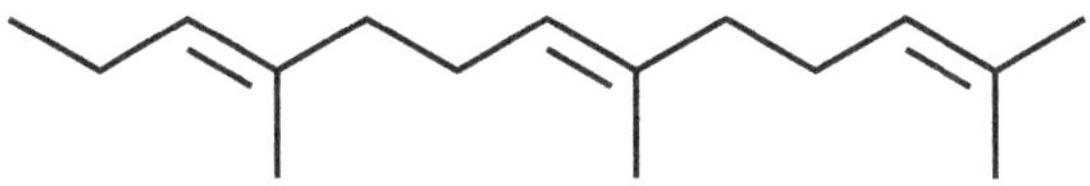

The tocotrienols have three unsaturated bonds near each of the methyl side chains.

The double line in the diagram shows that not all the possible positions are occupied by hydrogen. This is called a carbon double bond and what is meant in chemistry by the term **unsaturated**.

This gives a total of eight different structures produced by nature. Vitamin E is always found as a mixture in nature, never in only one molecular form. There must be a reason, but unfortunately, no one has the answer at this time. What is known is that in trials since 1938, when alpha-tocopherol was first manufactured in a laboratory, inconsistent benefits have been demonstrated for vitamin E.

Recent research into the family of vitamin E molecules has shown that the ring structure that makes up the head performs the antioxidant work. The heads are identified as alpha, beta, gamma, or delta depending on where the methyl groups are attached. The tail determines whether the molecule is a tocopherol or tocotrienol. Both tails anchor into cell walls; the walls are composed of fat molecules that form lipid membranes. Tocotrienols have shorter and more flexible tails because they have fewer atoms compared to tocopherols. Tocotrienols have the effect of lowering total cholesterol and LDL cholesterol, which tocopherols do not do. This difference in vitamin E molecules came to light after the discovery by Barrie Tan, PhD, that the annatto plant produces only tocotrienols, which allowed studies of the various molecules. Prior to this, the major source of vitamin E was wheat germ, which produces all eight molecules, and they are difficult to separate.

How to Read a Study Involving Vitamin E

Big Pharma has used this confusion to its advantage to pooh-pooh any benefit to vitamin E. But now that you know what the difference is, you will know how to read a study involving vitamin E. What is the definition of vitamin E in the study? Nearly all studies reported in the family of AMA journals and the *New England Journal of Medicine* do not use vitamin E in the eight forms in which Mother Nature produces it.

The second factor to consider is the amount of vitamin E. Very often, the amount will be less than the recommended dietary allowance (RDA). Traditionally, vitamin E is measured in units, and this is what you look for when you go to the store to buy it. Some studies will add to the confusion and report it as milligrams (mg), micrograms (mcg), or, still more confusing, millimoles (mmol). You have no idea how a study relates to a bottle of vitamin E that you hold in your hand. In an attempt to use the same unit of measurement for vitamin E, modern researchers are favoring the unit of measure as the milligram. A unit of vitamin E is so close to a milligram of vitamin E that they are basically interchangeable. Researchers are leading the way on milligrams, and it will soon be the more common unit of measure in the products found in stores.

Work of the Shute Brothers

From the 1950s to the 1970s, the Shute Brothers of Canada published five books on their experiences and the benefits of vitamin E. They came from a large family of physicians in several fields who all contributed much original work to the fields of obstetrics and gynecology, cardiology, and internal medicine. Dr. Wilfrid E. Shute worked with and wrote about vitamin E from 1933 to the 1970s. Much of his work is about heart attacks, or coronary thrombosis, in doctor language. Vitamin E prevents the abnormal clotting of the blood that is responsible for heart attacks, strokes, and blood clots in the legs and lungs. In his book *Dr. Wilfrid E. Shute's Complete Updated Vitamin E Book*, he discusses heart attacks going from an almost nonexistent disease in 1910 in America to more than 700,000 heart attacks a year in the 1970s.

According to Shute, in 1900, the disease of coronary thrombosis, a heart attack caused by a clot obstructing an artery of the heart, or a coronary artery, was unheard of. He did cite an uncorroborated report by Dr. George Dock, in 1896, of four cases of heart attacks. The first formal description of a myocardial infarction, or heart attack, was by Dr. J. B. Herrick in 1912. Dr. Paul Dudley White, who was one of the first cardiologists in America and President Eisenhower's doctor, said that when he graduated from medical school in 1911, he had never heard of a coronary thrombosis or heart attack.

So how did something so rare become so common? A disease that was almost impossible to get now affects one in four people. What changed in America? What has the medical community ignored? Who continues to be oblivious, even after the suggestion and demonstration by the Shute brothers?

Dr. Wilfrid Shute suggested that it may be the way we process our food. Prior to 1900, wheat was ground up and the wheat germ and cotyledon packaged together. This combination of embryo and cotyledon is the whole seed. The embryo is the new plant, and the cotyledon is the food for the plant before photosynthesis can take over. The problem with this process is that the wheat germ, or embryo, contains fats, proteins, and vitamins, including vitamin E, that can be oxidized and become rancid. This gives the cotyledon or flour, the processed material from wheat, a short shelf life.

The technology of the 1900s could separate the wheat germ from the cotyledon, which is mostly carbohydrates. This white flour has been stripped of the high-nutrient embryo with its proteins, fats, and vitamins. The white flour can be packaged and kept on the shelf without the more perishable components oxidizing, breaking down, and going rancid. So much of the nutrients are removed in the milling and processing that natural and artificial vitamins are added to the final product to try to bring it back to some form of a useful product. The industry calls these products **fortified**.

Wheat germ contains the largest amount of vitamin E of any food.

Vitamin E Content of Foods	
100 g of food	**Vitamin E content(mg)**
Wheat germ oil	216
Sunflower seeds	90
Sunflower oil	88
Safflower oil	72
Almonds	48
Sesame oil	45
Peanut oil	34
Corn oil	29
Wheat germ	22
Peanuts	18
Olive oil	18
Peanut butter	11
Oatmeal	3
Carrots	1
Peas	0.99
Eggs	0.83

In the last century, the processing of food has undergone major changes. This includes how we grow food, process food, and protect it for distribution. Food has been denatured, adulterated, irradiated, gassed, and colored to visual perfection. Unfortunately, it is not healthy. Bread was a staple for centuries, but now it has been stripped of its nutrient value. Bread is not only robbed of its value in the processing, but farmers also take some blame as well. The farming goal today is bushels per acre. Not quality. Potassium, ammonium, and phosphate are used liberally to grow large grains, fruits, and vegetables, but they lack in mineral content and nutrient value.

Dr. Wilfrid Shute's most significant finding in the initial use of vitamin E is the vitamin's ability to inhibit abnormal clotting, such as the clots that cause heart attacks and peripheral blood clots in the legs. In his many books, he credits **alpha tocopherol** with two important characteristics: its ability to **inhibit clots** and its ability to **dissolve clots**. This was also reported by Zierler in 1948. In 1964, Alton Ochsner from Tulane University School of Medicine wrote to the *New England Journal of Medicine* that "alpha tocopherol is a potent inhibitor of thrombin that does not produce a hemorrhagic tendency and is therefore, a safe prophylactic agent against venous thrombosis."[158]

Tocotrienols and the Work of Dr. Barrie Tan

Initially, the study of vitamin E focused on the tocopherols, namely alpha-, beta-, gamma-, and delta-tocopherol. This is because in the natural source, wheat germ, these are the majority of vitamers produced. The form found mostly in the blood is alpha-tocopherol; the other forms are in or on the cell walls or in the cytosol. Alpha-tocopherol is what the Shute brothers spoke most about. Recently,

---

[158] Shute, W. E., *Dr. Wilfrid E. Shute's Complete…Updated Vitamin E Book*, Pivot Health Books, 1978, 91.

the discussion has moved to the tocotrienols because it has been discovered that tocotrienols, which were difficult to separate from the more abundant tocopherols, can now be obtained from the **annatto** plant, which does not produce significant amounts of tocopherols, thus avoiding a costly and difficult separation of the tocotrienols from the tocopherols. Having a natural source of alpha-, beta-, gamma-, and delta-tocotrienols has permitted new investigations into their properties and opens new knowledge.

The story of the discovery of tocotrienols began in 1983, when on a visit to his homeland of Malaysia, Barrie Tan, PhD (chemistry), was invited by a friend to visit a palm oil manufacturer. On analysis of the oil, in 1984, he found tocotrienols. In 1986, he began to publish his findings that 50% of the vitamin E in palm oil is delta- and gamma-tocotrienols. In 1995, he discovered that 35% of the vitamin E in rice is tocotrienols, and in 1999, he discovered the **annatto** plant in South America that contains only delta- and gamma-tocotrienols. The annatto plant is also called the lipstick plant because of the fatty red pigment in the seeds of the flower, which are a bright, deep red.

Tocotrienols are derived from three sources: rice, palm oil, and the annatto plant. They produce different ratios of tocopherol to tocotrienol. Recent data shows that the ratio in rice is 50:50; in palm oil, 25:75; and in the annatto plant, 0.1:99.9. That means that the annatto plant produces 99.9% tocotrienol and opens up a new area of study, as a near pure form of tocotrienols is available for study.[159]

Observing this natural group of vitamers has allowed Dr. Barrie Tan to study the effects of tocotrienols on the body. He has found that tocotrienols have a good anti-inflammatory ability to inhibit the COX-2 enzyme. Delta-tocotrienol, the smallest molecule of vitamin

---

[159] Vasanthi, H. R., Parameswari, R. P., and Das, D. K., "Multifaceted Role of Tocotrienols in Cardioprotection Supports Their Structure: Function Relation," *Genes & Nutrition*, 2012, 7(1), 19–28, https://doi.org/10.1007%2Fs12263-011-0227-9.

E (with gamma-tocotrienol being the next smallest), has significant antioxidant, antithrombotic, and cholesterol-lowering abilities as well as antitumor effects.[160]

As a group of molecules, the tocotrienols are smaller and more flexible and can cover more membrane area, providing antioxidant protection. One might consider the tocotrienols a stealthier molecule, because they are generally found on or in the cell, unlike the tocopherols that are readily found in the blood. This quality has allowed them to go unnoticed by researchers for years. Most research is performed on blood, as it is easy to obtain and generally easy to analyze. Tissue samples are more difficult to obtain. A piece of tissue must be cut out of the person, fewer candidates avail themselves for study, and sample sizes are generally much smaller. However, with micro techniques, studies are advancing, yielding new information.

Tocotrienol's anticancer effect is attributed to its anti-inflammatory nature. Delta is slightly more effective than gamma. By reducing inflammation, delta-tocotrienol has shown to have a positive effect in reducing cancer of the breast, pancreas, and colon. Pretreating cancer patients 24 hours before undergoing radiation with delta- and gamma-tocotrienols has improved survivability and protects the normal cells. The lining of the stomach, the gastric mucosa, is also protected with delta-tocotrienol because it inhibits the COX-2 enzyme. Almost any process that involves inflammation as the nasty culprit can be improved with delta-tocotrienol, including osteoporosis.[161]

Tocotrienol and Cardiac Protection

Let me tell you the story of my patient, Cheryl. She is a nurse, currently 70 years old, and five years ago, she experienced chest pain.

---

[160] Tan, B., and Trias, A. M., "Vitamin E Tocotrienols: Quenching the Fires Within," *Townsend Letter*, October 2013, no. 363, 86–93.
[161] Ibid.

She had the usual cardiac workup: history, physical, blood tests, EKG, echocardiogram, stress test, and a nuclear study. The discomfort was still present after all the usual studies, and the only test left was to undergo cardiac catheterization to look at the condition of the arteries.

She underwent a full catheterization. It was found that she had a 50% stenosis of the left anterior descending (LAD) artery of the heart. The general rule is that stents are put in only if the narrowing is 70% to 99%. When Cheryl awoke from anesthesia, she was informed that she was in great shape and had only a 50% narrowing and did not need a stent. As a nurse she was primed for a stent, but she was upset that she had a 50% stenosis with no stent! She was doomed to statin drugs, and she knew how dangerous of a proposition that it was. More than anything else, the idea was in her head that she had a 50% lesion and that it could get worse over time. She was committed to exercise, diet, and statins. This solution was unacceptable to her.

Cheryl was on a journey to do everything she could to help herself. She was on vitamins, minerals, thyroid replacement, bio-identical hormones, and a diet that offered no comfort or taste. Every time I saw her in the office or socially, she lamented the 50% lesion and said she needed a new catheterization because she knew it was getting worse, even though, at this time, she had no pain. She searched online and through all the reading material she could find, looking for an answer to her problem. She was a woman on a mission. She started looking at vitamin E and bumped into a form that she did not know about before: tocotrienol.

She asked me about it, and I knew about the anticancer effect, but at the time, I knew little about the cardiac protection. I did not give it much thought, but I did not think it would do any harm.

As all little seeds can grow into big trees, the idea in Cheryl's head grew to a size that was all consuming. She kept running to her cardiologist saying that the 50% stenosis was getting worse and that she did not want another nuclear study to fill her body up with radioactive material that is difficult to remove—she wanted another catheterization. Her nagging, complaining, and phone calls paid off. The doctor could not go to the hospital without bumping into Cheryl and having to hear her story of impending doom. To give himself a break, he capitulated to her wish for a repeat catheterization.

Cheryl could not get onto the procedure table fast enough. Finally, the day came, and she had her invasive cardiac study. To the surprise of everybody, including the cardiologist, the original stenosis was gone. Nowhere to be found! Not a trace! In fact, nowhere in the cardiac arteries could any plaque buildup be found.

The only thing that could explain this was that for one year prior to the catheterization, she had been taking tocotrienols, two 125 mg gel capsules twice a day. Neither she nor I had heard of this before.

From Cheryl's experience and all its new questions, it is obvious that the story of vitamin E and its biochemistry is incomplete. This vitamin was discovered more than 100 years ago, and we still do not know what power this vitamin has. In the last 20 years, its ability to treat cancer and heart disease has been added to its list of benefits. I am sure that this is not the end to the chapter of vitamin E.

Functions of Vitamin E

Vitamin E is a fat-soluble antioxidant that is stored in the liver and fatty tissue. It promotes fatty acid metabolism and enhances the action of enzymes. It destroys free radicals, the unstable oxygen molecules of metabolism that damage cells. It appears that its antioxidant affect may be its dominant function. It prevents the production of toxic, oxidized, unsaturated fatty acids that promote problems such as heart disease.

Cardiovascular Benefits

Vitamin E has an anticlotting benefit to prevent heart attacks, as reported by Dr. Shute. This advantage is not limited to clots in heart vessels. Vitamin E has the ability to prevent strokes and thrombosis in the legs and pelvis and even to help dissolve blood clots. Blood clots in the thigh and pelvis are the most dangerous and can travel to the lung, and if of sufficient size, can totally obstruct all blood flow to the lung and cause death. Smaller clots can be dissolved if sufficient vitamin E is given daily in a dosage of 2,400 mg or more. It is better to take vitamin E to prevent unwanted clots than to have treatment after the damage is done.

I have interviewed vascular surgeons on this subject, and their response is that vitamin E causes minor problems with prolonged bleeding during an operation. They say aspirin is far more problematic than vitamin E. Nevertheless, I still see surgeons advising patients not to take vitamin E prior to surgery. If you stop five days before surgery, you will still have the advantage of reducing your chances of developing a thrombus. Most vitamin E is in the cells and lipid layers of the cell wall; the majority of it is not circulating in the blood, though it can be found there.

Antioxidant Effects

Vitamin E has an antioxidant effect and the ability to decrease the demand for oxygen in the tissues. It can reduce the need for oxygen in the tissues of the lung and retina, but it does not eliminate the need for oxygen. When oxygen is not available to the tissues in sufficient amounts, for example, at a higher altitude, vascular obstruction from local edema can develop. When leg cramps or claudication develop, blood vessels do not dilate in response to a greater demand for oxygen. Under these conditions, vitamin E in the range of 400–800 mg once, twice, or three times a day will give relief. Vascular leg cramps that occur after getting into bed are relieved with a bedtime dose. Any condition that may involve reduced oxygen in the tissues would benefit from vitamin E.

Capillary Permeability and Vasodilation

Capillary permeability and vasodilation are improved with vitamin E. Treated early on, capillary function can be improved, but chronic conditions do not respond as well. The chronic condition should be neither neglected nor ignored; it too will benefit, but it may take much longer to see its effect.

Keloids

Keloids are an exuberance of scar tissue. These scars can be provoked by a minor injury to the skin, causing raised, reddened tissue that will not recede and flatten to the level of the normal surrounding tissue. In fact, it may expand and slowly deform the normal local tissue. Application of vitamin E to the scar will promote healing with a minimum of fibrous scarring. It is often used after plastic surgery or on any area where less scarring is desired. Scar-reducing preparations often include other elements in the formula, but the key ingredient is vitamin E.

Nonalcoholic Fatty Liver Disease

Vitamin E can help prevent damage on the outside of the body, such as scarring, and repair damaged skin. The inside of the body can also be damaged by disease or by what we eat. Fructose is a sugar made from corn and now being used where cane sugar was once used. It is cheap; it is gooey at room temperature, not crystalline, giving food a sticky quality. Unfortunately, it is now used in sodas and baked goods. It is the major component of breakfast cereals and can be found in most candies. Eating more than 15 g per day is a major cause of obesity and can lead to **nonalcoholic**

steatohepatitis (NASH), a form of cirrhosis, or hardening, of the liver, caused by the scarring of fat deposits. This is not a well-known disease, but it soon will be. It can progress from cirrhosis to liver failure and death. This form of cirrhosis is now more common than alcoholic cirrhosis. Eating fructose is more damaging than drinking alcohol. Fortunately, vitamin E has been shown to help arrest and even reverse this form of liver damage.

The findings of two studies have supported the treatment of NASH with vitamin E and noted that fat deposition, oxidative stress, and symptoms of liver disease improved.[162] Additionally, treating with vitamin E reduced triglycerides and lipid peroxides in the liver and prevented liver fibrosis (scarring).[163] Both these studies used Mother Nature's mixture of tocopherols and tocotrienols.

Alzheimer's Disease

The risk of the development of Alzheimer's disease is reduced by vitamin E. In 1998, Martha Clare Morris was the lead author of a prospective study, funded by the National Institute of Aging, on the development of Alzheimer's disease and its relationship to taking either vitamin E, vitamin C, or both antioxidants. The study, which ran for 4.3 years, involved 633 people aged 65 years and older. In the group that was not taking vitamins E or C, 91 cases of Alzheimer's developed. In contrast, no one in the treatment groups developed Alzheimer's disease. It was predicted that the vitamin E group would have 3.9 cases and the vitamin C group 3.3 cases—the

---

[162] Sumida, Y., et al., "Role of Vitamin E in the Treatment of Non-alcoholic Steatohepatitis," *Free Radical Biology and Medicine*, 2021, *177*, 391–403.

[163] Yachi, R., et al., "Effects of Tocotrienol on Tumor Necrosis Factor-A/D-Galactosamine-Induced Steatohepatitis in Rats," *Journal of Clinical Biochemistry and Nutrition*, 2013, *52*(2), 146–153, https://doi.org/10.3164%2Fjcbn.12-101; Medical News Today, April 25, 2013.

frequency found in the general population.[164] This prospective study suggests that taking either vitamin E or vitamin C reduces the risk of Alzheimer's disease. To me, this is significant. Taking these vitamins is very protective. The benefit is great and the risk low. This study alone is enough reason to take either vitamin E, vitamin C, or both.

Skin Repair

Fatty deposits in the skin around the eye that usually have a yellow appearance are called **xanthomatosis**. Once, the only treatment was surgical removal, but Dr. Wilfred E. Shute reported that they may be removed by ingesting a combination of vitamins E and C. Vitamin E has been reported to reduce Dupuytren's contractures and reduce scarring from burns.[165]

Cancer

Not all research is politically motivated. There is good research into vitamin E that has shown it is effective in promoting spontaneous cell death, a process called **apoptosis**. This is significant when it comes to its effect on cancers such as acute lymphoblastic leukemia HL-60 and adenocarcinoma of the colon.

Gabriella Calviello and her team at the Catholic University of Rome have shown that gamma-tocopherol has an oxidative metabolite called **gamma-tocopherol quinine** that is toxic to lymphoblastic leukemia, promyelocytic leukemia cells, and colonic

---

[164] Morris, M. C., et al., "Vitamin E and Vitamin C Supplement Use and Risk of Incident Alzheimer Disease," *Alzheimer Disease & Associated Disorders*, 1998, 12(3), 121–126, https://doi.org/10.1097/00002093-199809000-00001.
[165] Shute, W. E., *Dr. Wilfrid E. Shute's Complete…*, 220.

adenocarcinoma WiDr cells.[166] It is suggested that this quinone is of a fatty nature and activates the mitochondrial pathway, activating caspase-9 and the release of cytochrome *c* in the cytosol of the cell (the fluids of the cell) to promote apoptosis. The gamma-tocopherol quinine is less toxic than the commercial cytotoxic chemotherapy quinones such as doxorubicin, mitomycin C, and menadione that are used to treat leukemia and breast cancer.[167]

Prostate Cancer

In October 2011, the news reported on a study that said that giving men vitamin E with or without selenium increased the risk of prostate cancer. That was the sound bite and just about what the general public and the professional medical community understood as the take-home message. This was reported on the airwaves, on cable TV, and in newsprint. I remember one doctor reading this article directly from *The New York Times* in the hospital, accepting this information without question. This was followed by a disparaging remark that vitamins are not always good for you.

I knew this did not sound right. The mass media, including the *Times*, did not understand the story they were reporting on and did their readers a great disservice. I was not at the time ready to challenge my colleague, as I felt some facts were missing, but I knew they did not use Mother Nature's vitamin E and probably used some laboratory-produced form of vitamin E.

I found the original article written by Dr. Eric A. Klein, "Vitamin E and the Risk of Prostate Cancer: The Selenium and Vitamin E Cancer Prevention Trail (SELECT)," in the October 12, 2011, edition of the *Journal of the American Medical Association*.[168] The

---

[166] Calviello, G., et al., "Gamma-Tocopherol Quinone Induces Apoptosis in Cancer Cells via Caspase-9 Activation and Cytochrome *c* Release," *Carcinogenesis*, 2003, 24(3), 427–433, https://doi.org/10.1093/carcin/24.3.427.
[167] Ibid.
[168] Klein, E. A., et al., "Vitamin E and the Risk of Prostate Cancer: The Selenium and Vitamin E Cancer Prevention Trial (SELECT)," *JAMA*, 2011, 306(14), 1549–1556, https://doi.org/10.1001/jama.2011.1437.

study involved a total of 35,533 men in the United States, Canada, and Puerto Rico, in 427 centers, who were followed for 7 to 12 years.

The first thing I looked for: What was their definition of vitamin E, and what forms did they use? Remember, my very first paragraph in this chapter is on what is the definition of vitamin E. What molecules are we talking about? In this report, Dr. Klein noted that the vitamin E used was ***rac-alpha*-tocopheryl acetate**. This is not a natural product, but a laboratory-produced compound that to be utilized in the body must be broken down to produce alpha-tocopherol. This is only one of the vitamers produced by nature. It is never found alone, and it does **not** offer the same beneficial effects as when all eight molecules are working together.

After mentioning his definition of vitamin E once in the abstract and once in the body of the report, he never informed the reader of any other form of vitamin E. By the investigator's omission, he hid the fact he was not using Mother Nature's vitamin E. I do not feel that this was a report by ignorant researchers—the report was designed to mislead the public. The purpose of the report was to caution people not to take vitamins, and in this case, vitamin E. The conclusion of this report was written to be a sound bite: "Dietary supplementation with vitamin E significantly increased the risk of prostate cancer among healthy men."[169] Can you believe that 21 doctors coauthored and signed their names to this misinformation that leads to confusion and not clarity?

From this article, it is easy to see that even doctors can be fooled into toeing the party line and espousing information that is neither true nor correct. Remember, articles undergo peer review by experts in the field before publication for relevancy and accuracy. They either did not understand the article or were in on the ruse. Journals often demand clarification or a rewrite as a condition to publication.

---

[169] Ibid.

This is just one of many examples of why it is important to read the original article and evaluate it for yourself.

Lung Cancer

The report on prostate cancer was not the only piece of misleading information published. You have probably heard of this article that was originally reported in the prestigious *New England Journal of Medicine* in April 1994. The article is 30 years old and is still being quoted. It has been referred to many times, and I do not know of anybody who read the original article. In summary, the article had to do with a study that said adding vitamin E or beta-carotene to the diet of smokers did not reduce the incidence of lung cancer. In fact, the supplements may have been harmful.

This does not align with what I know about vitamin E, or any vitamin, for that matter. So I got a copy of the original paper, "The Effects of Vitamin E and Beta-Carotene on the Incidence of Lung Cancer and Other Cancers in Male Smokers."[170] Epidemiologic studies have shown that cancer rates are lower in people who take vitamins and eat fresh vegetables than in those who do not. To confirm this hypothesis, a study was developed called the Alpha-Tocopherol, Beta-Carotene Cancer Prevention Study. A study group of 29,133 male smokers aged 50 to 69 were divided into four groups and given the following:

- 50 mg of alpha-tocopherol
- 20 mg of beta-carotene
- 50 mg of alpha-tocopherol and 20 mg of beta-carotene
- Placebo (a pill that contained no vitamins)

The materials and methods are questionable from the outset. They used a synthetic vitamin E and not Mother Nature's blend of

---

[170] Alpha-Tocopherol, Beta-Carotene Cancer Prevention Study Group, "The Effects of Vitamin E and Beta Carotene on the Incidence of Lung Cancer and Other Cancers in Male Smokers," *New England Journal of Medicine*, 1994, *330*(15), 1029–1035.

eight vitamers. For vitamin E, the quantity may be correct, as you do not need much vitamin E—as little as 30 mg a day would be sufficient—but the molecules are the wrong ones. They did follow the US Pharmacopoeia, which in 1949 declared that all research should be done using the pharma-created vitamin E as the industry standard.[171] This is just one mistake after the other.

In the second arm of the study, using beta-carotene, it was shown that there were more cancers in the men taking beta-carotene than in those not using beta-carotene. This, they explained, may be due to selection bias, the inadequate duration of beta-carotene, the wrong dose, or inadequate interventions.[172]

If the men smoked and had a higher beta-carotene level, cancer was more likely than in a nonsmoker. This higher incidence of lung cancer was again noted in a 2005 French study involving adult females, and it was reported in the *Journal of the National Cancer Institute*.[173] The combination of beta-carotene and smoke may form a substance, as yet unidentified, that promotes cancer of the lung. This should not be taken as beta-carotene being bad for your health. This is not true. The risk of lung cancer is lowest in the nonsmoker group with the highest beta-carotene level. It is the product of smoke and beta-carotene that causes an increased incidence of lung cancer.

The lung cancer may have the ability to cut or cleave the beta-carotene in the wrong location. Normally, the beta-carotene is cut in half, producing two molecules of retinol, which is how vitamin A is formed. The cancer produces not two molecules of retinol, but some

---

[171] Robinson, M. D., and Miles, H., "Vitamin E Propaganda: More of the Same Old Thing," *A.C. Grace Company*, 2005, *4*(1), 3.
[172] Alpha-Tocopherol Beta Carotene Cancer Prevention Study Group, "The Effects of Vitamin E."
[173] Zielinski, S. L., "Press Release: Beta-Carotene Associated with Higher Risk of Tobacco-Related Cancers in Women Smokers but Not in Nonsmokers," *Journal of the National Cancer Institute*, 2005, *97*(18), 1315, https://doi.org/10.1093/jnci/dji335.

other product or products that are harmful to the healthy cell. It is interesting that beta-carotene is not harmful to normal tissue that is cancer free.

Back to our discussion of vitamin E. It is clear that the type of vitamin E, specifically what molecules we are talking about, must be defined. The public and the medical profession have been fooled too long about vitamin E. Shame on the doctors—they are the ones who studied organic chemistry in preparation for medical school and should have picked up on this.

Vitamin E Deficiency

Vitamin E deficiency is rare, but it can be potentiated by either **fat malabsorption syndrome** or a **genetic abnormality of the alpha-tocopherol transfer protein**. This deficiency leads to neurological symptoms such as loss of muscle coordination called ataxia, paresthesia-like tingling sensations, and loss of deep-tendon reflexes (i.e., no knee jerk when the patellar tendon is hit with a reflex hammer). This is because the large sensory neurons of the dorsal root ganglia are affected morphologically by vitamin E deficiency. The chemotherapy agent cisplatin produces the same effect in patients who receive it for the treatment of ovarian, lung, or prostate cancer, and it can be prevented if these patients are treated with vitamin E. Oncologists have been reluctant to provide vitamin E with chemotherapy, as they think it will make the treatment less effective. Recent studies have shown that this is not the case. In fact, the ability of the chemotherapeutic agents to promote apoptosis, or programmed cell death, is increased with the addition of vitamin E. Additionally, higher doses of chemotherapy can be given with fewer side effects.[174]

---

[174] Mustacich, D. J., "Vitamin E and Chemotherapy," *Linus Pauling Institute Research Newsletter*, Spring/Summer 2010, 8–9.

Vitamin E Supplements

Vitamin E is a fat-soluble antioxidant that can donate electrons, thus reducing oxidation. We do not take in much dietary vitamin E, but it can be rejuvenated by the water-soluble antioxidant vitamin C. Vitamin C will donate an electron pair to vitamin E, in effect renewing it.

Structure is important. I started this chapter with the structures of the molecules or vitamers of vitamin E. Though the structures are similar, they are still different. There is the double-ring aromatic portion, called the chromanol ring, which has hydrogen or methyl groups in the R1, R2, or R3 positions. This determines whether the structure is alpha, beta, gamma, or delta. The side chain is the fatty or aliphatic tail, called the phytol chain. It is significant in that the tocopherols consist of the carbon atoms with all four of the binding sites attached to two carbons and two hydrogens. Tocotrienols have six fewer hydrogen atoms in the chain, producing three double bonds located at the carbon numbers 3, 7, and 11. Having six fewer atoms in the chain means that the chain, or tail, is much more flexible or fluid and can get close in to and align with the fatty molecules of the cell wall. Tocotrienols become part of the cell wall and structure. In fact, it was thought until recently that tocotrienols were quickly consumed, as they were not found in the blood. Now, researchers are looking not only at the blood but also at the tissues and finding that the tocotrienols are very much involved with the fatty cell walls and the contents of the cells.

With the availability of tocotrienols in their pure form, new observations and new information are emerging. An example is the effect that tocotrienols have on reducing vascular plaque.

When I tell my patients to start taking vitamin E, I tell them to look for a formulation that includes all four vitamers. If the formulation contains only alpha-tocopherol, it will not yield any benefits. You want Mother Nature's form that contains alpha-, beta-, gamma-, and delta-tocopherol. Even better is a product that contains both tocopherol and tocotrienol. Recent research has shown that tocotrienols have excellent cancer-fighting abilities. The tocotrienols also have a tail or side chain that is not fully saturated. It is shorter and more flexible, allowing them to engage with other chemicals and cells.

Recommended Dietary Allowance (RDA) of Vitamin E

The current RDA for vitamin E is shown in the table below.

Recommended Dietary Allowance (RDA) for Vitamin E			
Life stage	Age	Intake	
		mg/day	Units (IU)/day
Infant	0–6 months	4	6
	7–12 months	5	7.5
Child	1–3 years	6	9
	4–8 years	7	10.5
	9–13 years	11	16.5
Adolescent	14–18 years	15	22.5
Adult	18 years and older	15	22.5

This was adjusted upward for adults in 2000 by the **Food and Nutrition Board** of the **Institute of Medicine**, from 8 mg per day for women and 10 mg per day for men to the current 15 mg per day.

The adult blood level of vitamin E reported by BioReference Laboratories is from 600 to 1,700 micrograms/deciliter (mcg/dL). This test does not explain whether it is measuring all forms of vitamin E or only the alpha form.

But where do the reference values for RDA for vitamin E come from? Why did the Institute of Medicine pick these levels of vitamin E for infants, children, and adults? In 1962, Horwitt performed studies in an attempt to show the depletion of vitamin E in humans.[175] He found that vitamin E levels fall only after months of a diet being deficient in vitamin E. Maintaining a measurable amount of vitamin E without symptoms requires only 10–30 mg of vitamin E daily. Some things would alter this requirement; for example, a diet rich in unsaturated fatty acids requires more vitamin E to keep the level up, whereas vitamin E is preserved if the diet is rich in antioxidants, selenium, amino acids that contain sulfur, and chromium compounds.

The Food and Nutrition Board was under the National Research Council in the 1960s, when in 1968, vitamin E was added to the list of recommended nutrients for the first time—30 international units (IU) for men and 25 IU for women.

Natural versus Synthetic Vitamin E

Initially, vitamin E from wheat was the most abundant source. This was also the source of vitamin E for the Shute brothers. They produced their own in the office, pressing wheat germ for oil, which they bottled and stored in the office refrigerator before dispensing

---

[175] Horwitt, M.K., "Status of Human Requirements for Vitamin E_1," *American Journal of Clinical Nutrition*, 1974, *27*, 1182–1193.

it to patients. They were aware of tocopherols and tocotrienols but focused on tocopherols, as these were readily found and measured in the blood. It appeared that tocotrienols were metabolized and were not found when performing blood analyses. The results of the treatment were pronounced and readily apparent—and much better than anyone else's. Commercially produced vitamin E was not as good as theirs, and theirs was certainly much better than synthetic alpha-tocopherol. Using no preservatives, additional chemicals, or excessive heat during processing, in my opinion, protected the tocotrienols from destruction.

Tocotrienols were ignored until they were biochemically found to be a strong antioxidant around and in the cell walls. Tocotrienol is an electron donor and can help repair the cell wall and protect the contents of cells from oxidation.

The vitamin E molecule of alpha-tocopherol is primarily a fat molecule with a hydroxyl (-OH) group on the head of the molecule or the chromanol ring. This hydroxyl (-OH) group determines that the **tocopher*ol*** is an alcohol, and it is designated in the name by the *–ol* suffix. Natural vitamin E can become oxidized. In common terms, it becomes rancid if not protected by a sealed container or refrigerated. Oxidized vitamin E is of no value health wise and smells bad. Natural vitamin E has a shelf life and must be stored at room temperature or lower, in a capped bottle that protects it from light.

Natural vitamin E is a thick, sticky, oily dark reddish-brown liquid that is usually sold in gel caps for oral administration. It is also sold in bottles as a liquid for oral and topical use. For convenience, it is available in pump dispensers.

Synthetic vitamin E capsules are much lighter in color and are not alcohols. There are two commonly found esters of vitamin E: **alpha-tocopher*yl* acetate** and **alpha-tocopher*yl* succinate**. The ester form of tocopherol has an *–yl* suffix, not an *–ol* suffix. Less commonly found esters are linoleate, palmitate, and nicotinate, which are typically used in cosmetics. Synthetic vitamin E is manufactured as an ester to avoid oxidation of the alpha-tocopherol. An ester is formed by the chemical combination of an alcohol and a carboxyl acid.

In plain English, synthetic vitamin E is not an alcohol, but an ester. The alcohol form is the active antioxidant protector. The acetate form is a yellow-amber oil and is usually sold in gel caps and as a liquid in bottles and pump dispensers. Alpha-tocopheryl succinate is a powder and usually the form used in the manufacture of tablets and capsules.

I recommend the tocopherols and tocotrienol of Mother Nature, not the synthetic forms. They can be taken as gel caps or liquid. For topical use, gel caps can be punctured or cut open to apply the oil directly to the skin to promote the healing of cuts, surgical incisions, and burns and to reduce the size of keloids.

Available Forms

Plastic surgeons use a product called **Scarguard** to reduce scar formation. Its composition is 12% silicone, 0.5% hydrocortisone, and an unstated amount of vitamin E that is listed as an inactive ingredient. If it is inactive, why put it in the mixture? It does reduce scar elevation and improves scar color and texture. Similar products come in gels and gel sheets. The silicone reduces the scar production, and the steroid reduces itching. If you wish, add vitamin E, or use a standalone vitamin E product.

The premier brand of vitamin E is **Unique E**, manufactured by A.C. Grace Company, founded by Roy Erickson, who himself had coronary disease. After Roy's doctor said that there was little they could do for him after his heart attack and subsequent heart failure, he went to Canada to seek the help of the Shute brothers. He learned about vitamin E from them and returned to Texas in 1962 to establish his company, which is devoted to producing all the natural vitamers of vitamin E. His health improved with Unique E, and he worked for another 43 years running A.C. Grace.[176]

Another producer of natural forms of Vitamin E is Life Extension, with their *Gamma E Tocopherol with Sesame Lignans*. This product contains all the vitamers of tocopherol—alpha, beta, gamma, and delta—plus lignans that Life Extension says boosts antioxidant levels.[177]

I advise my patients to read the fine print and look for the vitamer gamma when shopping for vitamin E. If only alpha-tocopherol is listed on the label, it is probably the inferior synthetic form. If both alpha- and gamma-tocopherol are listed, it is probably the better one. If it lists all four vitamers, it is a good product. Synthetic vitamin E is light yellow; the natural vitamin E is a dark reddish-brown color.

The Allergy Research Group produces tocotrienols from palm oil that contains the natural balance of alpha-, beta-, gamma-, and delta-tocotrienols in a product called Tocomin SupraBio Tocotrienols, available in 100 mg and 200 mg soft gels in either 60- or 120-count bottles. They produce this from virgin red palm oil using low-temperature distillation with high vacuum. They say that with this process, other beneficial substances from the red palm, such as squalene, phytosterols, carotenes, and coenzyme Q10, are also carried over into the product. The product is 100% non-GMO and is kosher.

Barrie Tan also offers an excellent tocotrienol product. In fact, he is the source supplier to many producers of this vitamin E preparation. The ingredient he sells, called **DeltaGold**, consists of 90% delta-tocotrienol and 10% gamma-tocotrienol. Look for it in any brand you buy. If you would like to buy his product, look for **EAnnato DeltaGold** in either 125 mg or 300 mg soft-gel caplets.

---

[176] Interview with the stepson of Roy Erickson, November 2012.
[177] *Life Extension*, April 2009, *15*(4), 20.

Solgar sells both d-alpha-tocopherol and d-alpha-tocopheryl succinate. Do not just pick up any bottle. Read the label to make sure you buy the one you want—the alpha, beta, gamma, and delta formula. Solgar sells both the natural and synthetic forms. The softgel capsules contain Mother Nature's mixtures. Other good brands are Twinlab and the Vitamin Shoppe.

If you are looking for the tocotrienols from the annatto plant, a good source is **Unique Tocotrienol** (tocopherol-free). Each gel cap contains 125 mg of 90% delta and 10% gamma. The Quantum Nutrition Labs product is Quantum Delta Tocotrienol; each 100 mg gel cap is 84% delta and 8% gamma. Advanced Bionutritionals produces Delta-Tocotrienols; each 250 mg gel cap is 90% delta and 10% gamma.

Most of these tocotrienol products are similar because they are based on DeltaGold from Barrie Tan's company, American River Nutrition. DeltaGold is produced from the annatto plant, which naturally produces less than 1% alpha-tocotrienol, 10% gamma-tocotrienol, and 90% delta-tocotrienol.

The Tocovid SupraBio 200 mg capsule formulation is produced from virgin crude palm oil. Palm oil has a natural distribution of alpha-tocotrienol of 32% (62 mg), gamma-tocotrienol of 56% (112 mg), and delta-tocotrienol of 13% (26 mg) for a total of 200 mg of tocotrienol. But it also produces 92 mg of alpha-tocopherol.[178]

---

[178] Tan, G. C. J., et al., "Tocotrienol-Rich Vitamin E Improves Diabetic Nephropathy and Persists 6–9 Months after Washout: A phase IIa Randomized Controlled Trial," *Therapeutic Advances in Endocrinology and Metabolism*, 2019, *10*, https://doi.org/10.1177/2042018819895462.

Vitamin K

Benefits of Vitamin K

- Promotes clotting of blood
- Reverses arterial calcification
- Prevents osteoporosis
- Reduces the risk of coronary heart disease
- Prevents liver cancer from viral hepatitis
- Increases cancer cell death of myeloma cells
- Facilitates anticoagulant control with warfarin
- Inhibits breast and endometrial cancer growth
- Protects bone from the destructive forces of steroids
- Protects arteries from calcification provoked by warfarin
- Preserves sensitivity to insulin in older men and women

History of Vitamin K

Vitamin K is a fat-soluble vitamin discovered in 1929 and found to play a significant role in the clotting of blood. The anticoagulant warfarin (Coumadin) can block its effect, as it inhibits the clotting of blood. Warfarin is helpful for people with peripheral vascular disease, coronary disease, and atrial fibrillation and to prevent or treat pulmonary embolism or phlebitis. Most people know little else about vitamin K, and many multivitamins do not include it. Vitamin K has multiple benefits beyond this simple function of clotting the blood.

Vitamin K was first described and isolated by Danish biochemist Henrik Dam. Dam was studying a disease in chickens that tended to bleed. When he examined blood, he found that the blood took longer than usual to clot. In 1929, he determined that this disease was caused by a lack of antihemorrhagic factor in the diet. Five years later, he showed that this factor was a fat-soluble molecule that he named vitamin K for the Danish word **koagulation** (coagulation). By 1939, Dam had isolated the pure form of vitamin K, which allowed more studies and the immediate clinical use of it in medicine. Vitamin K controls the production of not only prothrombin but also the clotting factors II, VII, IX, and X.[179]

Functions of Vitamin K

Since the initial work performed by Dam, studies of vitamin K have demonstrated that it affects bone health, both repair and the prevention of osteoporosis; prevents atherosclerosis; returns calcium of arterial plaque and hydroxyapatite to bone; and protects against some cancers. Studies have shown that the different molecular forms of vitamin K have different effects and that they do not overlap, except for the clotting effect.

Like many other vitamins, **vitamin K** refers to a group of molecules with a similar fundamental structure and some variation of the attached side chain rather than a single molecule. Because each molecule has unique physiological effects, molecules are designated **K_1**, **K_2**, and **K_3**.

Let us look at the chemical structure of K_1, K_2, and K_3. Not everyone has to know this, but I find it interesting. It is like knowing that water is made up of H_2O; sometimes understanding the

---

[179] "Vitamin K," *Encyclopedia Britannica*, last updated August 16, 2024, https://www.britannica.com/science/vitamin-K.

molecular structure imparts a deeper understanding. After looking at many molecular structures, patterns and similarities develop.

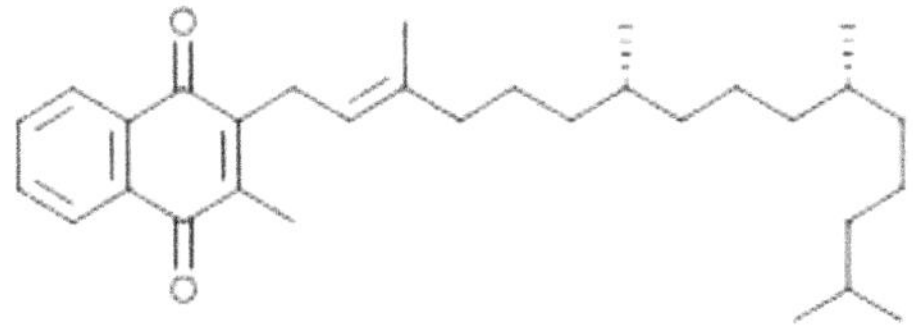

K_1, Phylloquinone

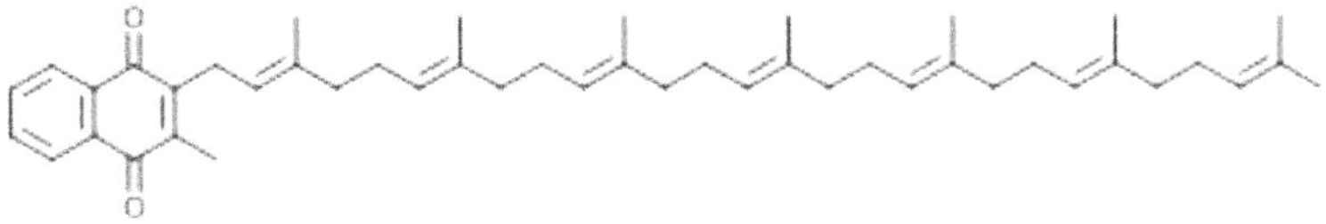

K_2, MK-7, Menaquinone

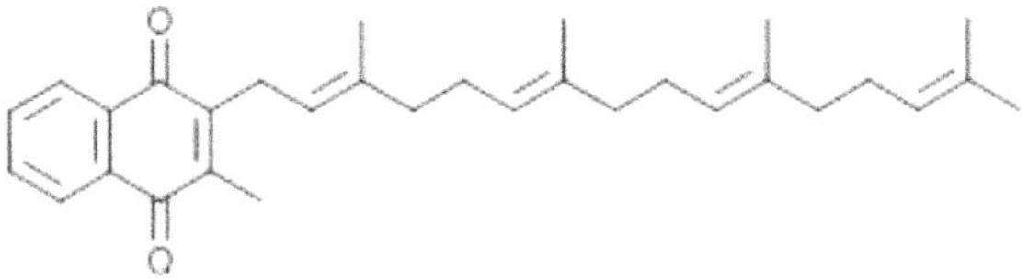

K_2, MK-4, Menatetrenone

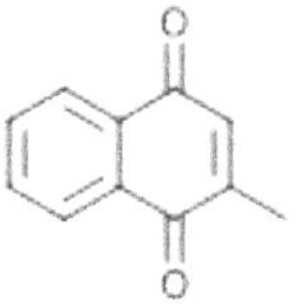

K_3, Menadione

The unifying body of the molecule in all the Ks is the **naphthoquinone** double-ringed structure, while the distinguishing feature is the side chain. K_1 has a simple short side chain of one **phytyl** unit. This is unique in that this is the only vitamin K produced by plants. K_1 is also called **phylloquinone (2-methyl-3-phytyl-1,4-naphthoquinone)** or **phytonadione**—three different names for the same molecule.[180] This can be confusing, but if you see any one of these names, we are talking about vitamin K_1.

---

[180] Goodman, L. S., and Gilman, A. (eds.), *The Pharmacological Basis of Therapeutics*, 4th edition, 2nd printing, Macmillan, 1972.

Vitamin K_1 is found in the chloroplasts of plants, the structures involved with photosynthesis. High levels are found in green leafy vegetables such as broccoli, cabbage, kale, lettuce, spinach, Swiss chard, turnip greens, brussels sprouts, and pistachios. This form is easily absorbed from food. Vitamin K_1 is also the only form prepared for medical intravenous use to correct prolonged bleeding problems, distributed under the name Aquamephyton.

Vitamin K_2 structurally has many forms; all the variations are in the one side chain. In fact, the length of the side chain defines the molecule. There is a repeating sequence of **prenyl** units, anywhere from two to nine units in a row. This gives rise to the nomenclature MK (*M* for **menaquinone** and K for vitamin K) and then a number that denotes the number of repeating units. **MK-7** is **menaquinone** with seven prenyl units and is a molecule in the vitamin K_2 group. Another important molecule in the vitamin K_2 group is **MK-4**, which has four prenyl repeating units in the side chain. This one is so unique that it also goes by the name of **menaquinone-4** or **menatetrenone**. The body can convert K_1, the plant form, to this specific K_2 form.

For many years, it was known that vitamin K_2 was produced in the bowel, primarily from gram-positive bacteria. New research has shown that soy natto and fermented cheeses are good sources of vitamin K_2 and that the benefits go beyond *koagulation*. The new benefits identified include preventing osteoporosis, preventing liver cancer, treating leukemia and myelodysplastic syndromes, lowering cholesterol, and balancing hormones.

Menadione is referred to as vitamin K_3, a synthetic form that has no side chains. It was once used in an injectable form to correct excessive bleeding from vitamin K deficiency. The practice was stopped because it caused liver and kidney toxicity, jaundice, and hemolytic anemia. It appears that K_3 interferes with the function of glutathione, a potent antioxidant, resulting in the oxidation and destruction of cell membranes.[181] The FDA has banned K_3 from nutritional supplements.[182]

Vitamin K and Blood Clotting

The only chemical function of vitamin K is to promote the carboxylation of glutamic acid. In simple English, this is the chemical reaction of adding carbon dioxide to glutamic acid. Glutamic acid is an amino acid. The final result is carboxyglutamic acid. This molecule has two acid side chains that are needed to bind the calcium needed for coagulation and to bind calcium to some proteins. Vitamin K is also needed for the liver to produce prothrombin and the other clotting factors, but it is not incorporated into the molecule of prothrombin.[183]

Warfarin

What I have just discussed about vitamin K is the main body of knowledge besides a warning to not eat green leafy vegetables when taking Coumadin (warfarin). This is the simple sound-bite warning about vitamin K. If this is what your doctor told you, get ready to expand your knowledge of this little-known vitamin. Eating spinach, kale, and broccoli rabe is not contraindicated with blood thinners; in fact, eating green leafy vegetables will make your prothrombin and INR clotting index much easier to control—besides giving you additional health benefits.

Instructing someone to avoid certain foods because they are on a particular medication is not good medicine when the data is there to support good nutrition. Good health comes from good nutrition.

---

[181] Higdon, J., et al., "Vitamin K," Linus Pauling Institute, Oregon State University, last updated May 2022, https://lpi.oregonstate.edu/mic/vitamins/vitamin-K.
[182] Pizzorno, L., "The Vitamin K Connection to Cardiovascular Health," *Longevity Medicine Review*, June 16, 2009.
[183] Ibid., Goodman & Gilman.

In most cases, drugs do not promote health but block something from happening. As doctors, we use drugs to try to tip the scale in one direction or another, to give the patient a physiological advantage. This is a short-term fix, but it does not correct the underlying problem. Recognizing and correcting nutritional deficiencies is a much better approach to diseases in that, generally, the normal physiology is enhanced.

The best example of this concept is the drug warfarin. It is used when patients have conditions of enhanced clotting, such as in atrial fibrillation and prolonged inactivity following orthopedic or abdominal surgery, and with diseases that develop vascular clotting, such as lupus, post heart attack, post stroke, and COVID-19. Telling someone to not eat a particular food group that is needed for more reasons than simply blood coagulation control is poor medical advice. As we will see, vitamin K is needed for bone health, the prevention of cancers, balancing the sex hormones, and the inhibition of the calcification deposited in the arteries.

Warfarin is used to inhibit the clotting of blood to decrease the complications of several medical conditions. Inhibition must be controlled in a very narrow window. Not enough warfarin and clotting will occur, causing a thrombus or clot to develop. A thrombus will impede or totally block the flow of blood at the site or dislodge and block the flow of blood at some other site downstream from the origin of the clot. Too much warfarin and bleeding will not stop.

Doctors use two tests to evaluate clotting when using warfarin: the **prothrombin level** and the **international normalized ratio (INR)**. These levels must be kept in a narrow window to avoid excessive clotting or bleeding. The job becomes more difficult if the patient's diet varies daily, introducing differing amounts of vitamin K into the system. Control is easier if the patient has a steady diet of green leafy vegetables or oral vitamin K on a daily basis. Adding as little as 150 mcg of vitamin K daily can **reduce the variability** in the response to warfarin.[184] A steady target is easier to hit than a moving target. Fewer complications occur and more benefits accrue, such as fewer fractures, less calcification in areas of inflammation, and less arterial calcification provoked by warfarin, and vitamin K prevents some cancers.[185]

Bone Health

Coagulation of blood is more a feature of vitamin K_1 than K_2, but both have this ability. Bone health is almost exclusively a feature of K_2, or more specifically of the MK-7 molecule. Some food groups such as fermented soybeans, known as natto, and fermented cheese have higher levels. Kaneki and colleagues in Japan measured the vitamin K levels in postmenopausal women with fractures and without fractures. The group with high MK-7 levels had fewer fractures compared to the group with low MK-7 levels. They found this most significant in comparing the women of Tokyo to the women of Hiroshima—the women of Tokyo ate far more natto than the women of Hiroshima. Incidentally, the women of Japan have far less osteoporosis and fractures compared to Western women who eat almost no natto. Fewer fractures, higher natto consumption, and higher MK-7 blood levels were found in Tokyo, with an MK-7 blood level of 5.26 nanograms per milliliter (ng/ml). In Hiroshima, the blood level of MK-7 was 1.22 ng/ml and only 0.37 ng/ml in British women.[186]

---

[184] Sconce, E., et al., "Vitamin K Supplementation Can Improve Stability of Anticoagulation for Patients with Unexplained Variability in Response to Warfarin," *Blood*, 2007, *109*(6), 2419–2423.

[185] Yoshida, T., et al., "Apoptosis Induction of Vitamin K_2 in Lung Carcinoma Cell Lines: The Possibility of Vitamin K_2 Therapy for Lung Cancer," *International Journal of Oncology*, 2003, *23*(3), 627–632.

[186] Kaneki, M., et al., "Japanese Fermented Soybean Food as the Major Determinant of the Large Geographic Difference in Circulating Levels of Vitamin K_2: Possible Implications for Hip Fracture Risk," *Nutrition*, 2001, *17*(4), 31–21, https://doi.org/10.1016/s0899-9007(00)00554-2.

In 1999, at Harvard Medical School, a prospective study showed that with a diet that is higher in vitamin K, fewer fractures occurred. A prospective study is a better quality of study in that better data collection is performed. The study group consisted of 72,327 women in the Nurses' Health Study. In the 10 years of monitoring, 270 hip fractures occurred from low to moderate trauma. Those women in the lowest quintile of vitamin K consumption (less than 109 mcg per day) had the most fractures.[187] The most common source of vitamin K in this study was lettuce.

Vitamin K_2 has been demonstrated to prevent bone loss and osteoporosis related to normal aging, in patients on kidney dialysis, and in patients with cirrhosis of the liver, with Parkinson's disease, and who were recovering from strokes.[188] Moreover, any drug that interferes with the normal recycling and function of vitamin K will affect fractures and osteoporosis. Warfarin prevents the recycling of vitamin K, lowers the amount of the vitamin in the body, and contributes to fractures. This was shown in the Framingham Heart Study, where the hip fracture rate in men went up as their vitamin K level went down.[189] Vitamin K deficiency is not limited to the ingestion of warfarin but can also be provoked by large doses of aspirin and cephalosporin antibiotics.[190]

This is a pretty good argument for the addition of vitamin K to the diet for someone on warfarin. It stabilizes the prothrombin level, making it easier to control; reduces fracture risk; and reduces the buildup of calcium in areas of inflammation. Patients treated with

---

[187] Feskanich, D., et al., "Vitamin K Intake and Hip Fractures in Women: A Prospective Study," *American Journal of Clinical Nutrition*, 1999, *69*(1), 74–79, https://doi.org/10.1093/ajcn/69.1.74.
[188] South, J., "Vitamin K2: More Than Just the 'Koagulation' Vitamin," *Vitamin Research News*, 2006, *20*(10),10–13.
[189] Barclay, L., "Vitamin K and Warfarin," *Life Extension*, June 2007, 59–63.
[190] Ibid., 63.

warfarin accumulate calcium in the arteries and damage valves at twice the rate of people who are not on it.[191]

Calcification

Soft tissue injuries, such as the bursa of joints, coronary arteries, heart valves that are damaged, and some sites of infection, are frequently areas of inflammation. Inflammation can lead to calcification. In the process of atherosclerosis of an artery, calcification of the plaque is stimulated by the inflammation of oxidized lipids.[192] The calcification then slows the inflammation and stabilizes the plaque. The amount of calcium is often "scored" or counted and used as an index of artery damage. Interestingly, these little areas of calcification in the arterial wall may develop into microscopic islands of bone structure.

Most of this calcium in arteries comes from bone; the calcium found in joints comes from bone, and the calcium of soft tissue injury comes from bone. All this misplaced calcium can be returned to the bone with the help of vitamin K_2. There is a relation here between arthrosclerosis and osteoporosis in that they both occur in the same person and with the same severity. In my opinion, osteoporosis is not a lack of calcium but a **loss of transporting factors**. Grandmother and granddaughter both eat the same meal together with the same amount of calcium, but the young girl has a more effective transport mechanism to carry calcium to the bone, whereas the older woman has a transport mechanism that is failing. A reversal of this failing mechanism can be achieved with the help of vitamin K_2.

---

[191] Schurgers, L. J., "Oral Anticoagulant Treatment: Friend or Foe in Cardiovascular Disease?" *Blood*, 2004, *104*(10), 3231–3232.
[192] Abedin, M., Tintut, Y., and Demer, L. L. "Vascular Calcification: Mechanisms and Clinical Ramifications," *Arteriosclerosis, Thrombosis, and Vascular Biology*, 2004, *24*(7), 1161–1170, https://doi.org/10.1161/01.atv.0000133194.94939.42.

Vitamin K_2 should be taken by someone on prednisone or cortisol, as it counteracts the bone-destroying effects of glucocorticoids.[193]

Transport of Calcium

Calcium is transported to bone with the help of progesterone, DHEA, vitamin D, and vitamin K. See my recommendation for Bone Health—a copy of my office brochure is included in the appendix. Each one of these compounds has multiple effects. Vitamin K_2 not only promotes transport of calcium to the bone but also influences osteoblasts and osteoclasts. Osteoblasts are the cells in bone that build new bone, and K_2 protects them from apoptosis. More blast cells mean more new bone or more repair of bone. This is in contrast to the effect of K_2 on the osteoclasts. These are the cells that destroy existing bone. K_2 increases the apoptosis of mature osteoclasts that become more numerous with age. Yet its benefits do not stop here. K_2 inhibits the production of inflammatory prostaglandin E_2 (PGE2), which works at the molecular level to dissolve bone.[194]

Cancer

Vitamin K_2 has beneficial effects on many cancers, including liver cancer, most lung cancers, prostate cancer, leukemia, and myelodysplastic syndromes. It is not a cure-all but something that can prevent or treat cancers without the negative effects of nausea, vomiting, weakness, and hair loss. The last thing someone with

---

[193] Yonemura, K., et al., "Protective Effects of Vitamins K_2 and D_3 on Prednisone-Induced Loss of Bone Mineral Density in the Lumbar Spine," *American Journal of Kidney Diseases*, 2004, *43*(1), 53–60, https://doi.org/10.1053/j.ajkd.2003.09.013.

[194] Hara, K., et al., "Menatetrenone Inhibits Bone Resorption Partly through Inhibition of PGE$_2$ Synthesis In Vitro," *Journal of Bone and Mineral Research*, 1993, *8*(5), 535–542, https://doi.org/10.1002/jbmr.5650080504.

cancer needs is a treatment that will make them sick, lose weight, and start describing their life in terms of good days and bad days.

I have not heard much of vitamin treatments for cancer by doctors in the United States, but a quick look at foreign literature yields many references. Most of these cancer preventions and treatments come from Europe and Japan. The most impressive vitamin is K_2. It was reported in 1994, by the Tokyo Medical University, that K_2 has the ability to treat various types of leukemic cells. Vitamin K_2 in the form of the menaquinones MK-3, MK-4, and MK-5 can help leukemic cells differentiate to the more normal adult cells.[195]

Cancers are essentially cells that in the course of development from the stem cell to the adult cell, such as a liver cell, white blood cell, or lung cell, stop their development and ignore the chemical signals sent to them. They begin to misbehave, grow large, consume most of the body's nutrients, and crowd out the normal cells, disrupting the orderly functions of the body. Sometimes, cancer cells resemble the adult cells, and sometimes they do not. Their normal development is, in a sense, arrested. Vitamin K_2 has the ability to coax these arrested cells into a more mature type of cell, to be more normal.

The ability to promote differentiation in cells is found with vitamin D as well. This ability to influence cells, to promote maturation and normalcy, leads me to think that these fat-soluble vitamins may be more hormone-like in nature than a vital amine. The effective concentrations are small, and the effects are large. Hormones enter a cell and affect the DNA, turning genes on or off, in this case, to a beneficial effect.

---

[195] Sakai, I., et al., "Novel Role of Vitamin K_2: A Potent Inducer of Differentiation of Various Human Myeloid Leukemia Cell Lines," *Biochemical and Biophysical Research Communications*, 1994, *205*(2), 305–310, https://doi.org/10.1006/bbrc.1994.2807.

Another benefit of vitamin K_2 is stimulating the death of abnormal cells without harming the normal cells. Besides influencing arrested cells to become adult cells, K_2 can promote the apoptosis of cancer cells.[196] **Apoptosis** is the built-in, preprogrammed spontaneous death of the cell. Normal cells in the body can undergo only so many cell divisions before they die. Vitamin K_2 has the effect of speeding up cell death by reducing the number of divisions for a cancer cell line.

In review, two effects of vitamin K_2 have been identified: maturation of arrested development and apoptosis. The reasons and the biochemistry behind this have not yet been identified with certainty. That will come with more research. The best part of treatment with vitamin K_2 is that there is nearly zero toxicity and no bone marrow suppression. It does not make you sick, and it will not stop you from making normal red and white blood cells.

The number of cancers affected by vitamin K_2 is impressive. Myeloma cells and B-cell lymphoma cells succumb to apoptosis from K_2.[197] Apoptosis appears to be induced by K_2 at the mitochondrial organelle of lung cancers: adenocarcinoma, small cell, large cell, and squamous cell carcinomas are affected.[198]

Viral Hepatitis and Liver Cancer

Viral hepatitis, both hepatitis C and hepatitis B, with cirrhosis of the liver predisposes someone to hepatocellular carcinoma, or liver cancer. Habu and his group at the Graduate School of Medicine in Osaka, Japan, set up a study to see the effects of vitamin K_2 on the development of this cancer from some incidental findings that were

---

[196] Miyazawa, K., et al., "Apoptosis/Differentiation-Inducing Effects of Vitamin K2 on HL-60 Cells: Dichotomous Nature of Vitamin K_2 in Leukemia Cells," *Leukemia*, 2001, *15*, 1111–1117.

[197] Tsujioka, T., et al., "The Mechanisms of Vitamin K_2-Induced Apoptosis of Myeloma Cells," *Haematologica*, 2006, *91*(5), 613–619.

[198] Yoshida, T., et al., "Apoptosis Induction of Vitamin K_2 in Lung Carcinoma Cell Lines: The Possibility of Vitamin K_2 Therapy for Lung Cancer," *International Journal of Oncology*, 2003, *23*(3), 627–632.

noticed in an earlier study with vitamin K_2 and its beneficial effects on osteoporosis.[199] The researchers noticed a drop in the development of liver cancer in women in the study.

In the new study, women with viral cirrhosis of the liver were given 45 mg per day of vitamin K_2, a usual, safe, and standard dose for osteoporosis in Japan.[200] The treatment group consisted of 21 women and the control group of 19 women. Most had hepatitis C, and one person in each group had hepatitis B. The study lasted eight years and yielded remarkable results. In the treatment group of 21 women, two developed cancer, whereas in the untreated group of 19 women, nine developed cancer. This converts to an odds ratio of 0.20—translation: If someone with viral hepatitis is treated with vitamin K_2, their risk of developing hepatocellular cancer is lowered by 80%.

Hormones

Sex hormones are kept in a youthful balance with vitamin K_2. Without this vitamin, testosterone is more rapidly converted to estrogen as we age, more so in men than in women. This promotes the accumulation of fat and enlargement of the prostate. K_2 inhibits the action of aromatase, the enzyme that is responsible for the conversion of testosterone to estrogen and that increases as we age.[201] K_2 preserves testosterone levels and may retard the aging process.

---

[199] Habu, D., et al., "Role of Vitamin K_2 in the Development of Hepatocellular Carcinoma in Women with Viral Cirrhosis of the Liver," *JAMA*, 2004, *292*(3), 358–361.

[200] Mizuta, T., et al., "The Effect of Menatetrenone, a Vitamin K_2 Analog, on Disease Recurrence and Survival in Patients with Hepatocellular Carcinoma after Curative Treatment: A Pilot Study," *Cancer*, 2006, *106*(4), 867–872.

[201] South, J., "Vitamin K2: More Than Just the 'Koagulation' Vitamin," *Vitamin Research News*, 2006, *20*(10), 10–13.

Insulin Sensitivity in Men

Insulin sensitivity for male diabetics in the 60- to 80-year-old range was serendipitously found to improve by researchers at the USDA Human Nutrition Research Center in Boston at Tufts University in a double-blind, controlled trial of vitamin K_1 designed for osteoporosis. Some effect for women was noted, but it was much less.[202]

Vitamin K Deficiency

The Food and Nutrition Board of the Institute of Medicine has established the adequate intake (AI) for vitamin K: 120 micrograms per day (mcg/day) for men and 90 mcg/day for women. Unfortunately, they do not provide guidance in terms of the amount of vitamin K_1 and K_2. For infants, AI is 2.0 to 2.5 mcg/day; children aged 1–13 years, 30–60 mcg/d; and adolescents aged 14–19 years, 75 mcg/day.

The best estimate of the daily needs of vitamin K was by Frick in 1967. He used starvation diets and antibiotics to deplete the body stores and then found the minimum amount of supplemental vitamin K to avoid the symptoms of vitamin K deficiency. The clinical signs of vitamin K deficiency are bruising, nosebleeds, blood in the urine, excessive bleeding from injury, and intracranial bleeding.

There are very few natural causes of vitamin K deficiency, and most cases occur in infants. The condition is known as **vitamin K deficiency bleeding (VKDB)** of the newborn, and it is divided into early and late forms. The early form affects infants from birth to two

---

[202] Yoshida, M., et al., "Effect of Vitamin K Supplementation on Insulin Resistance in Older Men and Women," *Diabetes Care*, 2008, *31*(11), 2092–2098, https://doi.org/10.2337%2Fdc08-1204.

weeks old. It was formerly called **hemorrhagic disease of the newborn**. The late form presents as an **intracerebral hemorrhage in infants** between the ages of two and twelve weeks of age that are breastfed. Both are treated with oral or injectable vitamin K. This has been the recommendation of the American Academy of Pediatrics (AA) since 1961. According to the most recent policy statement of the AAP, published in 2003, for the prevention of both the early and late VKDB, all newborns should be treated with vitamin K_1 as a single intramuscular dose of 0.5–1 mg.[203]

Very young infants less than two weeks old have little vitamin K available to them in either the diet or produced in intestinal bacteria. The vitamin does not easily pass into breast milk. Fortunately, not much of the vitamin is needed to maintain proper coagulation, as it is recycled and used many times to promote the production of prothrombin and bleeding factors.

Vitamin K Supplements

How safe is vitamin K? There is much evidence that both forms K_1 and K_2 are safe to what may seem high levels. Therapeutically, K_1 is given in a range of 0.5 to 1.0 mg for babies and up to 10 mg daily for adults, both intravenously and intramuscularly. K_2 has been used in many studies in the United States and Japan at 45 mg a day orally for two years, with the worst complaint being a slight rash that clears on discontinuance of the vitamin and no cases of increased coagulation.[204]

---

[203] American Academy of Pediatrics Committee on Fetus and Newborn, "Controversies Concerning Vitamin K and the Newborn," *Pediatrics*, 2003, *112*(1), 191–192.

[204] Asakura, H., et al., "Vitamin K Administration to Elderly Patients with Osteoporosis Induces No Hemostatic Activation, Even in Those with Suspected Vitamin K Deficiency," *Osteoporosis International*, 2001, *12*(12), 996–1000.

Vitamin K comes in tablets, gel caps, and liquids for oral ingestion. It can be found as K_1 or K_2, but the most common gel cap is a combination of 1,000 mcg of K_1, 1,000 mg of K_2 as menaquinone-4, and 100 mcg of K_2 as menaquinone-7 (MK-7). Vitamin K_1 is also available as Mephyton in a 5 mg scored tablet. Low-dose vitamin K_2 MK-7 is sold as a 45 mcg soft gel.

Topical vitamin K is used frequently to speed up the disappearance of bruising after plastic surgery. I often use it on the back of the hands and wrists on older patients who bruise easily and who hit their hands on doors and walls. It helps to speed recovery and reduces injury the next time by promoting good local bleeding control. Hopewell Pharmacy compounds vitamin K in a cream of K_1, K_2, K_3, or any combination of the Ks that I prefer in concentrations of 0.2%, 0.5%, and 1.0%.

Injectable vitamin K is often used to reverse coagulation and bleeding problems, subcutaneously or intravenously, if time permits, in the hospital setting. If immediate reversal is required in acute bleeding, vitamin K will not act fast enough, and doctors often resort to **fresh frozen plasma (FFP)** from blood donors to supply clotting factors that will work in an hour or two.

Vitamin K_3 is available to use in the intravenous form for the treatment of certain cancers.

Vitamin P

Benefits of Vitamin P

- Prevents allergies
- Enhances the effect of vitamin C
- Decreases capillary fragility
- Reduces varicose veins and hemorrhoids
- Reduces lymphedema
- Inhibits or slows the progression of cancers
- Controls asthma
- Reduces gout attacks
- Soothes insect bites

History of Vitamin P (Delisted)

Vitamin P was a designation for citrin, which was believed to affect the permeability of capillaries. Reduced permeability or leakage of fluid from the capillaries was observed by Stenz-Gyorgyi when natural sources of ascorbic acid, instead of laboratory-produced products, were used to treat scurvy. **Citrin** was isolated from lemons, originally called **hesperidin**, and thought to work independently from ascorbic acid, as it affected permeability. Hence, the **P** in vitamin P referred to permeability. Other substances such as **rutin** and **quercetin** had similar effects on permeability

Citrin, quercetin, and rutin all have the **flavone** molecule within their structures.

Citrin

Rutin

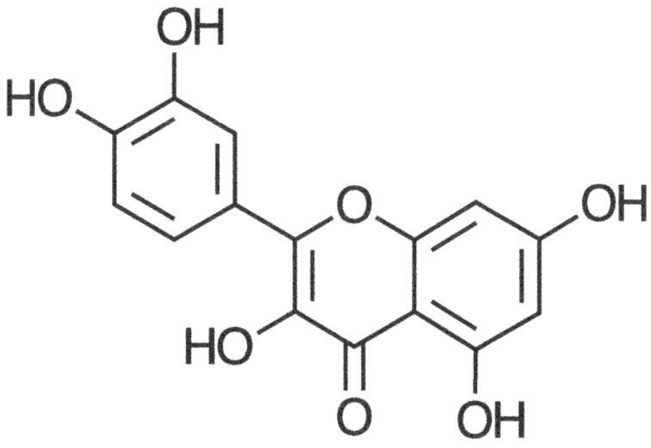

Quercetin

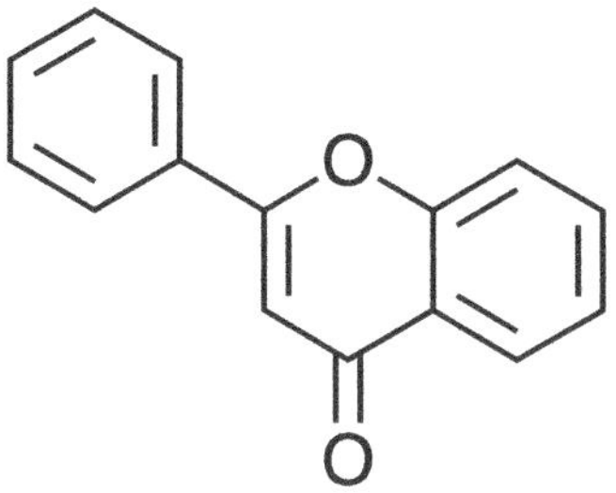

Flavone

Even though they affect the permeability of capillaries, their absence is not critical and they are not essential for life. Consequently, the **P vitamins have been delisted** because they are not "vital amines" and do not qualify as vitamins. Instead, they seem to potentiate the effects of vitamin C through oxidation-reduction reactions. In modern parlance, this is the antioxidant effect.

These are not vitamins, but they are related to each other through structure and their effects on oxidative systems. Because of this similarity, they are called flavone-like, or **flavonoids**. To add the meaning of "life" or "living things" to these plant-derived flavones they also are referred to as **bioflavonoids**. In the literature, the terms flavonoids and bioflavonoids are interchangeable.[205]

---

[205] Goodman, L. S., and Gilman, A. (eds.), *The Pharmacological Basis of Therapeutics*, 4th edition, Macmillan, 1971.

Bioflavonoids

Bioflavonoids are potent antioxidants, significantly more so than either vitamin C or E. Flavonoid and bioflavonoid are not the names of molecules but the names of the group of molecules that have the flavone backbone. An analogy would be fish is to trout as bioflavonoid is to quercetin. Bioflavonoids are found in soluble and insoluble pigments in fruits, leaves, and some nuts. Onions and apples are a good source of quercetin; rutin is found in buckwheat, black tea, and apple peels; and hesperidin is found in maritime pine bark and grape seed extract.

Vitamin C can be more effective with the addition of flavonoids because they prolong the effectiveness of the antioxidant effect of vitamin C, as they replenish the electron pairs in an equilibrium reaction favoring the reduced state of ascorbic acid. In this respect, they are referred to as **vitamin C sparing**. Often, vitamin C is prepared in combination with rutin, quercetin, or hesperidin and referred to as **vitamin C complex**.

Functions of Bioflavonoids

Rutin, quercetin, and hesperidin affect the permeability of blood vessels, stabilize cell membranes, lower cholesterol, are antithrombotic, contribute to the control of asthma, and have a significant effect on allergies.[206] The original and most significant effect bioflavonoids have is on the permeability of vessels and the loose, poorly defined term **capillary fragility**. Many conditions and diseases involve leaky blood vessels that contribute to morbidity. These include degenerative vascular diseases, allergic reactions,

---

[206] Holt, S., Wright, J. V., and Taylor, T. V., *Nutritional Factors for Syndrome X: A Wellness Guide*, Wellness Publishers, 2003, 96.

diabetes mellitus, macular degeneration, lymphedema, varicose veins, bleeding gums, and scurvy. Adding bioflavonoids to the diet decreases capillary bleeding and leaking. With vitamin C, bioflavonoids help repair collagen, strengthen tissue, and speed up wound healing.

Asthma and Allergies

The most remarkable effect of bioflavonoids I have seen is in controlling asthma and allergies. Quercetin is most effective in stabilizing the cell membrane of the mast cell. This is the cell that ruptures after allergic antigen-antibody complexes attack the cell membrane, releasing histamine that provokes most of the symptoms of allergies: runny nose, red injected sclera (white) of the eye (bloodshot eyes), swelling of the nasal passage, facial pain, and mucus production. For seasonal allergies, 500–1,000 mg of quercetin should be taken at least 15 minutes before venturing outdoors so that the allergic reaction is blocked and does not occur at all. Once the reaction has started and histamine is released into the mucus membranes, an antihistamine such as Benadryl (diphenhydramine) is more suitable to counteract the reaction. Antihistamines, however, have side effects such as drowsiness, dizziness, and impaired motor ability. We would like to avoid drugs as much as possible when a natural remedy is available. Bioflavonoids such as quercetin have virtually no ability to cause impairment even at 1,000–2,000 mg per dose.

I have treated asthma patients as young as nine months old on a continual basis with no problem. Bioflavonoids are not drugs but foods and come from diverse sources such as onions, apples, garlic, black tea, grapes, and the inner peel of citrus fruits. If breakthrough symptoms occur, additional doses can be given with no concern for toxicity or overdose. I have not found any drug interactions or side effects. In seasons when the pollen level is high, I usually start with 1,000 mg in the morning and add 500 mg if needed, usually because I am outdoors or going to the park. During the rest of the year, I usually take 500 mg once a day to benefit from the general anti-inflammatory and anticancer benefit.

Quercetin has been so effective for pollen allergies and asthma that most of my patients are on only this and vitamin C, B complex, and minerals to control the symptoms, and they experience no side effects. The longer this combination is taken, the more down regulation of the allergic response occurs and the less severe the symptoms if accidental exposure occurs.

Blood Vessels

Recently, quercetin and **epicatechin**, a bioflavonoid from green tea, were studied for their effects on blood vessels. Twelve men were given quercetin, epicatechin, epigallocatechin, or a placebo to determine whether these bioflavonoids have any effect on the endothelial function of blood vessels. Endothelial cells line the inside of blood vessels to keep the surface smooth, prevent clotting, and transmit substances to the muscular wall of the vessel to either contract to raise pressure and resistance or to relax the muscles, decreasing resistance and pressure in the artery. The production of **nitric oxide** by the endothelium causes the muscles to relax, dilating the vessel and lowering the resistance. A vasoconstrictor substance known as **endothelin-1 (ET-1)** also produced by the endothelium was measured.

Two of these substances, both bioflavonoids—quercetin and epicatechin—caused the endothelium to produce more nitric oxide for dilation of the blood vessels and reduced the production of endothelin-1, inhibiting constriction of the vessels. Both effects are considered beneficial to increase blood flow. The other two substances had no effect with constriction or dilation.[207]

---

[207] Loke, W. M., et al., "Pure Dietary Flavonoids Quercetin and (-)-Epicatechin Augment Nitric Acid Products and Reduce Endothelin-1 Acutely in Healthy Men," *American Journal of Clinical Nutrition*, 2008, *88*(4), 1018–1025, https://doi.org/10.1093/ajcn/88.4.1018.

Examples and Sources of Flavonoids

Other examples of flavonoids include the following:

- Procyanidolic oligomers, also called **proanthocyanidins**—pine bark and grape seeds
- **Anthocyanosides**—bilberry
- Polyphenols—**epigallocatechin-gallate (EGCG)** in green tea
- **Genistein**—antioxidants in soy that have effects similar to estrogen

There are thousands of colorful pigments in the plant world that are classified as flavonoids and antioxidants with no toxicity. They are best taken in a mixture to gain the best benefit. They prevent the breakdown of vitamin C, permitting lower doses to have a more lasting effect. Bioflavonoids are not stored in the body and are eliminated if they are not needed.

Eye health is supported with vitamin C and proanthocyanidins. Collagen and elastin in the eye are supported, as is capillary integrity, reducing capillary leakage in macular degeneration. Rutin from the citrus family can lower the intraocular pressure associated with glaucoma.

Citrus fruits such as oranges, lemons, grapefruits, limes, and tangerines contain a group of citrus bioflavonoids that includes citrin, which is also called **hesperidin**, and **naringin, naringenin,** and **eriocitrin**. This group of bioflavonoids reduces the permeability of capillaries, decreasing fluid leakage and swelling of the soft tissues, called edema. These are usually added to rutin, a flavonoid from buckwheat, to support healthy vessel function.

Two herbs that are not bioflavonoids but help with treating varicose veins are horse chestnut, which contains **escin**, and butcher's broom, which contains **ruscogenin**. Both these herbs are effective but should be used with caution with aspirin, anticoagulants, and antiplatelet drugs if you have either liver or kidney disease.

Silymarin is an extract from milk thistle, a member of the daisy family. The two major extracts are **silibinin** and **isosilybin B**. They support liver function with detoxification.

Food sources of bioflavonoids are oranges, lemons, grapefruits, cherries, plums, cabbage, grapes, tomatoes, broccoli, blackberries, cantaloupe, apricots, peppers, papaya, parsley, ginkgo, tea, wine, and dark chocolate. An optimal amount may be 900 mg per day.[208]

Vitamin P Supplements and Sources

Bioflavonoids are available in dry forms such as tablets and capsules and in some liquid preparations. Quercetin comes in 50 mg, 100 mg, 250 mg, and 500 mg tablets or capsules. Citrus bioflavonoids may be in a blend totaling 250–650 mg per tablet or capsule. Hesperidin and rutin also are found in the range of 200–600 mg per tablet or capsule. Polyphenols are found in green tea. To treat insect bites, mix powder with water to form a paste or use a damp tea bag.

---

[208] Null, G., *Get Healthy Now! A Complete Guide to Prevention, Treatment and Healthy Living*, Seven Stories Press, 1999.

Minerals

Boron

Benefits of Boron

- Slows the elevation of prostate-specific antigen (PSA)
- Protects bone from osteoporosis
- Reduces hot flashes
- Reduces the urinary loss of calcium and magnesium
- Improves mental alertness and cognition
- Reduces the symptoms of arthritis
- Maintains higher levels of estrogen and testosterone
- Improves hand-eye coordination
- Helps control the normal inflammatory response
- Lowers lipids
- Detoxes fluoride
- Mild diuretic

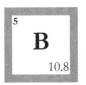

History of Boron

Boron is a metalloid (a nonmetal element) that influences such processes as bone development, inflammation, sex hormones, arthritis symptoms, and mental functioning and prevents the loss of minerals in the urine. It is listed as a trace mineral, as not much of it is found in the body or on earth. It has often been overlooked because of the focus on zinc, calcium, and magnesium. This little atom is found only in the more complete multimineral preparations.

The only time anyone has probably heard of boron is with the use of boric acid eyewashes. Some of your grandparents may have used this solution to treat eye irritation or infection. It is placed in an eye-wash cup, and then the head is tilted back and the eye opened. Beyond this, most people have not heard of boron.

Boron was first recognized in the salt form of borax by the Arabs, who called it *buraq*, and by the Persians, who called it *burah*.

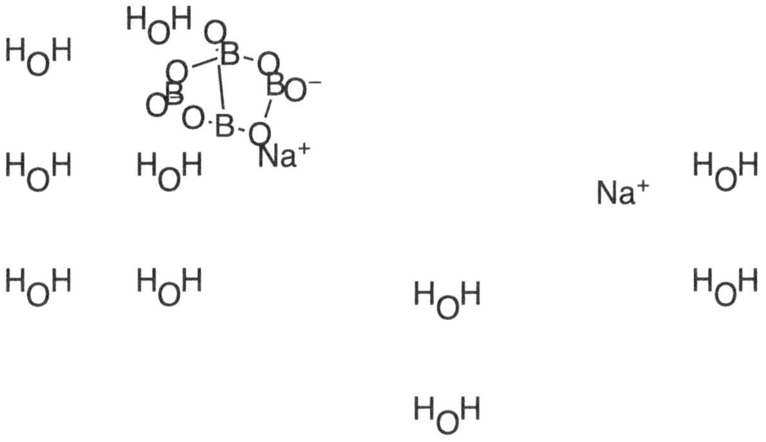

Borax

Borax ($H_{20}B_4Na_2O_{17}$) is associated with 10 molecules of water (H_2O). The basic form of this salt is sodium tetraborate ($B_4Na_2O_7$), depicted above, but it is hydroscopic (i.e., it attracts water) and is always in this form with the water. Hence, the structure is always depicted with 10 molecules of water around the borate.

Borax was first used as a cleaning agent because it emulsifies oil and grease. It is found in Tibet, China, Italy, and the United States.

$$HO-B(OH)-OH$$

Boric Acid

Boric acid was first discovered by W. Homberg in 1702. He reacted borax, a compound that contains boron and sulfuric acid, with heat to produce boric acid. The free element was first produced by Sir Humphry Davy in 1808, when he produced a brown precipitate of boron by passing an electrical current through borate solutions. He also produced it chemically by reducing boric acid with potassium. He coined the name boron for this new element. Confirming experiments in the same year by Joseph Louis Gay-Lussac and Louis Jacques Thénard showed that boron was a newly discovered element.[209]

$$H_2N-C(=O)-O-BH_2$$

Boron Glycinate

With an amino acid attached, boron has organic qualities. It is more easily absorbed and able to be utilized in the body much better than the inorganic forms.

The symbol for boron is **B**; its atomic number is 5 for five protons, five electrons; and its atomic weight is 10.811. It has two stable isotopes, 10 and 11, and three short-lived radioactive isotopes of less than one second, isotopes 8, 9, and 12. It is not found as a pure element but as a compound in the form of boric acid, borax, or borate and a mineral. Pure boron as a powder is black, but in mass form it is a dull metallic color. Because of the five electrons, bonding

---

[209] "Boron," *Encyclopedia Britannica*, last updated August 2024, https://www.britannica.com/science/boron-chemical-element.

to other elements and molecules is weak. Its physical properties derive more from how it fits into crystalline structures with other materials than its chemical bonding.

Uses of Boron

Modern uses of boron include in borosilicate glass, which has a low amount of thermal expansion, making it resistant to thermal shock. Two examples are Pyrex and Duran glass, which can go from hot to cold to hot without cracking if unevenly cooled or heated. The 200-inch mirror of the Mount Palomar telescope is made of Pyrex to limit distortion by thermal expansion and contraction. It is used as an additive to case harden steel, but it is too brittle to be used alone as a cutting edge or drill bit.

Boron is harder than carborundum and just below diamond in hardness (9.4 Mohs). It is used as a polishing agent and can withstand more heat than diamonds. It is used in high-strength fiberglass, semiconductors, and as a component of the very strong neodymium magnets ($Nd_2Fe_{14}B$). It is combined with ceramics used in tank armor. When combined with polymers, it gives added strength to bulletproof vests and can absorb nuclear energy to slow down reactions. Boron carbide is used in the nuclear field for shielding, control rods, and shutdown pellets. In March 2011, South Korea sent its reserve supply of boron, 310 tons, to Japan to help limit the nuclear reaction at the Fukushima Nuclear Power Plant.[210]

Boric acid was employed as an antiseptic and cleansing agent from the mid-1800s to the 1960s, when an unfortunate accident happened in a hospital. Until then, it was used by medical professionals in ointments, eye washes, and irrigating solutions. It

---

[210] "South Korea to Send Boron to Stabilize Japan Reactor," Reuters, March 16, 2011, https://www.reuters.com/article/world/south-korea-to-send-boron-to-stabilize-japan-reactor-idUSTRE72F0KG/.

could be found in many home medicine cabinets. Wong and his colleagues reported fatalities in a hospital nursery where boric acid was used in place of distilled water in infant formulas. Other reports appeared of illness or death from too much topical application of boron products, such as baby powder with boric acid and ointments, and the irrigation of closed cavities.[211]

Functions of Boron

Minerals, unlike vitamins, have an optimal range of daily intake and concentration in the body for the best effect. Boron is an essential mineral, and without it you die. With too much, you die. What we are trying to do is take the right amount for the healthiest outcome. There is no daily recommended intake of boron, as it is considered a trace element. For adults, the ideal range appears to be between 1 milligram (mg) and 10 mg of boron per day. The toxic level has been reported to be at and above 20 mg per day. Personally, I advise my patients, for bone health and as an anti-inflammatory, to take 2–4 mg of boron per day.

Even the plant world needs boron. If plants are deprived of boron, they first develop a condition called dry rot, then they die.

Sources of boron include fruits such as apples, pears, avocados, and grapes, vegetables, beans, almonds, peanuts, wine, and coffee. The bioavailable form of boron found in plants is called **calcium fructoborate**.[212] Boron is essential for the rapid cell growth of the fetus, and it protects bone growth in concert with vitamin D. It boosts sex hormone levels, supports the immune system, and is

---

[211] Goodman, L. S., and Gilman, A. (eds.), *The Pharmacological Basis of Therapeutics*, 4th edition, Macmillan, 1971, 1041.

[212] Scorei, R., Cimpoiasu, V. M., and Iordachescu, D., "In Vitro Evaluation of the Antioxidant Activity of Calcium Fructoborate," *Biological Trace Element Research*, 2005, *107*(2), 127–134, https://doi.org/10.1385/bter:107:2:127.

needed for a healthy nervous system. Men with prostate cancer have lower levels of boron in their diet than men without cancer. The food you eat influences your prostate. It is not known if the prostate protection is from the boron itself or its effects on the immune system or the level of testosterone. It is interesting that no molecular function has been identified for boron, and there are no known metabolites that contain boron, yet we know that it is required for cell division.[213]

Prostate Health

Good prostate health is something that can be fostered at home. This was pointed out by the Cancer and Epidemiology Training Program at the UCLA School of Public Health in 2001. They showed that dietary patterns predicted cancer when they compared 76 men with prostate cancer to 7,651 without prostate cancer. The men with prostate cancer had the lowest amount of boron in the diet, often from as little as one serving of fruit or less per day. The group in the upper quartile that had no cancer had the highest consumption of boron-rich foods, with a 64% reduction of prostate cancer. This upper group averaged 3.5 servings per day of boron-rich foods.[214]

Hormone Levels

The US Department of Agriculture studied boron and its effects on hormones. Twelve postmenopausal women were initially fed a diet that contained only 0.25 mg of boron for 119 days, and then their intake of boron was increased to 3 mg per day. The study showed that there was an increase of both testosterone and 17-beta-

---

[213] Cui, Y., et al., "Dietary Boron Intake and Prostate Cancer Risk," *Oncology Reports*, 2004, *11*(4), 887–892.
[214] Zhang, Z.-F., et al., "Boron Is Associated with Decreased Risk of Human Prostate Cancer," *FASEB Journal*, 2001, *15*, A1089.

estradiol.[215] Similar studies were performed on men, with similar results.[216] In effect, boron can raise hormone levels enough that if the level is low to begin with, the elevation will be felt as a positive effect. Taking boron may help alleviate vaginal dryness, hot flashes, and other symptoms associated with menopause. This is not limited to the sex hormones but also includes corticosteroids. People with rheumatoid arthritis who benefit from the use of prescription steroids will get the same benefit from boosting their own steroids with boron.

Kidney Stones

In this same study involving postmenopausal women, the researchers observed that boron supplementation reduced serum calcium concentration, and it reduced the urinary excretion of calcium and magnesium.[217] Further, boron reduced the urinary excretion of oxalate, which is significant because when excreted together, calcium and oxalate form kidney stones.[218] Taking boron is a good strategy to prevent calcium-oxalate kidney stones.

Bone Health

The function of vitamin D in promoting the transport of calcium into bone is enhanced by boron. This slows the

---

[215] Nielsen, F. H., et al., "Effect of Dietary Boron on Mineral, Estrogen, and Testosterone Metabolism in Postmenopausal Women," *FASEB Journal*, 1987, *1*(5), 394–397.
[216] Naghii, M. R., and Samman, S., "The Effect of Boron Supplementation on Its Urinary Excretion and Selected Cardiovascular Risk Factors in Healthy Male Subjects," *Biological Trace Element Research*, 1997, *56*, 273–286.
[217] Nielsen, F. H., et al., "Effect of Dietary Boron."
[218] Hunt, C. D., and Herbel, J. L., "Metabolic Responses of Postmenopausal Women to Supplemental Dietary Boron and Aluminum During Usual and Low Magnesium Intake: Boron, Calcium, and Magnesium Absorption and Retention and Blood Mineral Concentrations," *American Journal of Clinical Nutrition*, 1997, *65*(3), 803–813, http://dx.doi.org/10.1093/ajcn/65.3.803.

development of osteoporosis. This is just one more good reason to add boron to your list of supplements.

The World Health Organization (WHO) has studied the relationship of boron to osteoarthritis in a worldwide study and found that the more boron was found in the soil, the more boron was found in the local foods and the lower the incidence of osteoporosis in the local inhabitants. Jamaica, the country with the highest incidence of osteoarthritis, was found to have the poorest soil with the lowest concentration of boron.[219]

Boron inhibits inflammation by interrupting the cascade of mediators of inflammation: **cyclooxygenase (COX)** and **lipoxygenase (LOX)**. In areas where boron intake is less than 1 mg per day, the incidence of arthritis is estimated at 20–70%. The incidence of arthritis drops to 10% or less where the intake of boron is in the 3–10 mg per day range.[220]

The benefit of boron to bone works via many direct and indirect routes. The more direct effect is that it becomes part of the mineral crystallization that gives bone its rigid structure. When listening to current supplement sales pitches for calcium, one might get the impression that this is the only mineral required for strong bones. The fact is that many minerals participate with calcium in creating a strong mineral matrix. Other minerals, such as magnesium, boron, and strontium, are needed. This is akin to increasing the strength of iron with other metals to make it harder, stronger, and less able to fracture or crack. Adding differently sized atoms with different bonding characteristics improves cross bonding; it yields a more complex, and more durable, crystal structure.

---

[219] Bentwich, Z., et al., *The Art of Getting Well: Boron and Arthritis*, Foundation for the Eradication of Rheumatoid Disease, 1994.

[220] Traver, R. L., Rennie, G. C., and Newnham, R. E., "Boron and Arthritis: The Result of a Double-Blind Pilot Study," *Journal of Nutritional & Environmental Medicine*, 1990, *1*(2), 127–132, http://dx.doi.org/10.3109/13590849009003147.

Besides minerals, hormones and vitamins are required to help transport the minerals to the bone. I recommend to my patients that hormones are needed to direct the minerals to the bone and facilitate their journey. This is easy when you are young and Mother Nature and Father Time are on your side, but when you are older, help from supplemented hormones is needed. My formula for bone health includes DHEA and progesterone.

Vitamins that promote a good bone matrix are vitamins C, D_3, and K. Interestingly, for bone health, I do not recommend anyone take calcium. This may seem odd, but let me explain. You already ingest enough calcium in the food you eat and the water you drink. All foods that come from the ground contain calcium. Most water, including tap and spring water such as Poland Spring, contains about 100 mg of calcium per quart. Hard water from an artesian well such as Fuji Water contains 17 mg/liter of calcium, whereas a very hard mineral spring water such as San Pellegrino contains 208 mg/liter of calcium.[221] Many foods in the common American diet contain calcium: broccoli 90 mg/cup, whole wheat bread 30 mg/slice, white bread 73 mg/slice, ice cream 168 mg/cup, cheddar cheese 306 mg/1.5 ounces, and sardines 324 mg/3 ounces.[222] Normal eating will place most people above the 1,000 mg adequate intake (AI) recommended for adults for calcium.

Clearly, good bone health is not solely dependent on calcium intake but also on the supporting vitamins, hormones, and minerals such as zinc, magnesium, strontium, and boron. Calcium is the major mineral in bone, but much support is added by these minor players that are needed to create a strong amalgam with calcium.

---

[221] Mascha, M., *Fine Waters*, Quirk Books, 2006.
[222] http://www.nichd.nih.gov/milk/prob/other_foods.cfm, June 16, 2012; http://www.niams.nil.gov/health_info/bone/bone_health/nutrition/, June 16, 2012.

Mental Acuity

Mental alertness increases with boron. This was shown by both a randomized, double-blind, placebo-controlled study and by changes in an **electroencephalogram (EEG)**. Schauss designed a study with a group of students that tracked energy, the ability to stay focused, and alertness. This study lasted three months and had two arms: one group was treated with a placebo and the other with 3 mg of boron. The clinical findings were concurrent with the use of boron 92% of the time.[223]

Mental alertness was demonstrated to be lower with lower levels of boron and to increase with boron supplementation. Brain wave activity increased on the EEG in areas associated with alertness with additional boron.[224]

Cholesterol

This may be early information for humans, but studies have been performed on rats where boron compounds have lowered LDL, the bad cholesterol; raised HDL, the good cholesterol; and lowered triglycerides.[225] The complete study for humans has not yet been performed with boron but is worth doing.

---

[223] Schauss, A. G., "Boron: Higher Doses Necessary for Cognitive, Bone and Joint Health," *Vitamin Research News*, 2007, *21*(9), 12–15.

[224] Newnham, R. E., "Essentiality of Boron for Healthy Bones and Joints," *Environmental Health Perspectives*, 1994, *102*(Suppl. 7), 83–85, https://doi.org/10.1289/ehp.94102s783.

[225] Hall, I. H., et al., "The Effect of Boron Hypolipidemic Agents of LDL and HDL Receptor Binding and Related Enzyme Activities of Rat Hepatocytes, Aorta Cells and Human Fibroblasts," *Research Communications in Chemical Pathology and Pharmacology*, 1989, *65*(3), 297–317.

Topical Uses

Boron can be used to treat mold, candida, and yeast infections. It works well as a topical agent for athlete's foot. The best preparation is to make a paste with borax powder and water, and apply that to the foot and between the toes for a few minutes for two or three days. This will generally clear the infection in two weeks.

My patient, Ted, was not diabetic, but he was the athletic type, frequenting gyms, in and out of locker rooms, walking barefoot in many public spaces. He came to me with a yeast infection of one of his toes. This resembled the typical thickened nail with an exuberant growth of yeast on and in the nail. In most practices, this would be handled with a referral to a podiatrist and surgical removal of the nail. I recommended that he start by applying a paste of borax and water to the nail for a few days. This was followed by a daily spray of a saturated solution of borax in water and letting it air dry a few minutes before putting on his socks and shoes.

The first thing Ted noticed was that the local pain and irritation was relieved. Three weeks after starting this process, much to his surprise, while drying his foot with a towel, the mantel of yeast on the upper surface of the nail fell off with gentle action and with no pain whatsoever. A very thin and soft nail remained, preserving the nail bed. Over the course of four months, a healthy and perfectly normal nail grew back in. Ted was happy to avoid surgery. Now his gym bag contains a spray bottle of borax solution to avoid future yeast infections.

Boron Poisoning

There is much confusion about the use of boron or boric acid in current health recommendations. The acid itself if not very acetic and is on par with the neutrality of water. It seems that toxicity is caused by how much boron is absorbed or ingested. The average person does not have much exposure to boron, except through supplements, or to boric acid, and there is little risk of toxicity if directions are followed.

Boric acid is weak, but the word **acid** implies danger, like in the case of hydrochloric or sulfuric acid. But, in fact, boric acid is so weak that it will not turn litmus paper—paper impregnated with a dye that changes color when it comes into contact with acid—red. In fact, as an example for comparison, it is weaker than carbonic acid. If you place a glass of water on a table open to the air, in an hour or two it will absorb carbon dioxide from the air, and the water and carbon dioxide will chemically combine to form a weak acid: carbonic acid. The water will no longer be neutral, between an acid and a base, but will be slightly acidic. You can drink the water after pausing for a long conversation and never taste the change. As is the case with carbon dioxide, boric acid is weaker than carbonic acid because of the weak bonding of boron to hydrogen. It is not the acidity of boric acid that can be dangerous but rather the absorption of boron itself that gives it its toxicity.

The first symptoms of boron poisoning are nausea, vomiting, and diarrhea, progressing to a fall in body temperature, a red rash similar to scarlet fever, peeling of the skin and mucous membranes, and progressing to kidney and heart failure and death within five days. Lethal doses usually are 15–20 g (15,000–20,000 mg) for adults and 5–6 g (5,000–6,000 mg) for infants.[226] These lethal doses are high compared to therapeutic doses of 1–4 mg per day.

---

[226] Goodman and Gilman, *The Pharmacological Basis of Therapeutics*, 1041.

Nevertheless, because of incidents such as the fatalities in the hospital nursery, where boric acid was used instead of distilled water in infant formulas, boron use was curtailed and advisories issued despite it being essential to life. The new recommendations advised that boric acid be colored with a dye to distinguish it from water, that it should no longer be used as an irrigating solution, and that it should be labeled as poison.[227]

Is Taking Boron Safe?

After hearing these stories and descriptions of boric acid, most people are confused. Is it necessary for life? Can it hurt you? Is a substance that is essential for life a poison? The answer is yes, yes, and yes.

All substances have a concentration relative to human health. First, if it is essential, a minimum amount is necessary to sustain life. Second, there is an optimal range that is just right to provide the amount where the body thrives at the best rate of metabolism without wasting materials or energy. And third, there is a level where too much is toxic and can cause damage or death.

Let us look again at the lethal doses of boron for adults. Reported death from boron can occur from ingesting 15–20 grams (g). Watch the units here. That is 15,000–20,000 milligrams (mg) of boron. The usual therapeutic adult dose is 2–4 mg, with some protocols calling for 10 mg per day. The toxic dose is 1,500 times a heavy dose and 3,750 to 7,500 times the usual therapeutic dose. This element has a good safety margin between the therapeutic dose and the toxic dose.

All supplements are sold in the therapeutic range and are safe. I just wanted to review this with you so that you understand the concept of **essential** or **minimal intake**, **optimal intake**, and **toxic**

---

[227] Ibid.

amounts. I have no doubt that that when you discuss vitamins and minerals with your friends, they will question you on what safe amounts are. Good health is all about balance.

The intake of less than 0.3 mg of boron per day showed decreased brain EEG activity and symptoms similar to lead toxicity and protein-calorie malnutrition. This is compared to subjects who took 3.25 mg of boron per day. The latter group had better hand-eye coordination, manual dexterity, attention, perception, and short- and long-term memory.[228]

Boron is now being appreciated as a major player in health maintenance. More people are beginning to understand the benefits attributed to boron: the improvement in joint and bone health, cognitive improvement, the reduction in inflammation, and the conservation of calcium and magnesium. Prostate cancer can be avoided by having sufficient boron in the diet. I recommend that you check your supplements for boron, and if it is missing, add about 2 mg per day, minimum.

Boron Supplements

Boron comes in many forms. The three that have the most bioavailability are **boric acid**, **borax (the salt form)**, and the chelated form called **boron glycinate**. Glycine is an amino acid that is bound to the boron and that makes it much more absorbable. This is the new modern delivery preparation that does not cause stomach or intestinal irritation and has no complaints of diarrhea or constipation.

---

[228] Penland, J. G., "The Importance of Boron Nutrition for Brain and Psychological Function," *Biological Trace Element Research*, 1998, *66*, 299–317.

Boric acid comes as a powder or already in solution to be used as a contact lens cleaner. The contact lens cleaner made by Bausch and Lomb is a boric acid solution. Boric acid is used for vaginal yeast, candida, or mold infections, sold as a powder in a capsule or in a coco butter suppository for vaginal insertion. The usual dose of boric acid for capsules or suppository form is 600 mg used twice a day.

Borax is the salt taken from the earth. Most know it as 20 Mule Team Borax from Death Valley, California. It is not a detergent; it is a salt, referred to as a "**laundry booster.**" It helps dissolve oil in water because the molecule has a strong bonding to water. The borax box states, right on the side panel, that it is not to be placed in the eye or ingested. This is related to the incident in the nursery in the 1960s that I spoke of earlier. I would not put the salt in the eye, as the gritty power may scratch the cornea. Use either a dissolved solution of borax or the boric acid solution that is time tested. You can drink borax at the proper concentration. The salt can be taken directly from the box and dissolved in water.

Borax has a strong affinity for water, the salt picking up water, caking, and clumping. This does not affect the product. Break up the clumps with a spoon or the bottom of a glass prior to measuring out the powder. For a stronger concentration, add a quarter (¼) teaspoon of borax to one quart of pure water and drink it throughout the day. This delivers 110 mg of boron per day. For a weaker concentration, dissolve an eighth (⅛) of a teaspoon dissolved in one quart of pure water and drink it throughout the day. This delivers 55 mg of boron per day. I strongly suggest that you use the boron glycinate capsules that are safe and premeasured as cited below.

My experience is that at the higher concentration there may be a hint of a soapy taste. The lower concentration does not have a soapy taste. The drink can be taken five days a week; take two days off a week to permit any excess to be eliminated. The borax is slow to dissolve in the water, but within 15 to 20 minutes, the cloudy solution will be clear and ready to dilute to a full quart. Some prefer to warm the water to accelerate the process, but I find this unnecessary.

Boron glycinate is the combination of boron and glycine, an amino acid, that makes a very soluble molecule, readily absorbable with no stomach upset or irritation. The usual capsule size is 2 mg, and one to three capsules can be taken each day. Consider boron glycinate as an organic form and all the others above as inorganic forms. The organic form enters the body so much more easily that all of it is absorbed.

Other forms include **boron citrate**, which has no ill effects, and **boron aspartate**, which I do not recommend. Anything attached to aspartate may promote seizures and brain tumors.

Calcium

Benefits of Calcium

- Required for muscle contractions
- Essential for nerve conduction of electrical impulses
- Required for bone strength and rigidity
- Essential for blood clotting and to control bleeding
- Major buffering system for the chemistry of the body

History of Calcium

Calcium is an element with the symbol of **Ca**, an atomic number of 20, and an atomic weight of 40.08. The atom has a $^+2$ charge or valence. The Romans used lime since the first century and called it *calx*. It is considered a metallic element and is the fifth most abundant element on earth. It was not identified as an element until 1808, when both Davy and the team of Berzelius and Pontin produced it by the method of electrolysis. It is never found in an elemental state; usually, it is found as a compound of limestone ($CaCO_3$), gypsum ($CaSO_4 \cdot 2H_2O$), fluorite (CaF_2), or apatite, which is a fluorophosphate or chlorophosphite of calcium.[229]

---

[229] Hodgman, C. D., et al., *Handbook of Chemistry and Physics*, 44th edition, Chemical Rubber Company, 1962.

Functions of Calcium

Calcium is the most abundant mineral in the body. The body contains two to three pounds of calcium, with 99% of it in the bones and teeth. The remaining 1% is found in the fluids, tissues, and blood. It is required to give structural rigidity and strength to bones, but it is also needed for the transmission of nerve impulses, blood clotting, and enzyme function. The concentration of calcium is under the hormonal control of the **parathyroid hormone (PTH)**, which raises the blood level of calcium, and **calcitonin**, which is produced in the thyroid and lowers the blood level of calcium. Vitamin D promotes the intestinal absorption of calcium and the deposition of calcium into the bones. Magnesium (Mg) and phosphorus (P) both maintain a relation to calcium. The normal calcium to magnesium ratio is 2:1, and the normal calcium to phosphorus ratio is 1–2:1.

Sources of Calcium

Common food sources of calcium are dairy products: cheese, yogurt, calcium-fortified orange juice, winter squash, sardines, salmon, almonds,[230] beans, lentils, and leafy greens. Calcium is found in any food that is grown in the ground. It is so plentiful that between the food and water you consume, you ingest 1.5 g of calcium per day. Spring water may have a calcium content as low as 21 mg/L, whereas tap water may have a calcium content as high as 208 mg/L or higher.[231]

---

[230] Harvard T.H. Chan School of Public Health, "Calcium," last updated March 2023, https://nutritionsource.hsph.harvard.edu/calcium/.

[231] Morr, S., et al., "How Much Calcium Is in Your Drinking Water? A Survey of Calcium Concentrations in Bottled and Tap Water and Their Significance for Medical Treatment and Drug Administration," *Musculoskeletal Journal of Hospital for Special Surgery (HSS Journal)*, 2006, 2(2), 130–135, https://doi.org/10.1007%2Fs11420-006-9000-9.

Forms of Calcium

Calcium for consumption is a salt, such as calcium chloride. Larger molecules, such as calcium carbonate and calcium citrate, are also used.

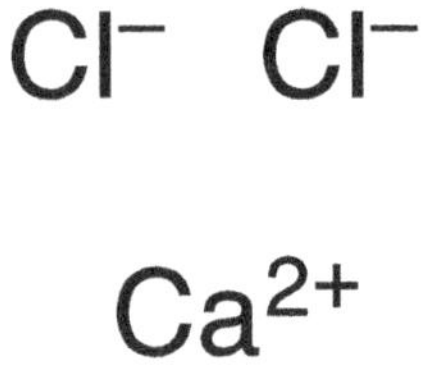

$$Cl^- \quad Cl^-$$

$$Ca^{2+}$$

Calcium Chloride

Calcium chloride has two chloride atoms for each calcium atom and is used in both oral and intravenous preparations.

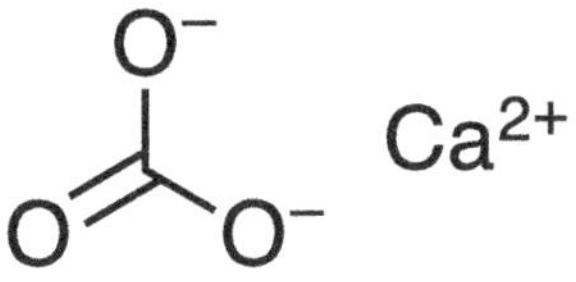

Calcium Carbonate

Calcium carbonate is the active ingredient in Tums that is used to balance stomach acid.

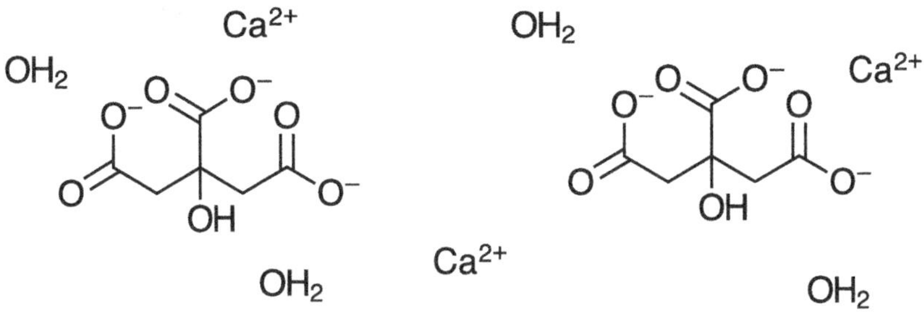

Calcium Citrate

In **calcium citrate**, with the chemical name calcium citrate tribasic tetrahydrate ($C_{12}H_{10}Ca_3O_4 \cdot 4H_2O$), three calcium atoms are balanced with two citrate bases. This molecule is a hydrate because it is hydroscopic, attracting four molecules of water.

Forms of Calcium in the Blood

Doctors generally refer to the three different forms of calcium in the blood as **ionized calcium, protein-bound calcium**, and **total calcium**. These terms do not refer to calcium in the bone.

$$Ca^{2+}$$

Ionic Calcium

Ionized calcium is what is dissolved and free in the blood. Protein-bound calcium is calcium in the blood that is bound to a protein, namely albumin. Total calcium is the ionized calcium plus the protein-bound calcium, which generally occurs in a 50:50 ratio. The total calcium is what is measured through lab analysis. The reference range is 8.6–10.4 mg/dL.[232]

Contraction and Relaxation of Muscles

Calcium is necessary for the contraction and relaxation of all types of muscles, of which there are three: **striated muscle** that is attached to bones for body movement, **smooth muscle** that is within the walls of the intestines and that provides parasitotic motion, and **cardiac muscle** that propels blood through the vascular system. Energy and calcium are required to elongate the filaments of **myosin** and **actin**, making the muscle longer before the next contraction. The contraction is initiated by a nerve impulse, permitting the filaments of myosin and actin to come together, interdigitating with force using the energy that was provided in the relaxation phase. Energy from the mitochondria and calcium will restore the muscle to the higher-energy relaxed level, ready for the next contraction.

---

[232] BioReference Laboratories, February 6, 2021.

Sufficient calcium is required to reset the muscle for the next contraction or the muscle stays in contraction. This is a painful condition called **spasm**. The normal range for blood calcium, simply called calcium, is narrow (8.6–10.4 mg/dL). It is kept in check with the help of the parathyroid hormone and calcitonin, while vitamin D assures that enough is absorbed from the intestines and it is properly distributed in the bones.

Blood Clotting

The coagulation system requires calcium to initiate the clotting mechanism. A series of molecules participate in the clotting of blood, of which calcium is an integral part. The first group is called the **intrinsic factors** because they are found in the blood; the **extrinsic factors** are found in the tissues of the blood vessels and supporting tissues. Both groups of factors use the **common pathway** to complete the clot.

Hypocalcemia and Hypercalcemia

Hypocalcemia refers to low levels of calcium in the blood. I have seen only one case of true hypocalcemia in my career in a woman named Molly, who had two parathyroid glands removed for hypercalcemia. Normally, there are four glands, two on the right and two on the left, above and below the wings of the thyroid gland. Unfortunately, she was not checked for the presence of four parathyroid glands prior to surgery and had her only two glands removed. She spent most of her day in and out of **tetany** (physiological calcium imbalance), which is characterized by muscle spasm in the hands, feet, arms, and legs. It was poorly remedied by taking Tums (calcium carbonate tablets) four to six times a day.

Hypercalcemia, or elevated calcium, is a much more common condition that causes abdominal pain, constipation, depression, fatigue, slowness of thought, sleepiness, and coma. The most common cause is not an overactive parathyroid gland but metastatic lesions of cancer to the bone, which dissolves the bone, liberating the calcium into the blood and causing hypercalcemia, provoking the symptoms. Other, less frequent causes are dehydration, kidney disease, and magnesium or phosphorus imbalances.

Recommended Dietary Allowance (RDA) of Calcium

The RDA of calcium, according to the Food and Nutritional Board of the Institute of Medicine, is set out in the table below by stage of life, age, and sex.

Recommended Dietary Allowance (RDA) for Calcium			
Life stage	Age	Male (mg/day)	Female (mg/day)
Infant	0–6 months	200	200
	6–12 months	260	260
Child	1–3 years	700	700
	4–8 years	1,000	1,000
	9–13 years	1,300	1,300
Adolescent	14–18 years	1,300	1,300

Adult	19–50 years	1,000	1,000
	51–70 years	1,000	1,200
	> 70 years	1,200	1,200
Pregnant	14–18 years	–	1,300
	19–50 years	–	1,000
Breastfeeding	14–18 years	–	1,300
	19–50 years	–	1,000

Calcium and Aging

There is much advice today to take calcium, but is this a wise thing to do? Experts suggest taking at least 1 g of calcium per day for strong bones to avoid osteoporosis. I do not see the evidence for it. In fact, the opposite is easy to see. Calcium intake is about 1.5 g per day from the food you eat and the water you drink. Any plant that grows in the soil has calcium; some plants have more than others. The only water that lacks calcium is distilled or reverse osmosis water. All others have calcium.

Calcium is found in all the wrong places the older you get. It is found in kidney stones and gallstones because of an imbalance with potassium or magnesium. This is obvious, and most patients and doctors do not attempt to figure it out or to take supplements to reverse the process. It is found in cholesterol deposits in the arteries in your heart, in the aorta, and even in veins. Calcium is found in your joint spaces, from your knees to smaller joints such as the shoulder and finger joints. It deposits along tendons, such as in a heel spur, which can be very painful, or in the cartilage between the ribs and breastbone, affecting the flexibility of the ribcage needed for breathing. It will deposit in soft tissue, such as the spleen, lung, and liver. Tumors may have deposits of calcium. The most carefully examined tissue is breast tissue—radiologists examine mammograms with a magnifying lens, looking for spicules of calcium that often deposit in breast tumors.

Most enzymes require a mineral such as magnesium or zinc as a cofactor to help them function. But with age and lack of energy, zinc or magnesium may be displaced by calcium. Even too much calcium from supplements can displace the other minerals. If zinc or magnesium is displaced by calcium, the enzyme is essentially turned off. This is aging. Do you still want to take calcium?

Restoring Bone Health

Supplementing with calcium promotes aging. Enzyme systems fail; joints become stiff, with pain and limited motion; arterial plaques become fixed obstructions to blood flow; and tissues harden.

The objective in treating osteoporosis is to stop calcium from leaving the bones and to promote the deposit of calcium into the bone structure. The clue lies in looking at youth. Grandmother and granddaughter may eat the same diet, but the physiologies of the granddaughter and grandmother handle calcium differently. The granddaughter may be in her teens, an anabolic stage of growing, assimilating all minerals, vitamins, and hormones, in a period when all systems are functioning, promoting growth. And this is often done without supplementing with calcium. Both are eating the same amount of calcium, but the younger woman has the advantage of being able to absorb vitamins, hormones are in abundance, and calcium and the supporting minerals are easily absorbed. The usual diet supplies 1.5 g of calcium daily from the food you eat and the water you drink. Unfortunately, the ability to absorb and transport calcium to the bones fails because of decreasing intestinal absorption, falling hormone levels, insufficient vitamins, and lack of supporting minerals.

Several things can be done to improve bone health and reverse osteoporosis. The approach to improving osteoporosis is improving vitamin levels, supplementing hormone levels, and providing minerals that contribute to a strong calcium crystal structure. The hormones required for producing strong bones are **progesterone, vitamin K, vitamin D**, and **dehydroepiandrosterone (DHEA)**. Yes, the fat-soluble vitamins are hormones—there are receptors on cells for these vitamins to direct the development and function of cells. They are directors, not cofactors of reactions.

Progesterone and DHEA are both steroid sexual hormones derived from cholesterol. These hormones not only have a stimulating effect on sexual structure and function but also affect the body's ability to thrive. They affect all tissues in the body for growth and function. They are involved in the absorption of calcium in the intestines, the transport of calcium in the blood, and the delivery of calcium to the bones. Vitamin D is produced by ultraviolet light shining on cholesterol under the skin, breaking one bond of the cholesterol molecule. That new molecule is called vitamin D. Said another way, vitamin D does not come from the sun—the energy to break the bond in cholesterol to produce vitamin D comes from the sun.

These hormones support the movement of calcium in the right direction from the intestines, preventing abnormal deposits of calcium in soft tissues and joint spaces and facilitating the transport of calcium to the bone for deposit. In a young woman, all these hormones work together to produce strong bones. In an older woman, the absorption of calcium might be impaired because vitamin K is not absorbed in the intestines, insufficient sunlight impairs the conversion of cholesterol to vitamin D, and menopause marks the end of the period of childbearing ability and lower production of progesterone and DHEA. The hormones necessary to support bone growth and maintenance begin to fade. It is not the lack of calcium that causes osteoporosis but the failing hormone support system, of which osteoporosis is only a symptom.

To produce strong bones, calcium is needed, but so are the supporting minerals. Crystal structures of calcium deposited on the protein skeleton of bone give little strength and rigidity. The flaky white deposits around a leaky water faucet are calcium. It is not strong and does not form a tough, durable solid. It crumbles, and by itself is not a great building product. It needs the support of other metals to form a firm crystal structure on the protein of the skeleton. When examining healthy bone, there is much calcium, but a significant number of other metals can be found, such as magnesium, zinc, copper, and manganese. But although they are discussed less often, strontium and boron are also present. Adding these minerals to the crystal structure of calcium supports the framework of the crystal lattice, like adding crossmembers to the structure, improving strength and rigidity. The additional minerals of strontium and boron should be added to any bone supplement. People usually take zinc and copper, or even magnesium for other reasons, not even thinking that they are needed for healthy bones. Manganese may be included in a multimineral, but it is rarely associated with bone strength.

Adding minerals to calcium creates an amalgam, a product that is stronger than calcium by itself. Similar to making steel, adding chromium to iron produces a product that is stronger and less brittle than iron.

Calcium receives more attention when it comes to bone because there is so much of it compared to the other metals. Also, it is the metal responsible for bones being visible on X-rays, so it gets all the attention by lighting up the bones. It steals the show. The other metals cannot be seen, and their value is not appreciated on simple observation.

Available Bone Health Formula

Calcium alone cannot prevent osteoporosis or prevent fractures; the supporting minerals are required to support calcium, and the vitamins and hormones bring the calcium to the bones. In formulating my bone health treatment, I did not add calcium to avoid aging. Most treatments for osteoporosis include calcium or are exclusively calcium and magnesium mixtures.

I started using my formula that I call **Bone Health** in my practice after 2000 (I wrote a patient information handout sheet in 2008, included in the appendix) as an alternative to drugs that were promoted by Big Pharma and prescribed by doctors to prevent osteoporosis. Boniva (ibandronate) and Fosamax (alendronate sodium) are in a class of drugs called bisphosphonates. Unfortunately, these drugs have significant side effects, such as heartburn, nausea, diarrhea, constipation, and spontaneous hip fractures. Fractures are what this class of drugs were supposed to prevent. It was further noted by an oral surgeon, Michael Erlichman, of Little Falls, New Jersey, in 2006, that bisphosphonates cause osteonecrosis of the jawbone (dying of the jawbone, with the teeth falling out), for which there is no known repair process.[233] It would take at least three years before this condition became apparent after the drug was started and deposited in the bone. It does not wash out easily and continues its destruction for years.

---

[233] Silverman, E., "Bone-Builders Linked to Bone-Rotting Side Effect," *Star Ledger*, June 13, 2006, 51.

I have patients who undergo **bone density scans** and **DEXA** studies to monitor or evaluate the development of osteoporosis. I do not recommend them, as I feel that osteoporosis and the dwindles are the opposite of growth and thriving. It is all part of the natural life cycle. Nevertheless, if a patient asks for the test, I will oblige and order the test. This became a learning point.

For my patients who took my Bone Health formula, the DEXA scans showed an improvement in bone density in one year's time. When the patients pointed out to the radiologist that the bone density improved, the most common remark by the radiologist was that the first scan may have been wrong. Never once did anyone ask, "What are you doing?"

Florence is an 82-year-old patient of mine with severe osteoarthritis of the hip. The pain was so bad that she elected to have a hip replacement to control the pain. Three years prior to the operation, I had placed her on my Bone Health formula for osteoporosis. I just started referring to an orthopedic surgeon because he complemented the general anesthesia for surgery with a nerve block to the leg to control pain post operatively. This nerve block lasted for three or four weeks, enough that the patient could begin physical therapy, with full range of motion the first day after surgery. This avoids frozen joints and blood clots and preserves muscle.

After the surgery, I encountered him in the hallway as we were going to the recovery room to see Florence. I did not ask him, but he volunteered this comment. He said that she had a significant amount of arthritis around the hip joint, but when he got to the bone, it was of good quality and much stronger than he usually sees in an 82-year-old.

Calcium Supplements

Calcium carbonate is found in Tums antacids at 750 mg per tablet. It neutralizes stomach acid on contact and is a good source of calcium. Calcium citrate is a mild cathartic and is used to support calcium levels with low doses. It comes in liquid, tablets, and capsules. Pure Encapsulations provides 300 mg of calcium in capsule form, Puritan's Pride offers 1,000 mg of calcium as a calcium citrate capsule, and NOW Foods provides 600 mg of calcium from citrate.

Copper

Benefits of Copper

- Prevents anemia
- Curtails the loss of weight
- Treats neuropathy
- Supports immune function
- Essential to produce collagen
- Promotes the absorption of iron
- Necessary for mitochondria to convert sugar to energy

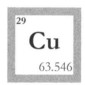

History of Copper

Copper has been known since prehistoric times, in both the elemental and the salt forms. The name *cuprum* is from Latin. The Roman supply is reported to have been largely from the island of Cyprus. It has been mined for at least 5,000 years.

Copper is a pinkish-red solid with a bright metallic luster. It is malleable, ductile, and a good conductor of heat and electricity. The chemical symbol for copper is **Cu**, and its atomic number is 29. It has an atomic weight of 63.546 and two stable isotopes, 63 and 65.

Copper is often used in alloys. **Brass** is an alloy of copper and zinc, and **bronze** is an alloy of copper and tin. Both zinc and tin increase the hardness of copper. Copper is also added to gold to create **rose gold**, giving the gold a more reddish color.

The most important copper compounds are oxides and sulfates. **Blue vitriol** is copper sulfate used as a fungicide and an algicide in water purification.

Functions of Copper

Copper is an essential element that has many functions. Many of the deficiencies of copper overlap with the deficiencies of other minerals and vitamins, so one must be knowledgeable about copper deficiency to differentiate problems related to a deficiency in copper from those related to other nutrients. Blood and tissue testing is necessary to identify a copper deficiency.

The body cannot produce copper, making it an essential element—it must be obtained from the diet. The total body content of copper is in the range of 100–120 mg. The suggested daily intake is 900 micrograms (mcg) per day, and copper is eliminated by the bile into the stool and through the urine.

Copper is necessary as an essential cofactor for four metabolic functions:

- Energy production from glucose
- Iron metabolism to avoid anemia
- The construction of collagen with cross binding of the fibrils
- The production of neurotransmitters to prevent neurodegenerative diseases

Energy production is promoted in the mitochondria by **cytochrome c oxidase enzyme** to produce the energy-rich molecule of **adenosine triphosphate (ATP)**. Cytochrome c enzyme is a copper-containing metalloenzyme needed for the final production of ATP. It helps shuttle electrons and is mostly found in the mitochondria.

Supplements of copper are **copper gluconate ($C_{12}H_{22}CuO_{14}$)**; **copper sulfate ($CuSO_4$)**, which was historically referred to in chemistry as blue vitriol; **copper glycinate ($C_4H_8CuN_2O_4$)**; and **copper citrate ($C_6H_8O_7Cu$)**. Copper glycinate is the most organic form of the metal and the easiest to absorb.

Copper Gluconate, $C_{12}H_{22}CuO_{14}$

Copper Sulfate, $CuSO_4$

Copper Glycinate, $C_4H_8CuN_2O_4$

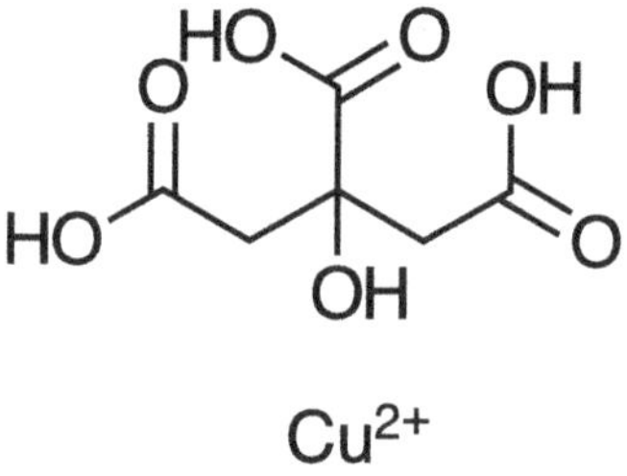

Copper Citrate, $C_6H_8O_7Cu$

Copper deficiency can produce fatigue that originates in the mitochondria. In addition, connective tissue structure will lose its strength; skin will wrinkle and sag; iron metabolism will be interfered with, promoting iron deficiency anemia; and neurological problems involving structure and function can result. Causes of copper deficiency include **insufficiency in the diet** or **poor absorption** at the intestines from prolonged diarrhea, celiac disease, malabsorption syndromes, and intestinal surgery for weight loss. Excessive zinc ingestion can cause the **increased elimination** of copper.

Production of Energy

Copper is necessary at the cellular level to produce energy in the mitochondria. The process does not require much, but without the copper-dependent enzyme *cytochrome c oxidase*, the packets of energy, or the ATP, will not be produced.[234]

Metabolism of Iron

Ingested iron is absorbed in the intestines and initially accumulated in the liver. Copper-containing enzymes are necessary to liberate the iron from the liver. If copper is not present, the iron will not be delivered to the bone marrow to be incorporated into

---

[234] Olivares, M., and Uauy, R., "Copper as an Essential Nutrient," *American Journal of Clinical Nutrition*, 1996, *63*(5), 791S-796S, https://doi.org/10.1093/ajcn/63.5.791.

new red blood cells. Copper deficiency will present as iron deficiency anemia. It is imperative to measure copper levels if iron deficiency anemia is not responsive to iron replacement. In copper deficiency, the blood smear will look like iron deficiency with microcytic, hypochromic red blood cells: small cells with less hemoglobin. It will not respond to additional iron, as there is plenty in the liver. Measuring the copper level will reveal the problem, and treating it with copper will correct the anemia, producing normocytic, normochromic cells. Keep in mind that we are talking about iron deficiency that is not related to bleeding, malnutrition, or cancer. Any time an unexplained iron deficiency anemia fails to respond to iron supplements, it might be helpful to test copper levels.

Neutropenia

A similar reduction in white cells called **neutropenia** occurs with depressed copper levels.[235] The chemical and genetic reason is not fully known at this time, but low copper levels are thought to delay proper development of progenitor cells into mature neutrophils, a type of white cell needed to fight infections. It is correctable with copper.

Construction of Collagen

Collagen is a unique protein that is connective tissue. It makes up 30–35% of the protein in the body. It is a substance that gives the body shape, form, strength, and resilience. Collagen is what makes up ligaments, tendons, connective tissue, and skin, and it gives form and shape to the eyeball. **Lysyl oxidase** is another copper-containing enzyme required for the cross-linking of fibrils of

---

[235] Lazarchick, J., "Update on Anemia and Neutropenia in Copper Deficiency," *Current Opinion in Hematology*, 2021, *19*(1), 58–60, https://doi.org/10.1097/moh.0b013e32834da9d2.

collagen or elastin. Copper enzymes give strength and maintain the form of the structures.

Collagen is made up of repeating sequences of amino acids: lysine—proline—X—glycine—lysine—proline—X—glycine—lysine—proline—X—glycine—and so on. In this sequence, X represents other random amino acids that give some variation to collagens that are slightly different and fulfil different functions. Molecules can be produced in a linear structure, as is found in ligaments and tendons, or the molecule can be folded to function like a glue that holds cells together in an organ. Copper does not become incorporated into the molecules of collagen, but like vitamin C, it is necessary for the assembly of the molecule.

Many people take collagen to improve the appearance and resilience of the skin. Unfortunately, these products contain little or no vitamin C. Without vitamin C, the amino acid building blocks will not be assembled into the appropriate structures or intercellular adhesives known as **ground substance**. Copper has a similar function to collagen as vitamin C.

Copper Deficiency

Copper deficiency is relatively rare, but it does occur in some people and under certain circumstances.

Copper Deficiency Caused by Medical Conditions and Treatments

Copper deficiency can occur in low-weight premature infants, in infants and children with prolonged diarrhea, in people with bowel diseases such as Crohn's disease or celiac disease, and in people who have undergone bowel resection where too much of the bowel was removed due to inflammation or cancer. It is also found in people on prolonged parenteral tube feeding, but new formulas contain trace amounts of copper to avoid copper deficiency.

Excessive Zinc Intake

Excessive zinc intake can block the absorption of copper at the intestinal level. This can be overcome by adding a little extra copper when taking zinc. To prevent copper deficiency, many formulators of supplements blend the two elements in a 15:1 ratio of zinc to copper.[236] If you are buying individual products, take 15 mg of zinc to 1 mg of copper, 30 mg of zinc to 2 mg of copper, or 60 mg of zinc to 4 mg of copper. The usual daily dosage of zinc is 30 mg and copper 2 mg. Zinc is now used to prevent and treat COVID infections, and that dose is usually 60 mg of zinc and 4 mg of copper.

Genetic Causes

Copper deficiency can have a genetic basis, but this is extremely rare. Causes in this category can be related to damage to the **ATP7A gene** and to diseases such as **Menkes disease, occipital horn disease**, and **Wilson's disease**.

ATP7A Gene

In very rare cases, copper deficiency is related to the **ATP7A gene**, the transporting ATPase enzyme that facilitates the intracellular transport of copper at the intestinal level, to vascular endothelial cells, and across the blood-brain barrier. Damage to the ATP7A gene results in systemic copper deficiency and accumulation of copper at the blood-brain barrier, with copper deficiency in the brain. The copper cannot traverse the blood-brain barrier, which can result in central nervous system demyelination and brain shrinkage, myelopathy or injury to the spinal cord, peripheral neuropathy (i.e.,

---

[236] Guo, C. H., and Wang, C. L., "Effects of Zinc Supplementation on Plasma Copper/Zinc Ratios, Oxidative Stress, and Immunological Status in Hemodialysis Patients," *International Journal of Medical Sciences*, 2013, *10*(1), 79–89, https://doi.org/10.7150%2Fijms.5291.

poor functioning of the nerves in the extremities), and optic nerve damage.

Menkes Disease and Occipital Horn Disease

Menkes disease and **occipital horn disease** present with low copper levels. Menkes disease presents with seizures, subdural hemorrhage, connective tissue disorders, and kinky hair. Occipital horn syndrome presents with muscle and connective tissue weakness and protrusions or bumps on the occipital bone.[237] Both diseases are treated with copper-histidine injections and must be treated early to be effective. Early infant screening of copper levels is necessary to detect Menkes disease so that treatment can be prescribed.

Wilson's Disease

Wilson's disease presents with too much copper in the tissues. This genetic childhood disease must be detected and treated early to avoid depositing too much copper in the tissues, which causes an early fatal end if it is not treated. The treatment consists of removing the excess copper by chelation. **Chelation** is a process whereby a chemical (in this case, penicillamine) is used to remove metals from the body. A large molecule surrounds the atom of copper, capturing it, preventing it from entering into other reactions, and transporting it to the kidneys for excretion. The usual dosage of penicillamine is 1 g orally per day in divided doses.

Wilson's disease is usually tested for during infant evaluations by testing for copper in the urine or serum. Alternative testing is to test the copper-protein complex **ceruloplasmin** or observe the **Kayser-Fleischer rings** at the border of the cornea and sclera. It is considered a childhood disease, but symptoms of hepatitis or

---

[237] Kodama, H., Fujisawa, C., and Bhadhprasit, W., "Inherited Copper Transport Disorder: Biochemical Mechanism, Diagnosis, and Treatment," *Current Drug Metabolism*, 2012, *13*(3), 237–250, https://doi.org/10.2174%2F138920012799320455.

neurological or psychiatric symptoms with elevated liver transaminase enzymes can occur between the ages of 5 and 50.

Biliary Cirrhosis and Cholestatic Conditions

Two other diseases that accumulate copper are biliary cirrhosis and cholestatic conditions. Ceruloplasmin binds to both copper and iron. The free atoms of copper and iron are potent catalysts of free-radical damage. Ceruloplasmin will bind to copper, preventing this oxidative damage. Ceruloplasmin facilitates the attachment of iron to its transport protein, transferrin, again avoiding oxidative damage.[238]

---

[238] Thackeray, E. W., et al., "Hepatic Iron Overload or Cirrhosis May Occur in Acquired Copper Deficiency and Is Likely Mediated by Hypoceruloplasminemia," *Journal of Clinical Gastroenterology*, 2011, *45*(2), 153–158, https://doi.org/10.1097/mcg.0b013e3181dc25f7.

Recommended Dietary Allowances for Copper

The recommended dietary allowances (RDA) for copper are displayed in the table that follows.[239]

Recommended Dietary Allowance (RDA) for Copper			
Life stage	Age	Male (mcg/day)	Female (mcg/day)
Infant	0–12 months	200	200
Child	1–3 years	340	340
	4–8 years	440	440
	9–13 years	700	700
Adolescent	14–18 years	890	890
Adult	19 years and older	900	900
Pregnant	All ages	–	1,000
Breastfeeding	All ages	–	1,300

---

[239] Food and Nutrition Board, Institute of Medicine, "Copper," National Academy Press, 2001, 224–257.

Food Sources of Copper

Copper is found in trace amounts in most foods, but it is most plentiful in liver, oysters, crabmeat, and cashews. The Food and Nutrition Board of the National Institutes of Health (NIH) has calculated the copper content in one serving size of common foods. It is presented below to give you a reference for food selection if you are trying to increase your intake of copper.

Food Sources of Copper		
Food	Serving size	Copper content (mcg)
Beef liver	1 oz.	4,128
Oysters	6 medium	2,397
Crabmeat	3 oz.	1,005
Clams	3 oz.	585
Cashews	1 oz.	622
Sunflower seeds	1 oz.	519
Almonds	1 oz.	292
Lentils	1 cup	497
Shredded wheat cereal	2 biscuits	167
Semisweet chocolate	1 oz.	198

Copper Toxicity

Acute copper poisoning has been caused by contaminated beverages stored in copper containers and by tainted water supplies, but these are rare events. Medications and supplements that contain copper have rarely resulted in acute poisoning. The symptoms of excess copper ingestion—nausea, vomiting, abdominal pain, and diarrhea—probably limit additional ingestion and absorption.

Chronic copper poisoning is also uncommon from high doses because the excessive ingestion may cause immediate symptoms. Long-term exposure to doses above therapeutic amounts may provoke more serious problems such as liver failure, kidney failure, coma, and death without provoking the symptoms of acute poisoning. The US Food and Nutrition Board has set the **tolerable upper intake level (UL) at 10 mg per day**, as no liver damage has been reported at this dosage. **Therapeutic dosages of 1–4 mg per day** are well below this limit. Your doctor can order copper blood testing to monitor your levels. Two tests are available: **serum copper levels** to measure the amount of copper in the liquid portion of the blood and **RBC copper**, which is a measure of copper in the red blood cells. RBC copper is a better measure of total body content in the tissues. The normal copper serum or plasma level is 63–121 micrograms per deciliter (mcg/dL). The normal RBC copper level is 80–180 mcg/dL.

Copper Supplements

The most readily absorbed form of copper is the **glycinate** form, also called **bisglycinate** because it has two molecules of glycinate for each copper atom. Glycine is a nonessential amino acid, an organic compound, and best paired with copper to give copper the optimal absorption. Suppliers include Pure Encapsulations, Throne, Solgar Chelated Copper, and Puritan's Pride. Another nonessential amino acid attached to copper is **glutamate**, which is sold by Swanson, Thorne, BoxNutra, and the Vitamin Shoppe. Copper citrate is sold in 2 mg capsules by Pure Encapsulations and Solaray.

Iodine

Benefits of Iodine

- Used for underactive and overactive thyroid
- Acts as a potent antioxidant
- Treats painful cystic breast disease
- Low iodine levels are more common with polycystic ovaries
- Beneficial for both cardiomyopathy and cardiomegaly
- Affects hypertension and arrhythmias
- Boosts mental ability
- Prevents goiter
- Deficiency increases incidence of stomach cancer and risk of breast cancer
- Increases child's IQ if the mother takes prenatal iodine
- Reduces the risk of diabetes
- Slows the growth of prostate cancer

History of Iodine

Usually, the medical field discusses iodine in relation to the thyroid or the therapeutic use of radioactive iodine to treat thyroid cancer. This is the limited understanding of most doctors of the thyroid and iodine. However, iodine, a nonmetallic element, is necessary for the production of energy in all cells of the body, not just the thyroid. As you will see, it has a profound influence on breast cysts and breast cancer, prostate cancer, cardiac function and hypertension, cholesterol levels, stomach cancer, cognitive ability and IQ scores, and water balance, and low doses are very effective free-radical fighters.

Iodine was discovered in 1811 by the French chemist Bernard Courtois. Iodine has the symbol of **I**, the atomic number 53, and an atomic weight of 126.9. It has 37 known isotopes with weights from 108 to 144; the most stable form is iodine-127. This is the iodine that is found in the natural state. Radioactive iodine-123 is typically used in thyroid imaging, and radioactive iodine-131 is used to treat thyroid cancer.

At room temperature iodine is a purple-black nonmetallic solid. It has a melting point of 114 degrees Celsius and a boiling point of 184 degrees Celsius. In its gaseous state, it is a deep purple, which prompted Joseph Louis Gay-Lussac to call it *iodine*, from the Greek word meaning "violet colored."

Functions of Iodine

Iodine is found in every cell of the body. It is a co-element of enzymes, an antioxidant, and a contributor to hormone production and immune function. Iodine is also a potent antibacterial, antiviral, antifungal, and antiparasitic agent. It is a mucolytic agent used to lower the viscosity of mucus, permitting its easy expectoration. It has anticancer effects and is used to treat the pain associated with and prevent the formation of fibrocystic breasts and ovarian cysts. A lack of iodine can result in cretinism, intellectual disability, goiter, hypothyroidism, increased infant and child mortality, and infertility.

Hypothyroidism and Hyperthyroidism

Hypothyroidism is the condition that results from an underactive thyroid, whereas **hyperthyroidism** is the condition that results from an overactive thyroid. Hypothyroidism is said to occur when the body's iodine level falls, leaving the thyroid gland unable to produce thyroid hormone. The normal serum iodine level is 40–80 micrograms per liter (mcg/L).

Goiter

Goiter is a well-established presentation of hypothyroidism and insufficient iodine. The goiter is produced by overstimulation of the thyroid by the hypothalamus, which detects too little thyroid hormone in the system. In turn, the hypothalamus produces thyroid-releasing factor and releases it to the pituitary gland, which produces more **thyroid-stimulating hormone (TSH)** to instruct the thyroid to produce more thyroid hormones, **thyroxine (T4)** and **triiodothyronine (T3)**. The thyroid, in an effort to capture more iodine, which is scarce, grows bigger.

Endocrine Disruptors

Iodine is in the group of elements known as **halides**. From lightest to heaviest, the halides are fluorine, chlorine, bromine, iodine, astatine, and tennessine. Any one of these elements can displace iodine from enzymes or from the thyroid hormones, thyroxine (T4) and triiodothyronine (T3), rendering the biological system nonfunctioning. These halides become **endocrine disrupters**. Endocrine disruptors can be anything from heavy metals; similar elements displacing another, as in the case of halides and iodine; plastics that have a similar structure to the hormone; or any chemical that increases or decreases the proper signaling of the hormone.

In 1924, Dr. David Marine, who was studying the problem of goiters in Ohio, demonstrated that young girls developed thyroid swelling after puberty because they need more iodine than boys do. Ohio is on the border of the American Goiter Basin, where there is less iodine in the soil, which translates into less iodine in the food. This was remedied by fortifying bread with iodine, which resolved the goiter problem. An added bonus was that the bread stayed fresher for longer. Unfortunately, as the years went by, the reason iodine was added was forgotten, and bread manufacturers started to look to save money by removing it. The fortification of bread stopped in the 1970s, and bromine, an endocrine disrupter, took its place. The result was weight gain from a slow metabolism, loss of energy, and an uptick in cancers of the breasts and prostate.[240] It is only logical that if higher iodine levels can prevent prostate or breast cancer, iodine should be used when treating either prostate or breast cancer.

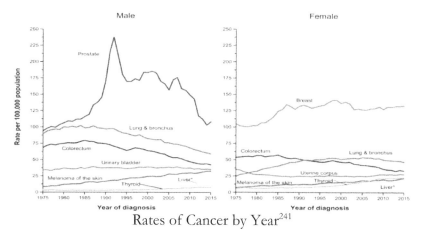

Rates of Cancer by Year[241]

Some foods are natural endocrine disrupters; before the term **endocrine disruptors** became popular, these foods were called **goitrogens**. While they are considered healthy foods, they do disrupt the functions of iodine and thyroid hormones. The strongest disruptors are the cruciferous vegetables: broccoli, arugula, cabbage,

---

[240] Farrow, L.
[241] National Cancer Institute, Statistical Research and Applications Branch, April 2006.

and brussels sprouts. Spinach and peaches are two of the weaker goitrogens.

Treatments for Iodine Deficiency, Hypothyroidism, and Hyperthyroidism

Lugol's Solution

Fortunately, changes to iodine levels caused by endocrine disruptors can be addressed to some degree by taking Lugol's solution or its tablet form. This overwhelms or upsets the balance just by increasing the concentration of iodine atoms so that they outnumber the fluoride, chlorine, and bromine atoms. Many people feel the boost in energy just from one dose of Lugol's. This treatment can be one, two, or three days a week or daily. Your energy level will increase and then level off. You will not develop hyperthyroidism. Once your body has enough iodine, it will eliminate excess iodine in the urine. Your body does not have a system to store iodine. This is one reason hypothyroidism is common.

Lugol's solution was developed by Dr. Lugol, a French physician practicing in Paris 200 years ago who treated his patients with thyroid issues with a solution of **potassium iodide** and **elemental iodine**. It worked well and for the next 150 years was the preferred treatment for both hypothyroidism and hyperthyroidism. The beauty of this preparation was that if a patient had hyperthyroidism, it worked on one mechanism in the thyroid, and if a patient had hypothyroidism, it worked through another mechanism to correct the condition. How good is that—it works in either case. So what happened? A new product, **Synthroid** (with the generic name **levothyroxine**), with an advertising budget and a higher price came on the market. Unfortunately, what replaced Lugol's solution was neither cheap nor more effective.

Levothyroxine (Synthroid)

Shortly after the commercial entry of Synthroid, two doctors at the University of California, Berkley, presented research on levothyroxine of such poor quality that today it would be called fake medical research. The **Wolff–Chaikoff effect** describes a transitory hypothyroid state that occurs when iodine is given to a **euthyroid** (healthy) person. It may last from a few days to a week or so and then return to normal. They used this information to discredit the use of Lugol's solution, saying that treating with iodine causes hypothyroidism. They talked only about transient hypothyroidism, never reporting the fact that it returns to normal. This is where the misinformation that treating with iodine causes hypothyroidism came from.

The dip in function occurs because the balance between thyroid hormone production and the tissues affected is changing. We see this today in clinical practice. An elevated **thyroid-stimulating hormone (TSH)** will transiently increase when medication is started and then settle down as needs and production are met. Because of this multifactorial balance, it may take six months after starting thyroid treatment for the TSH to reflect a true value. It is not a simple balance like a seesaw—it is more like an artist's mobile with multiple weights and beams. Touch one weight and it will need time to equilibrate.

The study itself was poorly designed. The researchers gave mice iodine and then measured their thyroid hormones, which showed that they were hypothyroid. They did not measure the thyroid levels prior to giving them iodine. And then they had the nerve to extrapolate this data from mice to humans.

This sloppy research was produced and passed through the old-boy network in the academic publishing machine known as **peer review**. This is a system in which articles for publication are reviewed for relevance and political correctness and to determine whether the author is of the correct pedigree. This also gives the members of the peer review panel the power to deny the publication of significant discoveries, pass the information on to their friends, or withhold the information from publication to alert the competition and give them time to publish first, and maybe even steal the concept of theory or data.

Thyroid Hormone Replacement

Thyroid hormone replacement is a treatment for hypothyroidism that comes in three forms: **bioidentical** hormone replacement, **chemical analogs** of thyroid hormones, and **desiccated** thyroid. Bioidentical hormones are the same molecules that the thyroid produces, and they function in an identical manner. These hormones are refined from natural products or manufactured, but the products are the identical molecules to those produced in the human thyroid. Chemical analogs are chemicals that may have similar effects, but their structure has been changed by removing, replacing, or adding an atom or functional group or otherwise changing the structure. Desiccated thyroid is thyroid tissue taken from pigs, sheep, or cows and prepared to serve as a replacement hormone.

Bioidentical hormones are the best replacement hormones. They are the least intrusive and do not develop antibodies, and it is only a matter of how much and when they are given. The structures of two molecules, **thyroxine** and **triiodothyronine**, are shown below. Each is followed by its chemical analog: Thyroxine is compared to Synthroid (levothyroxine) and triiodothyronine to Cytomel (liothyronine).

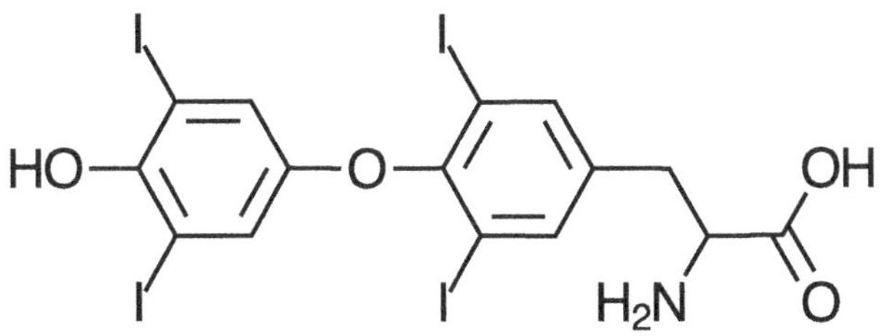

Thyroxine, T4

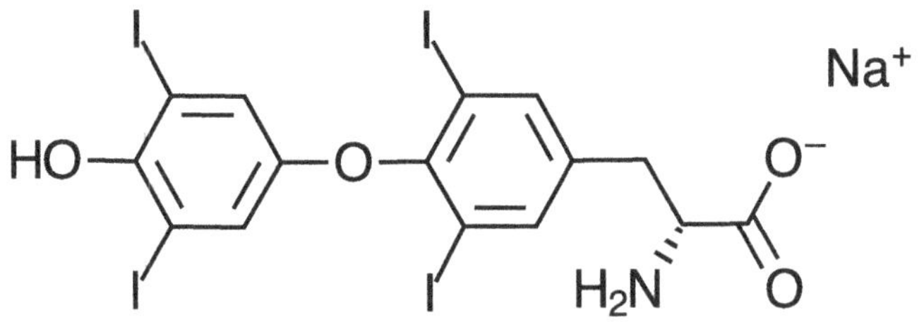

Levothyroxine, Synthroid

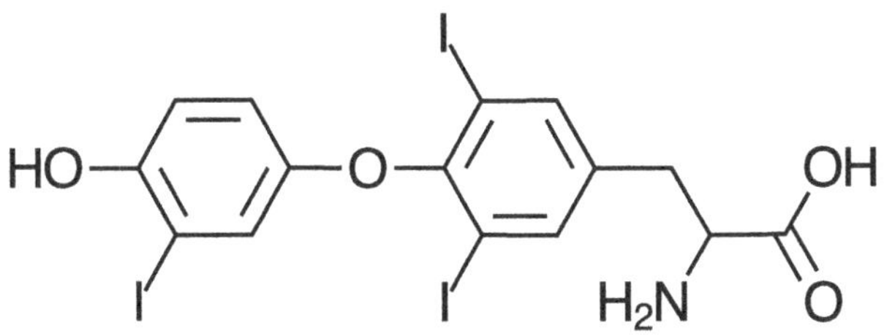

Triiodothyronine T3

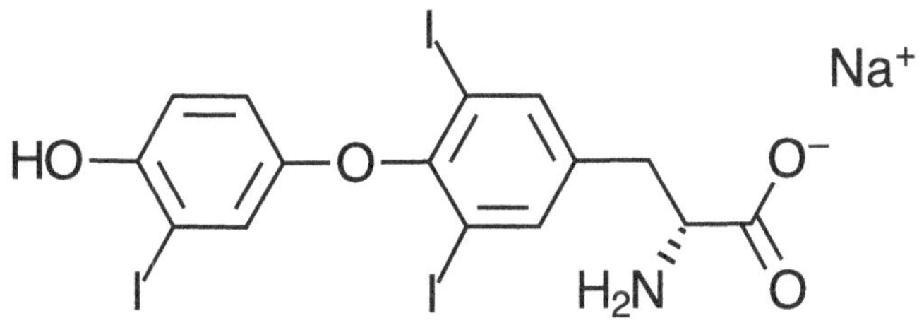

Liothyronine, Cytomel

The thyroxine molecule has been altered by removing a **hydrogen** atom in the **hydroxyl group (–OH)** and replacing it with **sodium (Na)**. This makes it an entirely different molecule. This exchange of atoms permits the manufacturer to patent the molecule, own it, and prevent others from making it. It was a new invention. It never occurred in nature before, and that makes it patentable. This molecule functions similarly but differently than the human molecule of thyroxine. Enzyme systems in the body may not be able to metabolize levothyroxine like they metabolize thyroxine. Synthroid is referred to as T4, but as you can see, it is different. This may explain why treatment with Synthroid may not be effective or even deleterious.

The illusion of Synthroid and Cytomel is that the manufacturers and academia have kept the doctors busy on the left side of the molecule, counting the number of iodine atoms and what ring they were removed from, when the real switcheroo was on the right side of the molecule. The substitution of hydrogen with sodium fundamentally changes the molecule.

Thyroxin (T4) is converted to **triiodothyronine (T3)** in the peripheral tissues (i.e., in the cells) and is the more metabolically active hormone. One iodine atom is removed from the far-left ring, transforming T4 to T3. The body also removes one iodine atom from the far-left ring of Synthroid, producing not T3 but **Cytomel (liothyronine)**. Again, liothyronine is a sodium-substituted product, and at times the body has difficulty with its metabolism.

Desiccated thyroid is the third form of thyroid hormone supplementation. It is derived from the whole thyroid and may have a therapeutic advantage in substances we may not know are in the product. It is reported that desiccated thyroid not only has T4 and T3 but also **T2** and **T1**, plus **thyroglobulin**.

Considering the three approaches to thyroid supplementation, the best and easiest to administer is the porcine, or pig, desiccated thyroid. The next is bioidentical T4 and T3. However, the most common supplementation for thyroid replacement is either the branded product Synthroid or the generic levothyroxine.

Beyond the Thyroid

Generally, when a medical doctor or even an endocrinologist discusses iodine, they talk only about iodine and the thyroid gland. This is the limit of the discussion. There is no discussion of iodine in relation to intelligence, breast health, ovarian function, alertness, the prevention of cancer by promoting the apoptosis (genetic self-destruction) of cancer cells, and the alkalization of the body to a higher pH level. Iodine is a great killer of pathogens: bacteria, molds, viruses, and protozoa. It promotes higher levels of oxygen in the tissues, supporting the immune system. It is required by all glandular systems to function and secrete hormones properly. Sadly, doctors not only overlook all these functions but also seldom even know about many of them!

I will take you beyond the simple knowledge of iodine that the medical community has and give you a better overview of some of the functions of iodine and why it is necessary to ingest more than the minimum amount of iodine.

The body contains about 1.5 g of iodine in total. This is what is in the thyroid hormones and what is captured in the enzyme systems throughout the body. There is no storage form of iodine in the body. If it is not utilized, it will be eliminated. This can be demonstrated in a simple storage test initiated by Guy Abraham, MD.

Fifteen years ago, I performed this test on 34 of my patients, aged 32 to 88 years. The test is performed by the patient ingesting 50 mg of iodine, and then the urine is collected for the next 24 hours. In a normal person, 90%, or more than 45 mg of the iodine, will be excreted in the urine. If there is a body deficit, the person will absorb more than 10% of the iodine, producing less in the urine. For my test, each person took 50 mg of iodine in the form of Iodoral tablets. The composition of Iodoral is 30 mg of iodine from potassium iodide (KI) and 20 mg of free iodine (I_2). This is the same formula as the original Dr. Lugol's solution.

The test yielded two interesting observations: First, only 2 of the 34 tests showed normal results, and second, the older the participant was, the greater the deficit for iodine. According to this data, only 6% of this population has sufficient iodine in their diet, and the older a person is, the more they need iodine in their diet.

Throughout medical literature, it is reported that 35–80% of the ingested iodine goes to the thyroid. But where does the rest of the iodine go? The majority of it goes to the breast, followed by the ovaries, uterus, nervous system, brain, and various enzyme systems throughout the body. Lactating breasts may absorb up to 43% of the newly ingested iodine at times, more than the absorption of the thyroid. Sufficient iodine is necessary for developing the nervous system and brain of the fetus. It is a well-known fact that without sufficient iodine, cretinism is the outcome. **Cretinism** is congenital hypothyroidism. Difficult to correct, it is characterized by neurologic impairments, short stature, an enlarged tongue, infertility, and hair loss. A woman properly supplemented with iodine three to six months prior to and during pregnancy can have children with higher IQs and better intelligence.

If you think iodine is all about thyroid function, read on. It has much to do with metabolism, alertness, energy levels, and immune system support.

Breast and Glandular Tissue Health

Iodine, which is needed by all the thyroid hormones, is accumulated in the thyroid, and this is where most of the medical attention has been focused. Surprisingly, this is not the gland that concentrates the most iodine: The breasts require and accumulate the most iodine. And the larger the breasts, the more they accumulate iodine. A low level of iodine in the breast is found in atypical tissue, dysplasia, and neoplasms.[242] The growth rate of breast cancer is inversely related to the amount of iodine in the breast. The less iodine in the breast, the faster the cancer grows.

Iodine is also required for the glandular functions of the breasts and prevents the formation of fibrotic cysts—and treats the pain if they do form. Lactating breasts require as much as twice the amount of iodine as nonlactating breasts. Moreover, iodine accumulates in the prostate, salivary glands, brain, spinal fluid, choroid plexus, substantia nigra, ciliary body of the eye, gastric mucosa, and ovaries.[243] All glandular tissue requires iodine to perform its function. It has also been suggested that iodine is required by the mitochondria in minute amounts for the production of energy.

The reason iodine is so important and necessary to breasts is that in the breast, iodine acts as a catalyst to transform the more active form of estradiol to the less active form of estriol.[244] Estradiol is the most active estrogen, and excessive estradiol levels that are not in balance with the other forms of estrogen—estriol and estrone, the storage form of estrogen—may promote breast cancer. In prescribing bioidentical hormones, a blend of hormones is always preferred over a single hormone application. Both estriol and estradiol bind to the hormone receptors to tell the cells how to behave. Estriol is a weak stimulator; instead, it acts more to protect the integrity of the receptors, preventing other chemicals and pollutants from sending the wrong signal to the cells.

Iodine is definitely required for healthy breasts and all glandular tissue. Adding iodine to breast cancer regimens helps to get the cancer under control. I have had good results with 12.5–50 mg daily

---

[242] Eskin, B. A., "Iodine and Mammary Cancer," In Schrauzer, G. N. (ed.), *Inorganic and Nutritional Aspects of Cancer. Advances in Experimental Medicine and Biology*, 1978, *91*, https://doi.org/10.1007/978-1-4684-0796-9_20.

[243] Adrasi, E., et al., "Iodine Concentration in Different Human Brain Parts," *Analytical and Bioanalytical Chemistry*, 2004, *378*, 129–133, https://doi.org/10.1007/s00216-003-2313-3.

[244] Kennedy, R., *Nutritional Protocols, Book Two*, 1997.

of **I-thyroid**. Take note that I am talking about iodine, not thyroid thyroxine or triiodothyronine, where iodine is incorporated in the thyroid hormone molecules. Non-thyroid tissues, such as breast, prostate, and gastric mucosa tissue, prefer iodine (I_2), whereas thyroid tissue prefers iodide (KI), the more soluble form.

Fibrocystic Disease of the Breast

Fibrocystic disease of the breast (FDB) describes the development of painful cysts of the breast. If left untreated, the cysts develop a fibrous stiff capsule, which makes it impossible for them to naturally dissolve. Iodine preparations such as Iodoral and I-Thyroid can reduce the pain and the size of the cysts by detoxifying the breasts. It may take several months to a year or two, but it is worth a try, as no other remedy is available besides surgery.

Fetal Development

Iodine is necessary for proper brain growth and development, the alert functioning of thought, and the transmission of neural impulses in both the central nervous system and the peripheral nerves. Fetal development takes place in the first 12 weeks of pregnancy. Iodine is critical for brain development. That is why it is critical that a woman ingest sufficient iodine before and during pregnancy. It is estimated that with a high-normal level of iodine, the woman will have a child with an IQ that is 10 points higher than that of the child of someone who is slightly deficient or has a low-normal level.[245] Prenatal vitamin supplementation should definitely include iodine.

---

[245] Bougma, K., et al., "Iodine and Mental Development of Children 5 Years Old and Under: A Systematic Review and Meta-Analysis," *Nutrients*, 2013, *5*(4), 1384–1416.

Antiseptic and Germicidal Properties

The exact mechanism of the germicidal action of iodine is unknown, but most bacteria are killed in one minute of exposure to a 1:20,000 solution of iodine. The spores of bacteria are also killed after 15 minutes of exposure to the same concentration of iodine. Even a dilute concentration of iodine at 1:200,000 will kill bacteria in 15 minutes. In addition, two drops of iodine tincture added to one quart of water will make the water drinkable after 30 minutes, killing viruses, funguses, and many protozoa.

Topical Iodine

Topical iodine, such as tincture of iodine (I_2 and KI dissolved in alcohol) can kill 90% of bacteria in 90 seconds, making it an extremely effective skin antiseptic for wounds and surgery preparation. Bacteria have not developed resistance to iodine like they have to some antibiotics. In the antibiotic era, after penicillin, various antibiotic ointments and creams have been developed and widely promoted, such as bacitracin, neomycin, and mupirocin. But still, the best by far is a preparation of iodine. The concentration is usually 2–7%. Its use is traced back to French surgeons as early as 1839, and it was in common use during the American Civil War for battle wounds. It is still the most efficacious, economical, and least toxic substance for germicidal action. It is cheap, effective, and nontoxic when used on the skin.

Potassium Iodine, Iodide, or Super Saturated Potassium Iodine (SSKI)

Potassium iodine (KI), also called **iodide** or **super saturated potassium iodine (SSKI)**, is an effective treatment for the herpes virus when applied to mucous membranes. A solution for gargling can be made using 10 drops of the potassium iodine solution in a glass of water. This is a safe therapy for both oral and genital herpes.

Iodoform

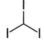

Iodoform

Iodoform, CHI_3

Iodoform is a methyl molecule with three of the four hydrogen atoms replaced with iodine. It is a lemon-yellow powder with which gauze can be impregnated for use as a topical dressing or, in strips, for packing into a wound to slowly release iodine. Infections that develop below the skin, such as an abscess or boil, when lanced and not fully drained will close up and continue to fester. Placing a strip of iodoform gauze into the pocket of the abscess with a small tail exposed to the outside permits the pus to be wicked out, keeping the skin from resealing the opening before the pocket is drained and sterilized. When the drainage of pus becomes clear serum, the wick can be removed.

Povidone-Iodine

Povidone-iodine (1-vinyl-2-pyrrolidinone polymer iodine complex), sold under the trade name Betadine, is a commercially made topical antiseptic solution designed to release iodine. It is primarily used as an antiseptic on the skin. Once the iodine is released, a polymer residue remains. If ingested, the polymer can injure the kidneys. It should never be swallowed, used to disinfect water for drinking, or be injected.

Nuclear Exposure

Potassium Iodate

Potassium Iodate, KIO_3

Iodate is the more common form of iodine found in Europe. It is also used for protection from radioactive iodine and to protect the thyroid gland after nuclear exposure. The idea is to saturate the thyroid gland with nonradioactive iodine so that when exposure to radioactive iodine occurs, the radioactive iodine will not be incorporated in the thyroid gland.

Poland dispensed potassium iodate to its people to protect them against the uptake of radioactive iodine from the fallout after the meltdown of the Chernobyl nuclear reactor in 1986. This protected the population against thyroid cancer. The Russians did not provide this protection to its people, and this negligence caused the Russian people to develop a significant number of thyroid cancers.

Food Sources of Iodine

Natural sources of iodine are seaweed, oysters, clams, lobsters, and some vegetables if the soil in which they were grown contained sufficient amounts of iodine. Some areas of the world have low amounts of iodine in the soil, and these areas are known as endemic goiter regions. They include the Great Lakes Basin of the United States, Switzerland, Austria, New Zealand and Australia, the Xinjiang Provence of China, remote areas of India, Zaire, and Kazakhstan.

The island of Crete also has low amounts of iodine in the soil, and a condition associated with iodine deficiency—**cretinism**—has been named after the island. The brain needs iodine for growth and development. If fetuses and children do not ingest enough iodine during the developmental stages, they can develop cretinism, which is characterized by hypothyroidism, dwarfism, extreme intellectual disability, and physical deformity. This effect is not genetic but is environmental, and it is avoidable.

The table that follows lists the iodine content of foods that contain iodine.[246]

Food Sources of Iodine			
Food type	Food	Serving size (g)	Iodine content (mcg)
Seaweed	Kumbu kelp	1	2,984
	Wakame	1	66
	Nori	1	43
Wild fish	Cod	85 (3 oz.)	99
	Shrimp	85 (3 oz.)	35
Egg	Whole egg	65	24

Kumbu kelp is found in Asia, wakame is found in the waters around Australia and New Zealand, and nori is the name of a group of Japanese seaweeds referred to as sea vegetables and used in sushi rolls.

The amount of iodine found in plants and animals is dependent on the amount of iodine in the area local to them. Most iodine is

---

[246] Berkheiser, K., "9 Healthy Foods That Are Rich in Iodine," Healthline, last updated February 1, 2023, https://www.healthline.com/nutrition/iodine-rich-foods.

found in the oceans, with little found in inland areas, as it may be washed down streams and rivers or may even evaporate. The iodine-deficient areas of the world are, for the most part, far from oceans or large mineral deposits.

Iodine Supplements and Products

Iodine is available as solutions and solid forms. The original therapeutic form of Lugol's solution, iodine and potassium iodide, is available in liquid and pill forms measured in both milligrams (mg) and micrograms (mcg). All the therapeutic strengths are in milligram amounts. The microgram amounts are too small to have any benefit, even though many products are in the microgram range. Lugol's solution comes in two strengths: 2% and 5%. The 2% solution contains 2.5 mg per drop, while the 5% solution contains 6.26 mg per drop. The table that follows sets out the total dosage of iodine by number of drops for Lugol's solution.

Total Dosage of Iodine per Drops of Lugol's Solution		
% solution	Number of drops	Total dosage (mg)
2	1	2.5
2	5	12.5
2	10	25
2	15	37.5
2	20	50
5	1	6.25
5	2	12.5
5	4	25
5	6	37.5
5	8	50

Iodoral is the tablet form of Lugol's solution. Each 12.5 mg tablet contains 7.5 mg of iodine from potassium iodide and 5 mg of free iodine. This does not include the potassium that is part of the potassium iodide. Iodoral can be bought in 12.5 mg, 25 mg, and 50 mg tablets. Similar concentrations in capsule form are sold as I-Thyroid by RLC Labs, Iodizyme by Biotics Research, and Tri-Iodine by VitaminLife.

Potassium iodide (KI) is used to thin mucus and loosen congestion in the sinuses and respiratory tract. Common product names are IOSAT (130 mg tablet), ThyroSafe (65 mg tablet), and ThyroShield.

Potassium iodate (KIO_3) is available from Medical Corps as an 85 mg or 170 mg tablet.

Iodoform gauze for wound packing and Xeroform dressing for wound application are sold by McKesson, Curad, and Cardinal Health.

Tincture of iodine is sold by Walgreens, Swan, Flinn Scientific, and Care+.

Iron

Benefits of Iron

- Corrects iron deficiency anemia
- Supports the transport and storage of oxygen in the body
- Required for energy metabolism in the mitochondria and other peroxidase enzymes

History of Iron

Iron, an element with the symbol **Fe** and atomic number 26, is in the first transitional series of metals. It has an atomic weight of 55.845. Iron was first found by humans in about 2,000 BC in Eurasia, and it began to appear in tools in about 1,200 BC, when furnaces could reach 2,730 degrees Fahrenheit (1,500 degrees Celsius) or higher. The body contains about 4 g of iron, mainly in the form of **hemoglobin** in blood and **myoglobin** in muscles.

Before discussing the importance of iron, I would like to point out a significant observation by Paul Carnot in 1906. Paul Carnot was experimenting with rabbits that were anemic. He injected the serum from anemic rabbits into healthy rabbits and observed the healthy rabbits did not become anemic but that their red blood cell (RBC) count actually increased. This led him to propose that a blood factor existed that caused the rabbits to make more red blood cells and increased the blood volume. He called this **hemopoietin**.[247]

It was not until the 1950s that researchers Reissmann, Erslev, and Jacobsen defined that the hormone, now called **erythropoietin**, controls red blood cell production based on oxygen levels and not iron levels. This hormone was found to come from the kidneys. Low levels of oxygen at the kidneys cause the kidneys to produce erythropoietin, stimulating the bone marrow to produce more red blood cells.

Subsequently, the gene for the production of erythropoietin was identified to be on human chromosome 7. This hormone is primarily expressed by the peritubular interstitial cells of the kidney during periods of low oxygen. It is now available, made synthetically and called epoetin alpha, under the trade names of Epogen, PROCRIT, or EPREX. It is administered as a subcutaneous injection of 50–100 units per kilogram of body weight one to three times a week. It is used frequently in people with renal failure or anemia of chronic disease. Much of this new form of erythropoietin is made by bacterial recombination.

Functions of Iron

Iron is an element that is needed for the transport and processing of oxygen in the body. Iron supplementation is recommended for children and pregnant women, and after significant blood loss. Generally, the body will take up iron and use it in a **red blood cell (RBC)**, and after the life of the RBC (usually 120 days), the body will recycle the iron and incorporate it in a new RBC.

---

[247] Kaushansky, K., and Kipps, T. J., "Hematopoietic Agents: Growth Factors, Minerals, and Vitamins," *Goodman & Gilman's the Pharmacological Basis of Therapeutics*, 12th edition, McGraw-Hill Medical, 2011, 1067–1099.

New RBCs are made in the bone marrow; they lose their nucleus and are released into general circulation as packages of hemoglobin that transport oxygen from the lungs to the body. They last about 120 days before becoming damaged from the physical stress of banging into the walls of the arteries, squeezing through capillaries, traveling through the veins, and having pressure applied to them as another go-around begins in the high pressure of the ventricles of the heart. They also undergo chemical stress from too much oxygen, from cytokines, and from chemicals as they pass through areas of inflammation. The cell membrane that keeps the hemoglobin within the cell becomes worn and may leak. The spleen is responsible for removing the worn-out cells, conserving the iron to return it to the bone marrow for the production of new RBCs. Iron is carried by a protein called **transferrin**, or **ferritin**, to the bone marrow or anywhere else it is needed, such as myoglobin in the muscles or heme-containing enzymes.

The body conserves iron and recycles it many times so that in stable times, little is needed to maintain the usual body content of about 4 g. It is needed for periods of growth—for example, during pregnancy and fetal growth, especially the last trimester. Iron is also lost due to blood loss during heavy menstrual flow and bleeding from trauma. Microscopic amounts are lost in the intestinal tract and from the gums, gastric irritation, bowel inflammation, and hemorrhoids.

This process of cycling iron from its incorporation in the bone marrow to RBCs, to the spleen, and back again to the bone marrow was understood in the 1950s. This helped with the understanding that under usual conditions, the body is efficient at iron conservation. The body needs little added iron. Adults need only 8–18 mg of iron per day.

In addition to iron, the body needs some hormone direction to maintain the proper level of hemoglobin and to maintain a stable blood volume. A hormone is a messenger chemical that tells, or instructs, one system or organ, such as the bone marrow, how much of something to produce—in this case, how many RBCs.

The function of hemoglobin is primarily the transport of oxygen in the blood, and that of myoglobin is the storage of oxygen in the muscles. Some respiratory enzymes in the cells also contain iron to support the oxidation processes. Respiratory enzymes that contain iron are **cytochromes, catalase, peroxidase, metalloflavoproteins, xanthine oxidase**, and the mitochondrial enzyme **alpha-glycerophosphate oxidase**.

Iron comes in two oxidation states: the **ferrous**, which has a **+2 charge (Fe^{+2})**, and **ferric**, which has a **+3 charge (Fe^{+3})**. All the iron in the body, such as that found in hemoglobin, myoglobin, or bound up with transfer proteins, is the ferrous +2 charge.

The table that follows shows the distribution of iron throughout the body in milligrams (mg) per kilogram (kg) of weight.[248]

Distribution of Iron in the Body in Milligrams per Kilogram of Body Weight		
Storage system	Male (mg/kg body weight)	Female (mg/kg body weight)
Hemoglobin	31	28
Myoglobin	6	5
Liver and bone marrow	13	4
Total	*50*	*37*

---

[248] Kaushansky, K., and Kipps, T. J., "Hematopoietic Agents: Growth Factors, Minerals, and Vitamins," *Goodman & Gilman's the Pharmacological Basis of Therapeutics*, 12th edition, McGraw-Hill Medical, 2011, 1077.

Anemia

Anemia is defined as a decrease in RBCs, hemoglobin (Hgb), or both because of impaired production, blood loss, or increased destruction. Each of these causes by themselves may cause anemia. Each cause has many factors; for example, impaired production may be caused by a lack of iron, poor nutrition, genetic causes, or environmental toxins.

Iron Supplementation

Iron glycinate is a form of iron that is relatively new for supplementation. The iron is not new—it is the attaching of the amino acid **glycine** to a metal that is new. The form of iron used by the body is the ferrous form (Fe^{+2}). It has a +2 charge and requires two molecules of glycine to balance the molecule electrically. The name of the chemical supplement is **iron bisglycinate**, with *bis* meaning two molecules of glycinate, but commonly it is referred to as iron glycinate.

Iron Glycinate

I have found this form of iron to be absorbed and incorporated into hemoglobin and to replenish body stores faster than any other. It can be both absorbed at the intestines and incorporated biologically into the body systems and structures faster and more completely than any of the available supplemental forms. I have noticed that when I treat with iron bisglycinate at a dose of only 30 mg, far more is absorbed faster, it raises the body stores, and it improves the hemoglobin level faster than any of the other oral preparations, **sulfate** or **gluconate**, used at the recommended dosage of 325 mg, or the intravenous **iron dextran** or **iron gluconate** of 100 mg.

That iron is attached to an amino acid, glycine, in iron glycinate implies that this form of iron is already in an organic form as opposed to an inorganic form. I believe this form of iron supplementation has two great advantages: First, it is in the proper oxidation state of +2, and, second, glycine is an amino acid, a compound needed for life. Because the metal glycinate is in an organic form prior to ingestion, the body does not have to spend time and energy to convert an inorganic form to an organic form of a metal. Consider it biologically ready, in a form that may be obtained from food. For example, a good plant-based form of iron is spinach, and an animal form is red meat—both represent biologically ready iron. Moreover, iron glycinate does not produce side effects such as stomach cramps, black stools, arthralgia, headache, or malaise.

Hooking a glycine molecule to a metal is an elegant method of increasing the absorption and body stores of most metals, making them organic minerals. Today, most minerals can be found in this form: magnesium glycinate, manganese glycinate, zinc glycinate, copper glycinate, boron glycinate, and iron bisglycinate.

Ferric Iron

As a point of practical information, ferric iron (+3) is the form used in intravenous injections and previously used in deep intramuscular injections to restore iron levels in iron deficiency anemia. It is difficult to use. The infusion time must be long, at least more than 20 minutes to avoid hypersensitivity, hypotension, and even an asthmatic attack. The iron will also leave a tattoo with a deposit of iron in the skin if some of the iron solution accidentally leaks into the skin during injection or leaks along the needle track after the needle is removed. Unfortunately, this treatment is given in multiple doses and is somewhat ineffective.

Limitations of Intravenous Iron

Contrary to what one might suspect, giving iron directly into the vein is not the most efficient method of quickly restoring iron. The ferric iron used for intravenous infusion must be converted to the ferrous oxidation state. This conversion requires significant amounts of vitamin C and enzymes that no doubt are already in short supply. This is a lengthy process, if it occurs at all. Side effects include headache, generalized lymphedema, fever, urticaria, arthralgia, and reactivation of rheumatoid arthritis. This ferric iron often is deposited in the liver and lymphatic tissue with little of it being incorporated in the red blood cells as intended.

I have treated several patients who were previously treated by hematologists with months of intravenous iron with no success. Once I started them on the oral organic iron glycinate, their hemoglobin quickly began to elevate, and most returned to normal levels. The oral route for the administration of iron is the best. It avoids iron overload in the liver and excess deposits of iron throughout the body that the body may not be able to remove due to being in the nonorganic, +3 oxidation state.

Iron Utilization

The conversion of iron into the organic forms of end products, such as hemoglobin, myoglobin, and oxygen transport molecules, requires the assistance of other minerals (cobalt, copper, and zinc) and the vitamins folic acid, vitamin B_{12}, thiamine, and vitamin C. The incorporation of iron into the complex molecules that are required for this life of ours depends on more than reducing the oxidation state of iron from +3 to +2. Iron utilization requires many factors and many steps to produce hemoglobin. The cause of iron deficiency anemia may not be the lack of iron but the supporting nutrients that participate in the absorption and conversion to the proper state of iron.

Heme Iron

Another form of iron that is significant for nutrition is the heme iron found in meat. It represents only 6% of the daily intake of iron, but because of its bioavailability, it is 30% of the iron that is absorbed.

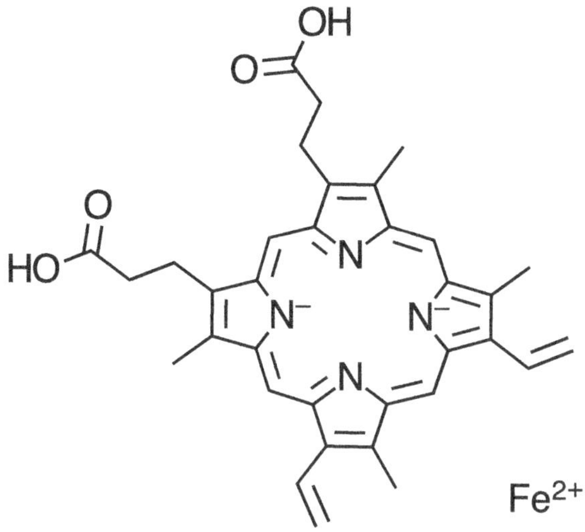

Heme

The iron atom with the +2 charge is held by electron attraction by the two negatively charged nitrogen atoms, and this molecule is called heme. This molecule can attract and hold a molecule of oxygen in a high-oxygen environment such as the lung and release it in a low-oxygen environment such as the peripheral tissues. The ring of nitrogen in the above structure is known as the **porphyrin ring** and is repeated in nature in proteins such as vitamin B_{12} and chlorophyll.

In 1962, M. F. Perutz and J. C. Kendrew of Cambridge University were awarded the Nobel Prize in Chemistry for demonstrating the structure of hemoglobin: four molecules of heme held together with the protein globulin.

Iron Toxicity

The conservation of iron is so efficient in the human body that poisoning, impairment of functions, and death are possible. This is why iron supplements should be taken only when indicated by laboratory tests and followed along with a doctor. Iron poisoning is most common in children less than six years of age, but fortunately, it is on the decline because of increased awareness and the FDA warning on all iron products:

WARNING: Accidental overdose of iron-containing products is a leading cause of fatal poisoning in children. Keep this product out of reach of children. In the case of accidental overdose, call a doctor or poison control center immediately.

The number for the Poison Control Center is **1-800-222-1222**.

The most common cause of iron poisoning is iron tablets, either from a supplement or leftover prenatal vitamin and mineral tablets. They usually are colored red and are attractive to children. Immediate symptoms that occur within 30 minutes of ingestion are lassitude (fatigue), drowsiness, pallor or cyanosis, hyperventilation, and cardiovascular collapse. As little as 1–2 g of iron my cause death.

A protein called the human hemochromatosis protein promotes the absorption of iron in the intestines. Iron is usually delivered to the intestines in small amounts. Another protein called **hepcidin**, produced in the liver, counteracts this as an inhibitor of human hemochromatosis protein, preventing an overload of iron. Both these systems can contribute to too much or too little absorption of iron. The liver can produce too much hepcidin in old age—up to 100 times the usual amount—and cause poor absorption, resulting in anemia. This overproduction of hepcidin can be caused by liver inflammation or iron overload in the liver. On the other end of the spectrum, too much iron can be absorbed by the over-ingestion of iron or a genetic mutation on chromosome 6 that causes overproduction of the human hemochromatosis protein.

Hemochromatosis is caused by a mutation in the gene that controls the amount of iron the body absorbs in the intestines. This gene is called the ***HFE* gene** (for high **Fe**). Hemochromatosis causes iron to be deposited in the liver, causing liver dysfunction; in the pancreas, producing diabetes; in the skin, giving it a bronze coloration; and in the heart, contributing to heart failure. Hemochromatosis is suspected when any of these conditions are found or when the serum iron or ferritin is elevated. The gene mutation cannot be corrected, but the excess iron can be removed through phlebotomy to keep the iron from depositing in the liver, pancreas, or heart, avoiding the deleterious effects. It occurs in men in middle age and is not apparent in women until after menopause when the monthly blood loss from menses stops.

Iron Intake

The recommended dietary allowance of iron, in mg per day, is set out in the table below.[249]

Recommended Dietary Allowance (RDA) for Iron			
Life stage	**Age**	**Male (mg/day)**	**Female (mg/day)**
Infant	0–6 months	0.27	0.27
	7–12 months	11	11
Child	1–13 years	7–10	7–10
Adolescent	11–18 years	11	15
Adult	19–50	8	18
	51 and older	8	8
Pregnant	All ages	–	27
Breastfeeding	All ages	–	9

---

[249] Food and Nutrition Board, Institute of Medicine, *Dietary Reference for Iron*, National Academy Press, 2001, 290–393.

Food Sources of Iron

The table below sets out several foods that are good sources of iron.[250]

Food Sources of Iron		
Food	Serving size	Iron content (mcg)
Oysters	6 medium	13.8
Spinach	1 cup	6.1
Mussels	3 oz.	5.7
Chicken liver	1 oz.	3.6
White beans	½ cup	3.3
Lentils	½ cup	3.3
Clams	3 oz.	2.4
Prune juice	6 oz.	2.3
Swiss chard	½ cup	2.0
Potato with skin	1 medium	1.8
Beef	3 oz.	1.6
Hazelnuts	1 oz.	1.3

---

[250] United States Department of Agriculture, FoodData Central, 2020, https://fdc.nal.usda.gov/.

Iron Supplements

Iron glycinate is the best organic form of iron for oral ingestion developed to date. Examples are Thorne Iron Bisglycinate, Solgar Chelated Iron, and Gentle Iron and the products available from California Gold Nutrition, Now Supplements, and Klaire Labs. Other names for iron glycinate are **chelated iron** and **Ferrochel**. The dosages are usually low compared to the traditional forms of iron salts: sulfate, gluconate, and fumarate.

The disadvantage of iron salts are that the dosages are usually about 30–325 mg per tablet or capsule and that they provoke symptoms of abdominal cramping, bloating, nausea, constipation, and, sometimes, black stools that may be confused with intestinal bleeding. Examples of iron salts are Feosol, Ferrous Sulfate 325 mg, Iron Gluconate, and iron attached to fumarate.

Another old favorite for iron supplementation is Geritol. It is in a class by itself for two reasons. First, it is the ferric iron in the +3 oxidation state that must be converted to the +2 oxidation state before it can be absorbed. Second, it is attached to Ferrex, which is a brand name for iron polysaccharide, also called polydextrose iron. The dextrose molecule is so large that in the intestines, it acts like a fiber and inhibits rapid absorption of the iron, making it a poor choice for iron replacement. It will do the job, but not efficiently.

The body also has difficulty incorporating intravenous iron into heme or myoglobin molecules because it too is in the +3 oxidation state and must be converted to the +2 oxidation state. Because it is delivered into the vein at a near neutral pH of 7.4, it is difficult for that conversion to occur, if at all. The best entry point for the +3, ferric state of iron is orally, to the stomach. The stomach acid, with the addition of vitamin C, will efficiently convert the iron to the +2 ferrous state.

Lithium

Benefits of Lithium

- Stabilizes the mood
- Reduces the rate of development of Alzheimer's disease
- Maintains the volume of the brain

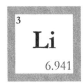

History of Lithium

Lithium is a soft, silvery white metal found in many rocks and soils in low concentrations. Its name comes from *lithos*, the Greek word for stone. It was discovered by the Swedish chemist Johan August Arfwedson from **petalite (LiAlSi$_4$O$_{10}$)** in 1817. It was first isolated as an element by Thomas Brande and Sir Humphrey Davy through the electrolysis of **lithium oxide (Li$_2$O)**. Today, it is refined from **lithium chloride (LiCl)**.

Lithium is the lightest metal and is easily made into light alloys with aluminum, copper, manganese, and cadmium. **Lithium hydroxide (LiOH)** is used to remove **carbon monoxide (CO)** from the capsules of spacecrafts. **Lithium stearate (LiC$_{18}$H$_{35}$O$_2$)** is a lubricant used in high-temperature applications. In recent years it has become an industrial commodity because of its use in rechargeable batteries.

Lithium is represented by the symbol of **Li**, it has the atomic number of 3 and the atomic weight of 6.94, it is the lightest of all the metals, it is soft and white in color, and it is never found in an elemental state, usually in a form with other minerals.

Uses and Benefits of Lithium

Treatment of Manic-Depressive Disorders

Lithium carbonate (Li_2CO_3) is used in the medical field for manic-depressive disorders.

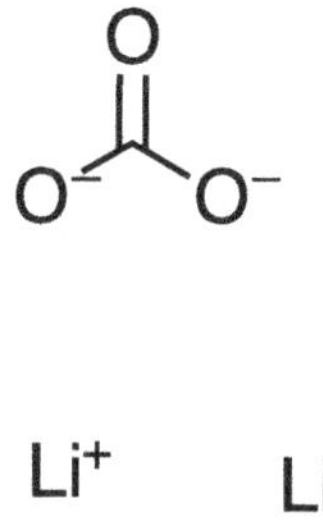

Lithium Carbonate

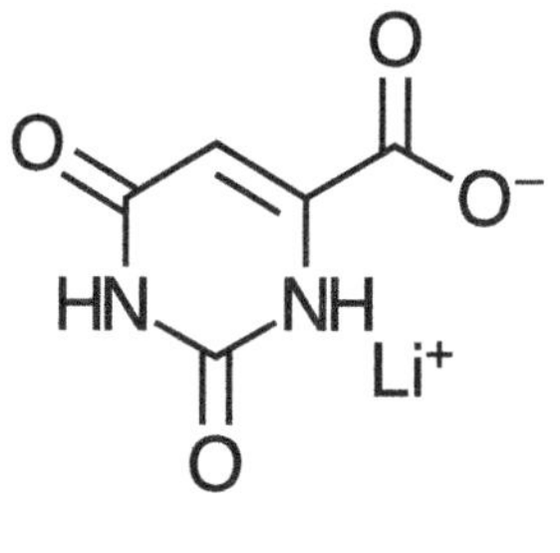

Lithium Orotate

Lithium has been used in psychiatry only since 1949. This rather recent event stems from an observation made by Cade while working with guinea pigs. He noticed that lithium carbonate in the water would sedate guinea pigs and reasoned that lithium would calm manic patients. Starting with this anecdotal observation, he gave lithium to 10 manic patients, whose symptoms were under control within a week.[251]

Since then, numerous studies, including double-blind studies, have demonstrated that lithium is better than a placebo and superior to phenothiazines in both manic and hypomanic conditions. Unlike other antipsychotic drugs, it does not cause sedation. To clarify, **manic psychosis** presents as a social emergency and requires hospital confinement for the administration of lithium and monitoring. **Hypomania** still refers to manic psychosis, but the severity is less intense, and it can be managed in an outpatient setting.

In practice, lithium carbonate is given as 300 mg two or three times a day until a serum level of 0.8–1.4 milliequivalents per liter (mEq/L) is reached. It usually takes 7 to 10 days to reach this therapeutic level. Frequent blood testing is necessary to ensure that the lithium level does not go beyond 1.5 mEq/L to avoid the symptoms of lithium toxicity: tremor, increased deep-tendon reflexes, headache, mental confusion, seizures, vomiting, cardiac arrhythmia, and poor kidney function. Within one week, the necessary dosage and a steady serum level are typically obtained, with stable clinical results.[252]

Alzheimer's Disease and Dementia

In the 1950s and 1960s, the treatment of bipolar disorders and depression with lithium carbonate for protracted periods became common, and it became apparent that those treated with lithium experienced a lower incidence of dementia. This observation was

---

[251] Cade, J. F. J., "Lithium Salts in the Treatment of Psychotic Excitement," *Medical Journal of Australia*, 1949, *2*(10), 349–352, https://doi.org/10.1080/j.1440-1614.1999.06241.x.
[252] *The Merck Manual*, 14th edition, 1982, ch. 146, 1460–1461.

first tested by treating a group of 66 elderly patients with bipolar disorders with lithium, with a control group of 48 similar patients who were not treated with lithium. The group treated with lithium experienced a 5% incidence of Alzheimer's disease, and the control group experienced a 33% incidence of Alzheimer's disease.[253]

In Denmark, two studies of more than 21,000 patients demonstrated a similar reduction in Alzheimer's and other dementias.[254] More recent findings in Texas, in 2018, showed that higher levels of lithium in the water correlated with fewer cases of Alzheimer's disease, and areas with less lithium in the water had a higher incidence of Alzheimer's disease.[255]

Brain Shrinkage and Neuroprotection

When I started to care for patients more than 45 years ago, I was fortunate to have a residency at a hospital that had a CT scanner—initially, only for heads. We were the only non–university hospital in the area to have a CT scanner. At that time, when a head CT was performed, the brain filled the entire skull cavity. Diets were different—not totally organic, but they were in the process of changing to the standard American diet, or SAD diet, which is nutritionally poor. The medical community was still fumbling about a clear definition of what constitutes Alzheimer's disease. But what developed over the years was that some people had significant brain

---

[253] Nunes, P. V., Forlenza, O. V., and Gattaz, W. F., "Lithium and the Risk for Alzheimer's Disease in Elderly Patients with Bipolar Disorder," *British Journal of Psychiatry*, 2007, *190*, 359–360.

[254] Kessing, L. V., Forman, J. L., and Andersen, P. K., "Does Lithium Protect Against Dementia?" *Bipolar Disorders*, 2010, *12*(1), 87–94; Kessing, L. V., et al., "Lithium Treatment and the Risk of Dementia," *Archives of General Psychiatry*, 2008, *65*(11), 1332–1335.

[255] Fajardo, V. A., et al., "Examining the Relationship between Trace Lithium in Drinking Water and the Rising Rates of Age-Adjusted Alzheimer's Disease Mortality in Texas," *Journal of Alzheimer's Disease*, 2018, *61*(1), 425–434, https://doi.org/10.3233/jad-170744.

THE FORGOTTEN AND HIDDEN FACTS OF VITAMINS & MINERALS

shrinkage. The reduced size of the brain in the skull cavity did not always correlate with mental function, but sometimes it did.

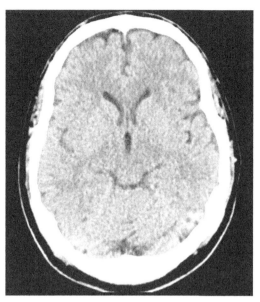

Normal CT of a 40-Year-Old Male

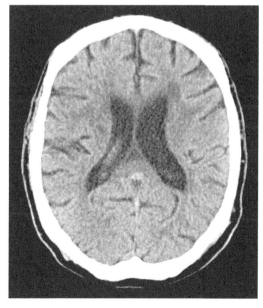

Age-Appropriate CT of the Brain of a 72-Year-Old Male

Interpretation: Cerebral atrophy, patchy, hypodensity in the periventricular and subcortical white matter bilaterally, consistent with the sequela of chronic microvascular ischemic change and ventricular dilatation.

Brain shrinkage progressed from white-matter atrophy and microvascular degeneration, and a simple determination whether the shrinkage was from diabetes, dementia, or vascular disease was nearly impossible to make. There is no doubt that, looking at the CT scan, there is wasting away of the brain, shown by less gray and white matter, the gyri outlined by the folds of the brain being more pronounced, with more fluid between the individual gyri and between the skull and the brain, and the central ventricles becoming major fluid-filled spaces. This is the radiographic picture that is compatible with Alzheimer's disease or dementia. This picture is not diagnostic of either disease, but it is compatible.

Not to cast any judgement on mental function, but the new term **age appropriate** is now found on many radiology reports. This may mean that the brain has shrunk anywhere from 10% to 30% of its volume. I do not see anything appropriate about a shrinking brain.

Lithium gives the brain neuroprotection by helping to maintain the length of telomeres. It promotes the synthesis of two proteins: **brain-derived neurotrophic factor (BDNF)** and **neurotrophin-3**. Telomere length is preserved by strengthening the endcaps on the chromosomes, increasing longevity and preventing diseases. Lithium reduces inflammation and oxidative stress. Dendrites that connect neurons to each other can be repaired. The neurotrophins promote higher volumes of gray matter through growth stimulation and the repair of brain cells.[256] Lithium lowers the concentration of abnormal *tau* **proteins** in cerebrospinal fluid that are associated with

---

[256] Moore, G. J., et al., "Lithium-Induced Increase in Human Grey Matter," *Lancet*, 2000, *356*(9237), 1241–1242.

dementia and Alzheimer's disease.[257] The **neurofibrillary tangles** and **plaques** found in Alzheimer's disease are produced less when lithium is present, reducing the enzyme called **glycogen synthase kinase-3 (GSK-3)** that is responsible for the tangles and plaques.[258] Some of these studies were performed on as little as 0.3–1.0 mg of lithium daily.

Lithium Supplements

A good dosage of lithium to take is 1–5 mg per day. No monitoring of blood levels is needed. Check with your doctor before taking lithium if you have a severe hypothyroid condition, renal failure, and dehydration.[259] Some unusual but reported side effects when starting lithium are dry mouth, metallic taste in the mouth, shaking hands, and tiredness.

Life Extension produces lithium in 1,000 mcg (1 mg) doses, with colostrum. Pure Encapsulations produces lithium orotate in 5 mg capsules. KAL lithium orotate is sold in 5 mg doses, as is Swanson lithium orotate. This is a much lower dose than prescription lithium, which is available in higher doses such as 150 mg, 300 mg, and 600 mg tablets and usually as lithium citrate or lithium carbonate, not as orotate. Orotate is usually reserved for over the counter, or OTC, preparations.

---

[257] Forlenza, O. V., et al., "Disease-Modifying Properties of Long-Term Lithium Treatment for Amnestic Mild Cognitive Impairment: Randomized Controlled Trial," *British Journal of Psychiatry*, 2011, *198*(5), 351–356.

[258] Takashima, A., "GSK-3 Is Essential in the Pathogenesis of Alzheimer's Disease," *Journal of Alzheimer's Disease*, 2006, *9*(3 Suppl), 309–317.

[259] NHS, "Lithium," n.d., https://www.nhs.uk/medicines/lithium/.

Magnesium

Benefits of Magnesium

- Protects against irregular heartbeats
- Relaxes muscles and tension
- Treats toxemia of pregnancy
- Improves premenstrual syndrome (PMS)
- Treats hypertension
- Reduces symptoms of fibromyalgia
- Treats migraine and cluster headache
- Improves exercise performance
- Alleviates leg cramps
- Relaxes the airways to relieve asthma
- Prevents kidney stones
- Promotes nerve conduction and treats seizures
- Required for bone and tooth structure
- Prevents osteoporosis
- Needed to treat and possibly prevent type 2 diabetes
- Relieves constipation

History of Magnesium

Magnesium is an alkaline earth metal with a symbol of **Mg**, an atomic number of 12, and a mass of 24.3. It may have come from a supernova with three helium atoms added to carbon to form the silvery white solid that makes up 2% of the earth's crust and is the third-most abundant element in seawater. It is often found in mineral waters and gives the water a sour or tart taste.

Magnesium is essential for all life. In plants, it forms part of the chlorophyll molecule and is necessary for the process of photosynthesis. In people and animals, it is necessary for the biological structures of DNA, RNA, and bones. More than 300 enzymatic processes require magnesium as a cofactor to function, including adenosine triphosphate (ATP) production.

Historically, magnesium was first described by the Greeks as *magnesia*, having been found in the district of the same name in Thessaly in northern Greece. It is found in mineral deposits of dolomite, magnesite, and mineral waters.

In 1618, a farmer had little luck in getting his cattle to drink water at Epsom in England because of the bitter taste from the high **magnesium sulfate (MgSO$_4$)** content of the water. However, he did observe that application of this water to rashes and scratches remedied the problems rapidly. Magnesium found other medicinal uses over time as a laxative, antacid, calming agent, and the first-line care for eclampsia, or toxemia of pregnancy.

Magnesium is found in seawater at about 12% of the concentration of sodium. Sea salt is not simple **sodium** and chloride (**NaCl**) but a mixture of the salts found in the water. Tropical water is saltier because of the evaporation of the water, the solvent. In temperate and cooler climates, the water is less salty from less evaporation, and near the poles, the addition of pure water from the icebergs melting into the ocean produces less salty water. Sea salts from different parts of the earth have different amounts of magnesium and other minerals, giving each variety its own claim to fame, such as salt from Okinawa, the Greek isles, and the Dead Sea.

Functions of Magnesium

The human body contains about 24 g of magnesium—60% is estimated to be in the bones to help give them rigidity and serve as a storage reserve of magnesium, 39% is intracellular, and only 1% is extracellular. The extracellular magnesium is mostly in the serum portion of the blood and has a concentration, normally, of 1.5 to 2.5 milligrams per deciliter (mg/dL). Unfortunately, measuring the concentration of magnesium in the blood does not accurately reflect or even estimate what is in the cells. This fact is apparent when simultaneous measurements of magnesium in both blood and tissue (hair analysis or red blood cells) are performed.

Magnesium comes in many forms and combinations with other anions. Magnesium is a +2 charged atom that often is found paired with chlorine, sulfate, gluconate, citrate, oxygen, and amino acids. Each product has its own characteristics, functions, and ability to interact or become part of the body. Each of these forms can be used as a function promoter, a supplement, or both. The most common and inexpensive form is magnesium oxide.

$$Mg^{2+} \quad O^{2-}$$

Magnesium Oxide

THE FORGOTTEN AND HIDDEN FACTS OF VITAMINS & MINERALS

This is found in cathartics, such as milk of magnesia, usually as a liquid, and it is irritating to the bowel. This promotes peristalsis of the bowel, encourages regularity, and is used to treat constipation. The most inexpensive form of supplemental magnesium is the oxide. **Magnesium oxide (MgO)** is really a lower dose and a pill form of milk of **magnesium hydroxide (H_2O_2Mg)**. Not much is absorbed, and it adds little to the serum or enzyme systems of the body.

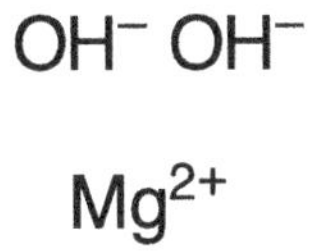

Magnesium Hydroxide

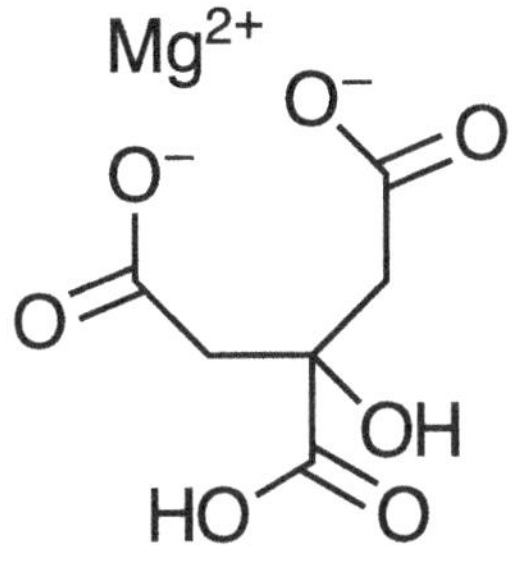

Magnesium Citrate

Magnesium citrate is a liquid form of magnesium, also used as a cathartic. It is better absorbed into the body, but not the best for raising blood levels.

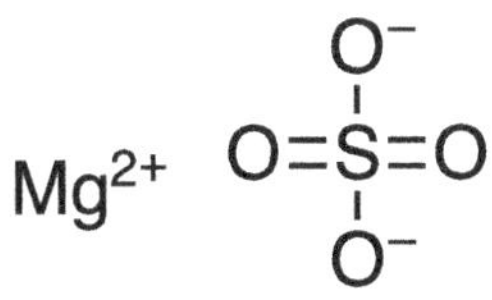

Magnesium Sulfate

Magnesium sulfate, also known as Epsom salt, has unique properties. It can be used topically to soak in, to be absorbed into the body to relax and soothe muscles. It can be ingested or injected to avert seizures and migraines and control heart rhythms and preeclampsia of pregnancy.

$$Cl^- \quad Cl^- \quad Mg^{2+}$$

Magnesium Chloride

Magnesium chloride has similar actions to those of sulfate, but the molecule is smaller.

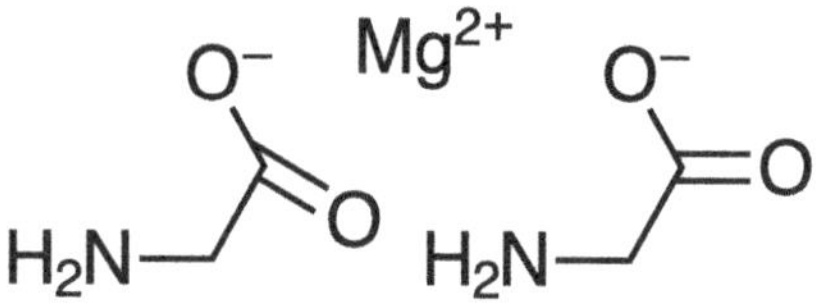

Magnesium Glycinate

The glycinate form of magnesium is a very absorbable oral preparation. It is a relatively new commercial preparation and is probably the most organic form of magnesium from the perspective of being easily absorbed and incorporated into enzymes. It is a unique preparation in that the anion portion of the molecule, glycine, is an essential amino acid. Essential amino acids are the building blocks of proteins. Absorption and assimilation are so efficient that the capsule form usually contains 120 mg of magnesium glycinate—compared to magnesium oxide, which is usually 500 mg in a compressed tablet.

Adenosine Triphosphate

Adenosine triphosphate (ATP) is the source or molecule that provides energy for most metabolic processes in the body. Magnesium is required to produce ATP in the mitochondria and is often made into an ATP magnesium complex to form **MgATP**. This is the mineral and energy packet that promotes many of the metabolic reactions in the body. It has a lot of influence on metabolic systems and, ultimately, on our health. A lack of magnesium has a significant effect on metabolic syndrome, hypertension, diabetes, heart rhythm, and nervous activity.

Magnesium at the Cellular Level

Magnesium is required for the assembly of DNA and RNA. It is necessary for the enzymes that produce nucleic acids and proteins. Enzymes that synthesize carbohydrates, lipids, and the antioxidant glutathione all require magnesium in one way or another.

Keeping our focus at the microscopic level, as pertains to magnesium, the cell and the cell wall are very much involved with this mineral. Besides being an element of intracellular concentration for enzyme activity, magnesium participates with what elements and molecules can pass through the cell wall. The cell wall is not just a barrier to define one compartment from another, but a membrane that controls a gradient of concentration of what is in the cell and what is exterior to the cell.

The cell wall is an active energy-consuming structure of the cell that maintains elements in the proper concentrations, both inside and outside of the cell. For example, in the wall of the cell is a pump that transports sodium out of the cell and a pump that transports potassium into the cell. Normal blood tests report the elements in the extracellular fluid to be 135–146 milliequivalents per liter (mEq/L) of sodium and 3.5–5.3 mEq/L of potassium. Inside the cell, the concentrations are nearly reversed. Intracellular sodium is 12 mEq/L, and potassium is 140 mEq/L. Other trace elements such as calcium, magnesium, manganese, and chloride move about to maintain a near-balanced electrical charge of the cell. Most cells normally have a net negative charge.

Calcium Channel Blockers

In addition to the sodium pump and the potassium pump there is a calcium pump. This pump has a significant effect on blood pressure and muscle contractility and an effect on many enzyme systems in the body. In the 1980s, a new class of drugs called calcium channel blockers was developed. They were called channel blockers for the blocking action they promoted at the cell wall. They were used for problems such as hypertension and angina, or chest pain, and to control aberrant rhythms such as tachycardia and flutter.

All these pumps are interrelated, and the action of one affects the others. The effect of channel blockers was not new—the only thing new was that now synthetic chemicals could do what magnesium could do. Magnesium is the ultimate calcium channel blocker. When there is not enough magnesium, calcium is permitted to enter the cell and interfere with the function of the cellular enzymes. Calcium takes the place of magnesium as the cofactor of enzymes and inhibits the normal enzymatic action. This is aging at the cellular level.

Proper magnesium levels must be maintained to correct problems such as hypertension, abnormal heart rhythms, muscle spasms, seizure activity, and bronchial spasm that produce asthma. Magnesium is also needed to prevent calcium deposits in arterial plaque and joint spaces and the development of osteoporosis. Aging is marked by calcium being in all the wrong places. Much of this can be prevented by supplying the body with the required magnesium.

Measuring Magnesium Levels

An indirect method of measuring magnesium is to do a blood-level test to check whether it is between 1.5 milligrams per deciliter (mg/dL) and 2.5 mg/dL. Hair analysis or red blood cell (RBC) magnesium analysis provides a much better evaluation of what is in the body. The RBC magnesium reference range is 3.9–5.9 nanograms per milliliter (ng/mL). Only 1% of the magnesium in the body is in the blood, and a small error here can be magnified 100 times if you are trying to judge the body stores. The body is always trying to keep the magnesium level in the blood in a narrow range at the expense of the bones, where 65% of magnesium is normally found.[260] Thirty four percent of the magnesium remains in the cells of the body to participate in the structure of DNA, RNA, ATP, and regulation of calcium and as a cofactor in enzymatic reactions.

Diabetes

Non-insulin-dependent diabetes mellitus (NIDDM; type 2 diabetes) and hypertension are both characterized by low intracellular magnesium concentrations and elevated calcium concentrations. This may suggest a common link to those problems, which are referred to as **metabolic syndrome**.

Magnesium is not known to be under the regulation of any specific hormone, but effects have been noticed. **Adrenaline** and **noradrenaline** affect magnesium uptake depending on the type of cell affected. An increase in either of these hormones causes fat cells to take up magnesium, where it reduces the uptake in heart muscle cells.[261] The net effect on heart muscle is increased excitability, promoting extra beats or rapid rhythms.

It has been demonstrated that insulin, after acting on its own receptor on the cell membrane, increases the entry of both magnesium and potassium into the cell. As insulin receptors are lost, intracellular magnesium diminishes, further inhibiting normal cellular metabolism.

Magnesium balance in and out of cells is regulated not by one hormone but by many. The most significant is insulin, with a lesser effect from adrenaline and noradrenaline. Vitamin D can slightly increase intestinal absorption of magnesium.[262]

---

[260] Paolisso, G., and Barbagallo, M., "Hypertension, Diabetes Mellitus, and Insulin Resistance: The Role of Intracellular Magnesium," *American Journal of Hypertension*, 1997, 10(3), 346–355.
[261] Ibid.
[262] Higdon, J., et al., "Magnesium," Linus Pauling Institute, Oregon State University, last updated November 2018,
https://lpi.oregonstate.edu/mic/minerals/magnesium.

Magnesium has been repeatedly demonstrated to affect both **insulin-dependent diabetes mellitus (IDDM; type 1 diabetes)** and NIDDM.[263] The Nurses' Health Study showed that taking magnesium decreased the incidence of NIDDM.[264] Laboratory studies designed to feed animals a magnesium-depleted diet have induced severe insulin resistance.[265] It is clear that in any way diabetes is approached—through diet, pills, or insulin—magnesium is a significant factor and should be monitored and supplemented as necessary.

Anyone with diabetes must measure their own blood sugar (glucose) levels. Portable instruments are cheap and easy to use and record the readings to help better design treatment plans. Besides measuring glucose and **hemoglobin A-1-C**, patients' magnesium levels should frequently be measured to obtain optimal control. In my own practice, I also stress other factors that influence glucose control, such as type of carbohydrates, gluten sensitivity, hormone replacement in the form of testosterone, and exercise.

Exercise

I myself am not a sportsman and have little interest in athletics. But I must say that from treating patients over the years, some sort of physical activity is necessary to keep the body functioning well and to maintain range of motion and flexibility to keep the joints free of pain. When I prescribe an exercise program, I do not expect someone to join a gym, spend money on exercise equipment, and spend hours in training. Life is too busy, and you have better things to do with your time.

---

[263] Djurhuus, M. S., et al., "Magnesium Deficiency in Patients with Type 1 (Insulin Dependent) Diabetes Mellitus," *Diabetes*, 1994, *4* (suppl 1), 259A; Schmidt, L., and Heins, J., "Low Magnesium Intake Among NIDDM Patients: A Call for Concern," *Diabetes*, 1993, *42*(suppl 1), 49A.
[264] Colditz, G. A., et al., "Diet and Risk of Clinical Diabetes in Women," *American Journal of Clinical Nutrition*, 1993, *55*, 1018–1023.
[265] Suárez, A., et al., "Impaired Tyrosine-Kinase Activity of Muscle Insulin Receptors from Hypomagnesaemia Rats," *Diabetologia*, 1995, *38*, 1262–1270.

My exercise prescription is that when you get out of bed in the morning, start the day with some quick stretches—fingers to toes, and reach as far as you can. Push-ups are good, but start with a small number, 5 or 10. If you are out of shape and even this is too much, do them on your knees, and then in maybe six months, graduate to 15 to 20 push-ups. Then, do them on your hands and toes.

The point is that this whole process should not take more than 5 to 10 minutes a day. You are not training for a marathon—you are keeping yourself in good enough shape that if you trip and fall on the floor, you can get up. If you have to move quickly to avoid danger, you can. As soon as you complete your five-minute exercise program, you can get your morning coffee or juice and start your day. If you do not prioritize exercise as the first thing you do each day, you will never find a place in your day for it.

My experience is that a modest exercise program is far more beneficial than any drug. It sounds too easy and inexpensive, but it is true. If you start modestly, it is nontoxic and has nearly no side effects.

Calcium Kidney Stones

Calcium kidney stones can be prevented with magnesium. Calcium stones form when too much calcium is excreted by the kidneys and precipitated in the urine-collecting system. The kidneys regulate the acidity of the body, in unison with the lungs. The lungs work on a more immediate balance, while the kidneys have a much slower and more long-term effect. If the body's pH or acidity must be reduced, the kidneys release a positive ion in the urine to achieve balance. There is a priority as to which positive ion is released first. The priority is based on the **electromotive force of the element**, known as its charge. The lower the charge, the more likely it is to be released. The table that follows lists the ions released by the kidneys and their electrode potential.[266]

Ions Released by the Kidneys and Their Electrode Potential	
Ion	Electrode potential (V)
Magnesium^{++}	2.40
Sodium$^+$	2.71
Calcium^{++}	2.87
Potassium$^+$	2.92

Normally, if sufficient magnesium is available, it would be released first, followed by sodium and then calcium. This happens continuously as the body tries to keep all the ions in their normal respective concentrations in the blood. If there is not enough magnesium to excrete, sodium will be pulled from the tissues; if not enough sodium is available, calcium will be pulled from the bones. A lack of magnesium in the diet will promote kidney stone formation at the expense of the bones, and taking calcium from the bones promotes early osteoporosis. Sufficient dietary magnesium is necessary because magnesium will always be eliminated first.

My experience of preventing kidney stones with magnesium has been successful. Kidney stones can easily be treated with 240 mg of magnesium glycinate daily.

Remember, there are two magnesium levels that must be watched. The most common one is the **serum magnesium** level; this is the blood level of magnesium. The most important one is **red**

---

[266] Hodgman, C. D., et al., *Handbook of Chemistry and Physics*, 22nd edition, Chemical Rubber Company, 1937.

blood cell magnesium (RBC magnesium). This is the tissue stores, or what is found in the cells that are available for enzyme function. It is possible to have normal serum magnesium and low RBC magnesium. Anyone with a history of kidney stones should know their levels and should be treated with magnesium glycinate.

Migraine Headaches

Magnesium recently has been used to treat migraine headaches. An oral dose is taken for maintenance, while a 1–2 g dose is administered intravenously for acute episodes.

Asthma

Asthma has many causes and just as many treatments. The most important factor to understand about asthma is the early and late phases of bronchial constriction. The general understanding of asthma is that it is a reaction to an irritant such as a gas, dust, or protein like pollen or dander or a reaction to an injection of pharmaceutical products. Today, doctors use therapeutics that are far more selective than aminophylline and theophylline, which were used in the past. The newer drugs treat only the **early phase of asthma**; this is called **bronchospasm**. The small muscles of the bronchial airways constrict, narrowing the diameter of the lumen, restricting the release of the trapped air. Magnesium helps relax the bronchial muscles, opening up the airways and giving some relief. Magnesium cannot do this by itself, but it does improve the efficacy of the newer drugs such as albuterol and isoproterenol.

The **late phase of asthma** occurs about 10 to 12 hours after the early phase. The wheezing in the chest sounds exactly like the early phase of asthma produced by the reduced airway diameter and restricted airflow. The cause is much different, and the newer drugs do not treat it. Typically, the inhaler will be effective at 9:00 a.m., but at midnight, the inhaler is totally useless. Many children died until it was recognized that the cause of the reduced airway diameter in the late phase was **bronchial wall edema** or swelling. The walls of the bronchus swelled to the point that the airway became restricted or totally obstructed, causing asphyxiation. This could have been prevented if inhaled steroids were given with the albuterol or isoproterenol in the early phase or the late phase could be treated with **epinephrine** to immediately treat the swelling.

In the earlier days of asthma treatment, aminophylline and theophylline treated both the early and late phases of asthma. The medical community did not realize this until more selective drugs were developed and the two phases were recognized.

Preeclampsia of Pregnancy

Preeclampsia of pregnancy is defined as the development of hypertension, albuminuria, and edema between the 20th week of pregnancy and the 1st week postpartum. **Eclampsia** is the term used if seizures or coma develops with the preeclampsia. These two conditions are treated with 2–4 g of magnesium sulfate ($MgSO_4$) in one liter of lactated Ringer's solution given rapidly until the relief of seizures, lowering of the blood pressure, and increase of urinary output.[267]

Magnesium Absorption and Intake

Gastrointestinal disorders and issues, such as celiac disease, malabsorption syndromes, Crohn's disease, and inflammation from radiation treatments, are usually responsible for poor magnesium absorption. Magnesium is absorbed in the small intestine and excreted in the urine or lost in the bowel. Unfortunately, less is absorbed with age, and more is excreted with age. Diuretics accelerate the excretion of magnesium, as does alcoholism, diabetes,

---

[267] *The Merck Manual*, 14th edition, 1982, 1727.

kidney disease, intense physical activity, stress, and agents such as cisplatin, a chemotherapeutic drug, and dietetics.

Low levels of magnesium affect diabetes. Taking too much zinc, in excess of 142 mg a day, will block the absorption of magnesium, as does too much fiber or a low-protein diet that includes less than 30 g of protein a day.[268]

When it comes to magnesium intake, our major problem today is our diet. Highly processed foods devoid of magnesium or food from magnesium-poor soils have no nutritional benefit. The soil is worked again and again, depleting it and reducing the mineral content, magnesium in particular. The **nutrition facts label** on cans and packages do not list magnesium, a reflection of the standard American diet (SAD). Most processed foods are nutrient depleted, with the nutrients washed out during processing. If you see the term **fortified**, it means that the damage of preparation was so severe that a feeble attempt was made to add some nutritional value to the product. This is common with breads and cereals.

Symptoms of low magnesium (below 1.0 mg/dL) are muscle spasms, high blood pressure, headaches, and loss of appetite, nausea, and/or vomiting.

Food sources of magnesium include green leafy vegetables such as spinach and kale, almonds, cashews, beans, and grains.

---

[268] Higdon, J., et al., "Magnesium," Linus Pauling Institute, Oregon State University, last updated November 2018, https://lpi.oregonstate.edu/mic/minerals/magnesium.

Recommended Dietary Allowance of Magnesium

The recommended dietary allowance (RDA) is the minimum intake of magnesium for good health. In fact, more may be needed to be at the optimal level of peak performance. This is just the starting point to avoid problems such as hypertension and to stop the development of diabetes, fibromyalgia, asthma, irregular heartbeats, seizures, menstrual cramps, migraine headaches, and osteoporosis. The table below is the RDA for magnesium by the Food and Nutrition Board of the National Academy of Medicine.

Recommended Dietary Allowance (RDA) for Magnesium			
Life stage	Age	Male (mg/day)	Female (mg/day)
Infant	0–6 months	30	30
	7–12 months	75	75
Child	1–3 years	80	80
	4–8 years	130	130
	9–13 years	240	240
Adolescent	14–18 years	410	360
Adult	19–30 years	400	310
	31 years and older	420	320

Magnesium Supplements

Common forms of over-the-counter magnesium are powders, tablets, capsules, creams, and ointments, and it can be found in water. Products can contain the following:

- Magnesium oxide (MgO)
- Magnesium sulfate ($MgSO_4$)
- Magnesium carbonate ($MgCHO_3$)
- Magnesium gluconate ($C_{12}H_{22}MgO_{14}$)
- Magnesium aspartate ($C_8H_{12}MgN_2O_8$)
- Magnesium citrate ($C_6H_6O_7Mg$)
- Trimagnesium dicitrate ($C_{12}H_{10}Mg_3O_4$)
- The chelated forms magnesium glycinate ($C_4H_8MgN_2O_4$) and magnesium orotate ($C_{10}H_6MgN_4O_8$)

Mineral waters that contain dissolved magnesium include the following:

- San Pellegrino (56 mg/L)
- Evian (24 mg/L)
- Fiji (13 mg/L)
- Perrier (3 mg/L)
- Poland Spring (1 mg/L)

Over-the-counter cathartics include the following:

- Milk of magnesia (MoM), which is magnesium hydroxide (H2MgO2)
- Magnesium citrate (C6H6O7Mg)

Magnesium sulfate ($MgSO_4$) is regularly used in the hospital and office settings, intravenously or intramuscularly, to treat eclampsia and preeclampsia (1–4 g intravenously), a complication of pregnancy. It is also used to treat a form of ventricular tachycardia known as **torsade de pointes** and rapid atrial fibrillation (1–10 g).

Several conditions and drugs may cause a loss of magnesium. If food is produced on land with a low mineral content or that has been over farmed, the produce will have low mineral content. The processing of food washes out magnesium. Diuretics, cisplatin chemotherapy, diabetic acidosis, and adrenal or thyroid overactivity also cause magnesium loss.

DermaMag is a magnesium skin lotion that contains 31% magnesium chloride that is absorbable through the skin. The topical application of this lotion prevents the unpleasant side effects of muscle cramping and diarrhea.

Potassium

Benefits of Potassium

- Helps lower blood pressure
- Normal levels prevent strokes
- Necessary to conduct nerve impulses and muscle contractions and regulate the heartbeat

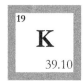

History of Potassium

Potassium is an element with the symbol **K** and atomic number 19. Its atomic weight is 39.10. In its elemental state, this soft white metal reacts almost instantly with oxygen from the air. It can split the water molecule to attach to the oxygen atom, in the process liberating the hydrogen atom. Potassium was discovered by Sir Humphry Davy in 1807 through the electrolysis of potash. Potash, or pot ash, is from the Dutch word *potasch* used to refer to wood ash or the ashes from the burning of wood.

Potassium is found in the body as a positively charged ion. It is a mineral that is classified as an **electrolyte** because it dissolves in water and conducts electrical current. It is necessary for many metabolic reactions, the passage of nerve impulses, and electrical signaling. It is found primarily in the cell and is less concentrated in the extracellular fluid.

Organic material is a good source of potassium because it is found in the cells of plants and animals. Adding water to ash in large iron pots liberates potassium as **potassium hydroxide (KOH)** and **potassium carbonate (K_2CO_3)**. Mineral sources of potassium come from the mines of Strassfurt in Saxony-Anhalt, Germany, as **kainite ($MgSO_4 \cdot KCl \cdot 3H_2O$)**, sylvan **(KCl)**, and **carnallite ($KCl \cdot MgCl_2 \cdot 6H_2O$)**.

Dietary sources of potassium include fruits and vegetables, nuts, seeds, and dairy products. Examples include potatoes, apricots, plums, prunes, raisins, lima beans, bananas, acorn squash, orange juice, grapefruits, and almonds.

Functions of Potassium

All life requires potassium for mostly intracellular function. Sodium provides an electrical charge outside of the cell, and potassium provides the internal charge. The difference between the two electrolytes creates potential in the cell wall, or an electrical gradient between the internal and external environment of the cell. This is key to the integrity and function of the cell and organism. Normal muscle and nerve cells have a range of -75 to -95 millivolts, with -85 millivolts as the average gradient between the interior and the exterior of the cell wall.[269] This gradient is maintained by **channels** in the cell wall that, with the expenditure of **adenosine triphosphate (ATP)** energy packets, pump sodium out of the cell and potassium into the cell. The cell wall is not just a bag to contain

---

[269] Guyton, A. C., *Textbook of Physiology*, 4th edition (illustrated), Saunders, 1971, 55.

the contents of the cell but an active **organelle**[270] that maintains the chemical balance and electrical charge.

The production of an electrical impulse is a passive event during which energy is given off from the charged state to the lower, less charged state. Sodium falls into the cell and potassium leaks out of the cell, releasing energy for a nerve impulse. The channels, often referred to as pumps, are where the sodium and potassium are pumped to increase their concentration and produce an electrical gradient. Other pumps have been identified in the cell wall besides the potassium channel and the sodium channel. An example is the calcium channel, which has been found to be a significant factor in blood pressure control. Channels have also been found for magnesium and trace metals such as manganese, silicon, molybdenum, and vanadium.

A lack of potassium promotes high blood pressure, low calcium levels, and kidney stones and worsens diabetes myelitis. It is also needed as a cofactor for enzymes and the maintenance of cell membrane potential.

Hypertension

A clinical trial comparing the **DASH (Dietary Approaches to Stop Hypertension) diet** to the **standard American diet (SAD)** demonstrated that a diet higher in potassium lowered blood pressure.[271] The DASH diet provides 8.5 servings per day of fruits and vegetables, which delivers 4,100 mg per day of potassium; the SAD diet provides only 3.5 servings per day of fruits and vegetables and 1,700 mg per day of potassium. In people with hypertension, the DASH diet lowered their systolic blood pressure by 11.4 mmHg

---

[270] A biological structure that performs a distinctive function inside a cell.
[271] Appel, L. J., et al., "A Clinical Trial of the Effects of Dietary Patterns on Blood Pressure. DASH Collaborative Research Group," *New England Journal of Medicine*, 1997, *336*(16), 1117–1124, https://doi.org/10.1056/nejm199704173361601.

and their diastolic blood pressure by 5.5 mmHg. In people without hypertension, systolic pressure decreased by 3.5 mmHg and diastolic by 2.1 mmHg. These are excellent results for a nutritional approach, and the outcome rivals results obtained by some commercial drugs.

Stroke

Strokes come in two basic forms: **hemorrhagic** and **ischemic (thrombotic or embolic)** strokes. A hemorrhagic stroke occurs when a blood vessel in the brain bursts and blood bleeds into the brain tissue, disrupting blood flow, the transport of oxygen, and brain function. The more common form of stroke is the embolic stroke, which occurs when a blood clot enters an artery of the brain, disrupting blood flow, the transport of oxygen, and brain function. A thrombotic stroke occurs when the blood clot in the artery of the brain developed in the artery that is affected; an embolic stroke refers to a stroke caused by a clot that develops in either the carotid artery or the heart and then travels to the brain.

Most studies of strokes are observational; they review the current medical condition and prior medical records to construct the conditions that were present before the stroke. Some of this data can be collected from **prospective studies**, in which groups of patients (we like to call these groups **cohorts**) are studied using regular exams and bloodwork to look for the development of conditions that would be expected at a certain age or stage of life. A meta-analysis[272] of nine prospective studies showed that people with a daily intake of potassium of between 3,510 mg and 4,680 mg had a 30% lower chance of a stroke.[273]

---

[272] A meta-analysis reviews previous research to form conclusions about the body of research.
[273] Aburto, N. J., et al., "Effect of Increased Potassium Intake on Cardiovascular Risk Factors and Disease: Systemic Review and Meta-Analysis," *BMJ*, 2013, *346*, f1378, https://doi.org/10.1136/bmj.f1378.

Potassium Levels

Medically, doctors take low levels of potassium and especially elevated levels of potassium very seriously. A normal potassium level in the blood is 3.5–5.4 milliequivalents per liter (mEq/L).

Potassium deficiency can be caused by a potent diuretic, diarrhea, or vomiting. Initial symptoms can be muscle weakness and nausea, and a deficiency can lead to the development of heart failure.

Excessive potassium can develop because of the failure of the kidneys to excrete potassium or the ingestion of too much supplemental potassium. Too much potassium will cause stomach irritation, progressing to nausea, and irregular heartbeats. Very high levels of potassium are dangerous. Irregular heartbeats can progress to cardiac arrest and death. To put the danger of elevated potassium levels in perspective, high concentrations of potassium chloride are used for execution by lethal injection.

Under normal conditions, the body can safely handle up to 18 g of potassium a day from fruit and vegetables. It is extremely difficult to reach toxicity from potassium-rich foods such as oranges, kiwis, bananas, and potatoes. Usually, kidney failure or excessive supplementation of potassium via pills or liquids taken orally or intravenous injection are necessary before this happens. The US Food and Drug Administration (FDA) limits over-the-counter (OTC) potassium to doses of less than 100 mg. A prescription dosage of potassium is 10 milliequivalents (mEq) or 20 mEq daily. The 10 mEq dose equals 750 mg of potassium, and 20 mEq equals 1,500 mg of potassium.

Potassium Supplements

The safest form of potassium is from fruits and vegetables. But before upping your potassium intake even with fruit and vegetables, check with your doctor and get a blood test to measure your potassium level. Having renal failure or even mild renal insufficiency can keep you from eliminating excess potassium. Several medications can increase potassium levels.

- **ACE inhibitors**, a class of blood pressure medication (e.g., captopril, enalapril, Acezide, lisinopril, and Lotensin), can provoke potassium levels above 5.4 milliequivalents per liter (mEq/L), a condition known as **hyperpotassium** or **hyperkalemia**.
- **Beta blockers** such as propranolol (Inderal), atenolol (Tenormin), metoprolol, and carvedilol (Coreg) also increase potassium.
- **Nonsteroidal anti-inflammatory drugs (NSAIDs)**, which include aspirin, ibuprofen, naproxen, indomethacin, and ketorolac, produce a slight elevation in potassium.
- **Potassium-sparing diuretics**, which include spironolactone (Aldactone), triamterene (Dyrenium), and amiloride (Midamor), have the unique ability to cause the kidneys to excrete sodium before excreting potassium.

A low blood level of potassium, below 3.5 mEq/L, is known as **hypopotassium** or **hypokalemia**. Potassium can be supplemented with fruits and vegetables as the first choice, but also with tablets, liquids, and powders.

Nature Made Potassium Gluconate capsules contain 550 mg of active ingredients, of which 90 mg is potassium and 460 mg is gluconate. Remember that only 99 mg can be sold over the counter without a prescription by order of the FDA. KAL produces Potassium 99 Chloride; each tablet, according to the label, supplies 99 mg of potassium. BulkSupplements.com produces potassium citrate in powder form, with 275 mg, equal to $1/10^{th}$ of an ounce of powder, delivers 98 mg of potassium.

Salt substitutes are potassium, although this is not implied in the name. These are formulated products designed for someone who wants to avoid sodium because they have hypertension. MySALT Substitute is 100% potassium chloride (KCl) and lysine with no sodium. It can be substituted 1:1 for table salt (NaCl), and ¼ of a teaspoon of MySALT is 1 g in weight but contains 356 mg of potassium and 644 mg of chloride and lysine. Additionally, MySALT produces its salt substitute with flavorings of garlic, ground ginger, green chili, coriander, horseradish, and lime peel.

Pharmaceutical manufacturers produce potassium in dosages greater than 100 mg that require a prescription and, I hope, monitoring and professional guidance. An example is Klor-Con Extended-Release Tablets, which are potassium chloride (KCl) in a wax matrix in dosages of 8 mEq (600 mg) and 10 mEq (750 mg). The wax matrix is part of the delayed-delivery system. It is not absorbed, so it slowly liberates the potassium for absorption; the wax is passed on to the stool. Sometimes, the potassium cannot be liberated from the wax matrix because of a lack of digestive juices and poor intestinal peristalsis. This delivery system may not serve all patients well, and blood monitoring is necessary to measure the results.

Potassium chloride comes in powder or sprinkle form, in 20–25 mEq doses. The powder should be dissolved in 4 oz. of water so that it does not cause local irritation. Liquid potassium chloride comes in a solution of concentrations of 10% (1.3 mEq/mL) and 20% (2.6 mEq/mL), and like the powder, it must be diluted in 4 oz. of water or juice. The unpleasant taste of this product makes it unpopular. **Potassium citrate** and **potassium gluconate** are other oral forms.

Potassium replacement is not a task for medical hobbyists. If you think you need potassium, I urge you to seek professional guidance and laboratory testing by your physician.

Selenium

Benefits of Selenium

- Converts thyroid T4 to T3; supports iodine metabolism
- Prevents prostate cancer
- Reduces the incidence of bladder cancer
- Prevents cataract development
- Helps with protein production
- Increases energy
- Delays degenerative diseases
- Reduces muscle pain
- Treats acute pancreatitis and supports the normal function of the pancreas
- Assists with heavy metal detoxification
- Required in trace amounts to activate antioxidant enzymes
- Prevents oxidation of lipids, reducing cardiovascular disease
- Protects against cold sores and shingles
- Protects against rheumatoid arthritis
- Reduces asthmatic attacks

History of Selenium

Selenium was discovered by a Swedish chemist, Baron Jons Jakob Berzelius, in 1817. However, significant medical interest in selenium did not begin with the discovery of selenium but stemmed from epidemiology studies. In some parts of northern Nebraska and the Dakotas, the selenium content of the soil is highly concentrated. Plants absorb selenium but do not require it for growth, and it has no effect on them. For livestock this is different—some areas are so high in selenium that the land is unfit for grazing.

Selenium has the symbol **Se**, an atomic number of 34, and a weight of 78.9. It is in the sulfur family; it is considered to be a nonmetal and has similar characteristics to sulfur. Its physical appearance can be amorphous, crystalline, or metal-like, and it ranges in color from red to gray. Produced as a by-product of copper refining, selenium is used commercially in the vulcanization of rubber and the production of glass and electronic components. It is unique among the elements in that it conducts electric current proportional to the amount of light shining on its surface. This property was first discovered in 1873 by Willoughby Smith.

Functions of Selenium

Selenium is a mineral that associates with enzymes to perform several well-defined functions in the body. It boosts immunity, prevents oxidation, reduces the development and growth of cancer, is required for hormone production, reduces muscle pain, and increases energy. It inhibits the cross-linking of proteins, which is responsible for loss of tissue elasticity and cataract formation.

Selenium is an essential mineral, required in trace amounts for health and disease prevention. It is obtained in the diet mostly from foods that come from the soil. The content of selenium in the food is directly related to the selenium content of soil. If farmers are using nitrogen, phosphorous, and potassium (NPK) fertilizers to increase yields from depleted soil, the grains, fruits, and vegetables produced will contain fewer minerals. They may be larger and take the blue ribbon at the county fair, but the nutritional value will be inferior. This classic example of this is the 200-pound pumpkin grown by the farmer's son after applying too much fertilizer.

The selenium content of soil varies even in two adjacent fields because of water runoff, farming, and the natural distribution of selenium. According to the 17th edition of *The Merck Manual*, Americans and Canadians consume 100–250 mcg of selenium per day. In contrast, the inhabitants of New Zealand and Finland average 30–50 mcg per day, and people in some parts of China may consume as little as 10–15 mcg per day.[274]

Nutritional studies were conducted in Lin Xian, China, to determine whether selenium added to the diet might reduce the incidence of cancer. Researchers in the original 5-year study tested beta-carotene versus beta-carotene and 50 mcg of selenium. The results were so impressive that the National Cancer Institute

---

[274] *The Merck Manual*, 17th edition, 1999, 54.

conducted a second 10-year study with 1,312 volunteers taking 200 mcg of selenium daily. The findings showed a 49% decrease in lung, prostate, and colorectal cancers.[275] After this second, attention-grabbing study, selenium garnered more interest.

Selenium is incorporated into many different enzymes called **selenoproteins**, or **selenoenzymes**. At least 35 proteins have been identified, but we know what only about half of them do. Enzymes help promote chemical reactions in the body at a low temperature, without resorting to adding heat like we would in a laboratory experiment. Usually, a chemical reaction either requires the addition of heat to make it happen or gives off heat. Human biological systems perform most chemical reactions at 98.6 degrees Fahrenheit. The chemical reactions are slower, and the process is more controlled.

Selenium is incorporated into amino acid molecules, such as **methionine** and **cysteine**, not as a salt but by substitution into the structure of the molecule. These are then incorporated into the DNA and RNA.

The importance of selenium to human health has been appreciated only in the last 30 years, and many conditions have been linked to low selenium levels. It may be regarded as a trace element, no doubt, but it is now considered an **essential trace element**. The recommended dietary allowance (RDA) is 55 mcg a day, but the optimal amount is above 200 mcg per day to yield a blood level above 135 mcg/L. Below 85 mcg/L is considered low. This optimal level has a positive effect on reproduction, growth, muscle function,

---

[275] Clark, L. C., et al., "Effects of Selenium Supplementation for Cancer Prevention in Patients with Carcinoma of the Skin. A Randomized Controlled Trial. Nutritional Prevention of Cancer Study Group," *Journal of the American Medical Association*, 1996, *276*(24), 1957–1963.

immunocompetence, controlling seizures, slowing cognitive decline, and Alzheimer's disease.[276]

Antioxidant Action

Selenoenzymes participate in many reduction and oxidation, or redox, reactions in the body. The main function of selenium, I would say, is that it is a super antioxidant, more powerful than vitamin E and C, but never working alone. The safety range of selenium from the daily recommended allowance (DRA) to the upper limit (UL) is narrow, whereas the latitude of vitamins E and C is broad in terms of micrograms and milligrams.

Selenoenzymes work in the cells to maintain the redox processes at a balanced and orderly rate. Too much oxidation, and early aging will occur; too much reduction, and the processes of living will fail. The best-known selenoenzymes are glutathione peroxidases, thioredoxin reductases, iodothyronine deiodinases, and selenophosphate synthetase.

Glutathione peroxidase keeps the glutathione in the reduced form. **Glutathione** is the body's number one molecule that protects against oxidation from peroxides. It maintains cell membranes and prevents the cross-linking of molecules that develops into loss of elasticity of collagen and cataract development.

Thioredoxin reductase rejuvenates **dehydroascorbate**, the oxidized form of vitamin C, to ascorbic acid. It has a similar effect on ubiquinol, reducing it to the active form of coenzyme Q10.[277]

---

[276] Rayman, M. P., "The Importance of Selenium to Human Health," *Lancet*, 2000, *356*(9225), 233–241.
[277] Passwater, R. A., "SeNRC," DrPasswater.com, accessed September 20, 2009, website no longer available.

Thyroid Hormones

Iodothyronine deiodinases, of which there are three forms, D1, D2, and D3, convert thyroid hormones to the appropriate form, and iodine is needed for activation and deactivation. Thyroxin, or T4 as it is referred to because it contains four atoms of iodine, is produced in the thyroid. T3, or triiodothyronine, is the more active of the two thyroid hormones. Small amounts of T3 are produced in the thyroid, but it is primarily produced outside of the thyroid by removing one iodine atom from thyroxin. This conversion of T4 to T3 is dependent on selenium in the form of selenoenzymes. Selenium deficiency leads to T3 hypothyroidism and poor processing of the thyroid metabolic products.

The selenium enzymes are also involved with thyroid-controlled processes of pregnancy, formation and function of the placenta, fetal development of the skin, and the central nervous system.[278]

Prostate Health

In a double-blind cancer prevention trial at the University of Arizona, reported in 1998, the researchers found that selenium supplementation reduced the incidence of prostate cancer by 63%. A total of 974 men were followed for over six years; 18 members of the treatment group developed prostate cancers, compared to 35 in the placebo group.[279]

Although selenium reduces the incidence of prostate cancer, it does not affect *prostate-specific antigen* **(PSA)** levels. Prostate cancer is diagnosed by taking a biopsy, or sample, of the tissue of the prostate, looking at it under a microscope to look for abnormal

---

[278] Ibid.
[279] Clark, C. L., et al., "Decreased Incidence of Prostate Cancer with Selenium Supplementation: Results of a Double-Blind Cancer Prevention Trial," *British Journal of Urology*, 1998, *81*(5), 730–734.

cells with abnormal and dark-staining nuclear material, and chemically staining the tissue to assess the chemical makeup. PSA is an enzyme produced by the epithelial cells of the prostate and referred to as a **tumor marker**. Its presence does not confirm a diagnosis of prostate cancer, but it is usually found with this cancer. In the SU.VI.MAX trial, the investigators showed that supplementation with selenium, vitamin E, or both decreased the incidence of prostate cancer but had no effect on PSA levels.[280] This is further evidence that PSA is associated with the prostate but does not indicate or measure cancer.

An often-overlooked risk factor for the development of prostate cancer, besides family history, age, and race, is having a low testosterone level.[281] The field of oncology has not addressed the subject of cancer and hormones beyond saying that men should not use hormones. In my experience with treating patients, if they have a good hormone profile, they are healthier. A prostate selenoprotein occurs in the prostate, and selenium participates in the production of testosterone and pituitary and adrenal hormones.[282]

Similar studies in Sweden, a country that generally has low soil selenium levels, found a higher risk for **benign prostate hypertrophy (BPH)** and prostate cancer in patients with low selenium blood levels.[283] Additionally, low selenium levels have been associated with spermatozoa with poor motility, where the midpiece

---

[280] Meyer, F., et al., "Antioxidant Vitamin and Mineral Supplementation and Prostate Cancer Prevention in the SU.VI.MAX Trial," *International Journal of Cancer*, 2005, *116*(2), 182–186.
[281] Morgentaler, A., *Testosterone for Life*, McGraw-Hill, 2008.
[282] Bedwal, R. S., et al., "Selenium—Its Biological Perspectives," *Medical Hypotheses*, 1993, *41*(2), 150–159; Potmis, R. A., et al., "Effect of Selenium (Se) on Plasma ACTH, Beta-Endorphin, Cortisosterone, and Glucose in Rat: Influence of Adrenal Enucleation and Metyrapone Pretreatment," *Toxicology*, 1993, *79*(1), 1–9.
[283] Hardell, L., et al., "Levels of Selenium in Plasma and Glutathione Peroxidase in Erythrocytes in Patients with Prostate Cancer or Benign Hyperplasia," *European Journal of Cancer Prevention*, 1995, *4*(1), 91–96.

of the tail breaks off and they are poor swimmers.[284] Likewise, low selenium has been found in idiopathic miscarriages of the first trimester and recurrent miscarriages.[285]

Selenophosphate synthetase catalyzes inorganic selenides with adenosine monophosphate (AMP) to a selenophosphate, and that becomes a donor of selenium to cysteine, to become selenocysteine.

Eight selenoproteins have been found in artery walls, eight in brain tissue, and nine in the testis. The medical community has little knowledge about their function at this time.[286]

Selenium Toxicity

Like other nutrients, especially minerals, selenium toxicity occurs if too much is taken. Selenium poisoning is known as **selenosis**. Symptoms include dermatitis, loss of hair follicles, abnormal nails, and peripheral neuropathy. Usually, these symptoms are associated with plasma levels greater than 100 mcg/dL (1 mg/L). That blood level can be achieved by ingesting more than 900 mcg per day. This is not much more than the adult optimal recommendation of 200–400 mcg per day.

When working with minerals, it is best to be knowledgeable about minimal amounts to prevent disease, referred to as the daily recommended allowance (DRA); the optimal amount (OA), which yields the best biological function; and the tolerable upper intake level (UL), which if continued, may lead to toxicity.

Selenosis has been reported from a manufacturing error in a preparation, taken by 13 people, that contained 27.3 mg (27,300 mcg) per tablet. The most frequent symptoms reported were nail

---

[284] Rayman, M. P., "The Importance of Selenium to Human Health," *Lancet*, 2000, *356*(9225), 233–241.
[285] Ibid.
[286] Qu, X.-H., et al., *Biological Trace Element Research*, 2000.

and hair brittleness and loss, skin rashes, intestinal upset, fatigue, irritability, nervous system effects, and a garlic odor to the breath.[287]

If someone works with selenium, like in copper refining, there are work exposure limits related to concentration and length of time of exposure before respirators, safety clothing, and gloves are required. These limits are set by the National Institute for Occupational Safety and Health (NIOSH), a US government agency, and change over time as scientific knowledge advances.

Death can occur from gram quantities of selenium. The table below lists the ULs, according to the Linus Pauling Institute, and the recommended dietary allowances (RDAs), according to the National Institutes of Health (NIH), for selenium.[288]

Tolerable Upper Intake Level (UL) and Recommended Dietary Allowance (RDA) for Selenium			
Life stage	Age	UL (mcg/day)	RDA (mcg/day)
Infant	0–6 months	45	15
	6–12 months	60	20
Child	1–3 years	90	20
	4–8 years	150	30

---

[287] Higdon, J., et al., "Selenium," Linus Pauling Institute, Oregon State University, last updated November 2023, https://lpi.oregonstate.edu/mic/minerals/selenium.
[288] Ibid.; National Institutes of Health, Office of Dietary Supplements, "Selenium: Fact Sheet for Health Professionals," accessed April 28, 2009, https://ods.od.nih.gov/factsheets/selenium-HealthProfessional/.

	9–13 years	280	40
Adolescent	14–18 years	400	55
Adult	19 years and older	400	55

The average American diet provides 100 mcg per day of selenium, and this must be considered when calculating the use of supplements. Dietary intake of selenium of 100 mcg should be added to a supplement of 200 mcg to provide the sum of a daily intake of 300 mcg. More could be taken, but it is advised to follow these guidelines and monitor serum blood levels. Monitoring the blood level is helpful to assess absorption, compliance, and toxicity.

Selenium Deficiency

Selenium deficiency is difficult to detect, as it is not characterized by a single condition or presentation. Hypothyroidism has many causes: primary glandular failure, hypopituitarism, autoimmune Hashimoto's disease, radiation exposure, iodine insufficiency, or selenium deficiency. Selenium deficiency certainly is not at the top of the list, and in most cases, not even on the list, of a differential diagnosis. A history that focuses on diet, location, work, and other medical problems may suggest but will not direct one to selenium deficiency. Laboratory testing of blood, urine, or toenail clippings would be needed to ferret out the answer. Hair analysis is available for selenium, but this method is unreliable, as some shampoos contain selenium sulfate. Blood levels are the most reliable method of analysis.

Three diseases have been associated with selenium deficiency: Keshan disease, Kashin–Beck disease, and myxedematous endemic cretinism. Keshan disease is characterized by an enlarged heart and heart failure in children who have low selenium levels and who may have had a viral infection as an instigating factor. It was first described in the 1930s in parts of China where the dietary intake of selenium is less than 19 mcg per day. Kashin–Beck disease is a form of osteoarthritis from selenium deficiency, and endemic cretinism results in intellectual disability.[289]

Modern medicine has created another condition that can cause selenium deficiency: **total parenteral nutrition (TPN)**. This is a formula of nutrients used to feed someone through an intravenous (IV) line. Supplementing TPN with selenium makes the patient less susceptible to stresses from infections and metabolic imbalance.[290]

Selenium investigation may be worthwhile in people with the following conditions:

- Intestinal malabsorption
- Crohn's disease
- Having undergone intestinal resection or lap banding procedures for weight loss
- Pancreatitis
- Weakened immunity
- Repeat infections
- An elevated, oxidized form of low-density lipoproteins (LDL; the bad cholesterol)
- Arthritis with joint swelling and stiffness
- Any form of hypothyroidism
- Cancer

---

[289] National Institutes of Health, "Selenium."
[290] Ibid.

DNA damage is reduced with higher levels of selenium.[291] The tumor suppressor gene p53 is also more effective with higher selenium levels.[292]

Selenium is a super antioxidant and may help in any condition in which free radicals play a part in the disease process. Any disease associated with inflammation or oxidative stress will be improved by selenium. A few examples are asthma, pancreatitis, chronic hepatitis B and C, and AIDS. The thioredoxin reductase helps to produce harmless water and alcohol from hydrogen peroxide and phospholipid hydroperoxides.[293]

Selenium Sources and Supplements

According to the Food and Nutrition Board of the National Academies of Sciences, Engineering, and Medicine, food sources of selenium include Brazil nuts, mushrooms, tomatoes, broccoli, garlic, asparagus, onions, and eggs.

Good sources of selenium are available from some of the better vitamin and mineral producers in the source guide. Selenium is available in tablet, capsule, and liquid form for oral ingestion and sterile liquid for intravenous administration. In addition, selenium is available in organic and inorganic forms. Organic forms of selenium include the following:

- Selenomethionine ($C_5H_{11}NO_2Se$)
- Selenium citrate
- Selenocysteine ($C_3H_7NO_2Se$)

---

[291] Waters, D. J., et al., "Effects of Dietary Selenium Supplementation on DNA Damage and Apoptosis in Canine Prostate," *Journal of the National Cancer Institute*, 2003, *95*(3), 237–241.
[292] Passwater, R. A., "SeNRC," DrPasswater.com, accessed September 20, 2009, website no longer available.
[293] Diplock, A. T., "Antioxidants and Disease Prevention," *Molecular Aspects of Medicine*, 1994, *15*(4), 293–376.

- Se-methylselenocysteine (SeMC), found in garlic and broccoli
- SelenoPrecise, a yeast-derived selenium that is 99% organically bound; absorption is more than 85%
- Selenodiglutathione

Inorganic selenium includes sodium selenite ($NaHSeO_3$) and sodium selenate ($NaHSeO_4$). Selenium for injection is selenious acid, in dosages of 40 mcg/mL in 10 mL vials. Topical applications include selenium sulfide (SeS_2), available as Exsel and Selsun, topical solutions for the treatment of dandruff, tinea (pityriasis) versicolor, and seborrheic dermatitis. Topical applications are *not* for use by ingestion.

Commercial forms of selenium may be a single form or a blend of forms. A capsule or tablet may contain only selenomethionine or selenium citrate. Some manufacturers, such as Life Extension, compound a blend of 75 mcg of methylselenocysteine, 50 mcg of sodium selenate, 50 mcg of selenomethionine, and 25 mcg of selenodiglutathione. Knowing that selenium works best with vitamin E, the manufacturer adds 30 units to complete the package. Life Extension also sells a liquid form of sodium selenite, where one drop delivers 50 mcg, for oral intake.

I have not seen any evidence that one particular form is better than another, but I suggest using a blend or mixture of forms. Nature presents many forms of vitamins and minerals, and usually it is best to give Mother Nature a choice of nutrients, as some are easier to use for different purposes. Not all of selenium's uses and chemical reactions are fully known.

Dr. Passwater, in his studies, used SelenoPrecise, his patented form of selenomethionine and selenium salts derived from yeast.[294] From a chemical point of view, I would like to point out that

---

[294] Passwater, R. A., "SeNRC," DrPasswater.com, accessed September 20, 2009, website no longer available.

selenomethionine is not a salt but a molecule of methionine in which selenium has been substituted for the sulfur in the carbon chain. This amino acid is then incorporated wherever the body uses methionine to make proteins. Selenomethionine is considered the easiest to absorb.

Most forms of selenium are good, both the organic and inorganic salts, but keep to a mixture. Plant-derived selenium, **methylselenocysteine (SeMC)**, contains a form of selenium that is not in a protein but available to be put into an enzyme such as glutathione peroxidase or iodothyronine deiodinase.

In 2000, the Food and Nutrition Board reduced the recommendation for selenium from 200 mcg per day to 70 mcg for men and 55 mcg for women. This does not make sense when new data shows that the 200–400 mcg per-day dose is more beneficial and safer.[295]

---

[295] Combs, G. F., "Impact of Selenium and Cancer-Prevention Findings on the Nutrition-Health Paradigm," *Nutrition and Cancer*, 2001, *40*(1), 6–11; Rayman, M. P., "The Importance of Selenium to Human Health," *Lancet*, 2000, *356*(9225), 233–241.

Sodium

Benefits of Sodium

- Necessary for balancing the proper amount of water in the body
- Used for the preservation of meat and fish
- Sodium chloride (salt) enhances the flavor of food
- Prevents hypotension in some cases
- Enhances water retention in dehydration

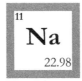

History of Sodium

Sodium is an element that is necessary to maintain cellular balance with other minerals and water in this system called life. It has a unique role within and outside of the cell—it distributes water in both locations.

Sodium is the sixth-most common element on earth. It is never found in the elemental state but is always associated with other elements or compounds. The symbol for sodium is **Na**, and it has the atomic number 11 and an atomic weight of 22.98. It was discovered by Humphry Davy in 1807, who isolated it from **sodium hydroxide (NaOH)** by electrolysis. Sodium hydroxide is also known as caustic soda, and sodium was for the **soda** in **caustic**

soda. The isolated element Na can react with, or ignite, the water molecule (H_2O) to produce sodium hydroxide (NaOH) and hydrogen (H_2).

Historical Consumption of Salt

Humans have eaten and used salt—that is, **sodium chloride (NaCl)**—almost forever, it seems. However, from Paleolithic times to about 5,000 years ago, it is estimated, people ate less than 1 g of salt a day. Initially, people ate fruit and vegetables, which provided 10 times more potassium than sodium. Meat did not add much sodium either, but salt was added to augment the flavor. The taste for salt probably started after people began to preserve fish and meat with salt.

The Chinese used salt for seasoning more than 5,000 years ago. The Egyptians used salt for seasoning, starting at around 3,000 BC, and for embalming. They used a salt known as **natron** to desiccate bodies for mummification prior to placing them in sarcophaguses. Natron is composed of **sodium carbonate (CNa_2O_3)** and **sodium bicarbonate ($CHNaO_3$)**, with lesser amounts of **sodium chloride (NaCl)** and **sodium sulfate (Na_2O_4S)**, a mixture harvested from dry lake beds in Egypt.

Human consumption of salt has varied over time, when used as both a seasoning and a preservative. While it has been estimated that people consumed less than 1 g per day in Paleolithic times, it is thought that this had increased to about 5 g per day by the 10th century. In 1500, Swedish consumption was 100 g per day because of the preservation of fish with salt. In the 1800s in Europe, the combination of both seasoning and preserving food with salt led to an estimated consumption of about 18 g per day. The invention of the refrigerator reduced the need for preserving food with salt, and consumption of salt in Europe and America dropped to 10 g per day.

Salt consumption stayed pretty much at that level until the 1980s, when the low-salt diet was resurrected for the control of hypertension and, more importantly, for the new interest in the treatment of chronic kidney disease with the new technique of hemodialysis. Water balance through the control of sodium in the dialysate fluid is critical for blood pressure, dehydration versus water intoxication, and the spacing of fluids in the legs, abdomen, and areas surrounding the brain.[296]

Louis Dahl presented a graph in 1960 that showed a positive linear relationship between hypertension and salt intake that reignited interest in the concept, but medications for hypertension remained the mainstay. Dahl showed that two important factors contributed to hypertension: salt and genetic predisposition. He also showed that when sodium is the cause of hypertension, blood pressure can be lowered with the addition of potassium to the diet.[297]

Functions of Sodium

The normal body content of sodium is about 100 g. Forty percent of the sodium is deposited in the bone matrix; the remaining 60% is distributed in the cells and extracellular fluid of the body.

One function of sodium is to maintain the balance of water within and outside the cell. The concentration of particles and water in the cell are kept equal to the particles and water outside of the cell, separated by a semipermeable membrane—in this case, the cell wall. This force of the fluid to move to the chamber of higher

---

[296] Roberts, W. C., "Facts and Ideas from Anywhere," *Baylor University Medical Center Proceedings*, 2001, *14*(3), 314–322.

[297] Bashyam, H., "Lewis Dahl and the Genetics of Salt-Induced Hypertension," *Journal of Experimental Medicine*, 2007, *204*(7), 1507.

concentration is called **osmotic pressure**. Other elements enter into the balance of water inside and outside the cell, but the primary element for the movement of water is sodium. Chlorine travels with sodium in many of the reactions, but sodium is the driving force that affects both ions. The imbalance of water results in either **dehydration** or **edema** (swelling).

Nerve impulses travel along a nerve at the cell wall when sodium enters the cell and potassium exits the cell. After the passage of the impulse, the potential of the cell must be reset by sodium pumps to remove sodium from the cell and potassium pumps to return potassium to the cell. The amount of sodium and potassium in a system is related to its energy. An imbalance of these two ions can cause weakness, fatigue, muscle cramps, and even seizures.

Experts cannot project how much sodium people need when they cannot agree on how much people are currently ingesting. The US Food and Drug Administration (FDA) currently estimates the daily intake of sodium in America at 3,200 mg and recommends an intake of 2,300 mg per day. The World Health Organization (WHO), in its report "Global Database of the Implementation of Nutrition Act, GINA," of October 6, 2022, reported daily intake of salt at 10.78 g. It recommends less than 2,000 mg of sodium or less than 5 g of salt (5 g = 5,000 mg). Salt by weight is 20% sodium and 60% chlorine.

Hormonal Control of Sodium Excretion

Aldosterone is a hormone that controls sodium retention to preserve blood volume and blood pressure during times of salt deprivation and reduced access to water. Water follows sodium, and the retention of sodium will retain water. Its third function is to promote the excretion of potassium by the kidneys to avoid high levels of potassium. The adrenal glands produce aldosterone. The overproduction of aldosterone by the adrenal glands may cause hypertension and fluid retention.

Recommended Sodium Intake

Daily sodium intake is difficult to judge. The Food and Nutrition Board of the National Academy of Medicine reported that it lacks the information needed to determine the daily requirements of sodium to formulate a recommended dietary allowance (RDA). Because we do not know the sodium intake of healthy people, recommendations are guesses at best. But the government did come up with an adequate intake (AI) for sodium in 2019.[298] The new AI is based on the **chronic disease risk reduction (CDRR)** intake. The Food and Nutrition Board does not provide a clear definition of CDRR intake and does not set out measurements or metrics. Have you got that clear?

Three-quarters of all the salt we eat is eaten in restaurants; the rest comes from preserved foods, packaged soups, stock cubes, gravy, canned meats, canned fish, condiments, salted nuts, sausage, bacon, ham, cured meats, commercial vegetable juices, and soy sauce. I list some popular dishes below. I find it difficult to believe that, if this is only one meal of the day, the total salt intake for the day does not exceed 5–10 g.

Salt Content of Common Food Items	
Food	Salt content (g)
McDonald's Big Mac	2.3
Reuben sandwich	6.4

---

[298] Food and Nutrition Board, National Academy of Medicine, *Dietary References for Sodium and Potassium* (uncorrected proofs), National Academies Press, 2019.

Corned beef sandwich	2.6
Arby's roast beef sandwich	1.9
Starbucks turkey pastrami	2.2
Spaghetti and meatballs	2.6
Ham and eggs	1.4
Tuna sandwich	2.6

Controlling salt intake is difficult. Even cardiac patients in the hospital who are on salt-restricted diets, in a controlled environment, somehow have salt packets appear on their trays. Surprisingly, the real problem is more pronounced with the kidney patients than the cardiac patients. The kidneys have a more difficult time excreting sodium than the heart does with fluid retention and too much sodium.

Hyponatremia

The collective mantra to reduce salt ingestion with hypertension has been so effective that I see more hypertensive patients with low sodium, that is, a blood level below 135 millimoles per liter (mmol/L), which is more harmful to the patient than high sodium, a level that exceeds 147 mmol/L. This hyponatremia, or low sodium, promotes weakness, confusion, brain fog, headaches, poor memory, light-headedness, and conditions that precipitate a fall. The patients find themselves worse off than when the hypertension was discovered.

Salt restriction aggravated by a diuretic to promote more sodium loss destroys the function of the nervous system. The nervous system runs on sodium and potassium. In the ready state, most potassium is within the axon, or the long arm of the nerve cell, and sodium is mostly exterior to the cell. The transmission of a nerve impulse along the axon of the nerve is like two rows of dominos—the sodium falls into the axon and the potassium falls out of the axon simultaneously, upsetting the electrical gradient across the cell wall of the axon and propagating an electrical signal to the brain. The cells pump this potassium back into the cell and pump the sodium out of the cell, preparing the nerve for the next transmission of a signal.

The treatment of hypertension is not the only cause of hyponatremia. Low sodium levels can be provoked by psychiatric medications and the misuse of medications in general. Medical conditions that cause low sodium include diarrhea, cirrhosis of the liver, endocrine disorders, sweating, and chronic kidney disease. The most common causes are behavioral and side effects from drugs.

David Brownstein, MD, believes the normal sodium level is 141–145 mmol/L.[299] The sodium level does not have to be 132 mmol/L to be considered low. I have seen a sodium level of 138 mmol/L causing weakness, headaches, or just being off center. This can be corrected with a quarter to half a teaspoon of either **Celtic Sea Salt** or pink **Himalayan salt** in 2–4 oz. of water. Within one hour, you will notice an increase in energy, alertness, and well-being. If you had a deficit of sodium for some time, you may have to drink saltwater for a week or two to replenish the body, not just the sodium in the vascular system. As a precaution, I advise my patients to stop by the office once or twice a week to monitor their blood pressure and do a blood draw for sodium and potassium to avoid overshooting the balance point. Question any sodium level below 141 mmol/L. Abnormal functioning can be found inside of the normal reference range of sodium.

The Salt Wars

The Salt Wars refers to an academic discussion that took place from 1904 to 1944 among doctors in France, the United States, and

---

[299] Brownstein, D., *Salt Your Way to Health*, 2nd edition, 2010, 68.

Germany as to the cause of edema and its treatment. In 1899, there were discussions that fluid retention might be caused by too much chlorine. In 1904, two French scientists, Ambard and Beaujard, promoted the idea that sodium was the cause of hypertension and fluid retention. They are credited for inventing the **salt–blood pressure hypothesis**. Over the years, the theory that chlorine was the cause of fluid retention kept being presented. This was countered by low-salt diets of 100–720 mg of sodium that failed to reduce blood pressure because they contained super high amounts of sugar.

In the United States, Meara promoted removing saltshakers from the reach of hypertensive patients. However, salt restriction was not successful for all patients with hypertension. It was successful in only 27% of essential hypertensives, and those without renal disease. Low-salt diets also provoked anorexia, loss of energy, and low urine output. Even the *Journal of the American Medical Association* in 1930 was not convinced that a low-salt diet was any more effective than a low-chlorine diet. The confusion was so great that by 1944, recommending a low-salt diet fell out of fashion, and the controversy all but died. The lack of controlled studies and consistent results ended the Salt Wars.[300]

Diuretics were on the horizon in the 1940s, and these new compounds would place pharmaceutical drugs ahead of dietary discretion for the control of blood pressure. The first diuretic was **mercuhydrin**, a mercury-containing diuretic administered by injection. It was, fortunately, replaced by **chlorothiazide** and **hydrochlorothiazide**.

Salt restriction for blood pressure control was never demonstrated in a double-blind cross-over study, and it is not a first-line approach to hypertension, but the mantra urging patients to

---

[300] DiNicolantonio, J. J., and O'Keefe, J. H., "The History of the Salt Wars," *American Journal of Medicine*, 2017, *130*(9), 1011–1014.

avoid salt keeps being repeated ad nauseum. It is hard to let go of an idea that sounds good once it catches on.

Most studies on salt intake in the diet are based on data collected by patients completing food questionnaires, the spot testing of urine for sodium excretion with extrapolation to 24 hours, and estimates of food ingestion. The study of salt intake and output is shrouded in sloppy science. Measuring salt in the laboratory is a difficult practical problem because it easily becomes a contaminate in the analytical solutions, all sources of water contain minerals in varying degrees, and controlling the sample purity and quantity is especially difficult with humans.

All Salts Are Not the Same

Morton Salt and **kosher salts** are made up of sodium and chloride. Morton does put out a product that has added **iodine (I_2)** to avoid goiter, but kosher salt is only sodium and chloride (NaCl). Kosher salt is known for its large granules and ease of application to meat. Both salts can be considered inorganic and bring only sodium chloride to the table.

Sea salts are harvested from the sea. Ocean water is pumped into shallow ponds and the water permitted to evaporate. These salts contain not only sodium and chloride but also every other mineral found in the water. That list of minerals may be up to 90 or more. The concentration of these other minerals is low, but they are essential for supporting enzyme function and the crystalline structure of bone, and they act as cofactors for vitamins. Pink **Himalayan salt** comes from mines in Pakistan and, like sea salt, contains multiple additional minerals, classifying it as a nutrient. Unfortunately, it does not contain iodine.

The salt-only products, like Morton's and kosher salts, are often referred to as dead salts, as opposed to live salts, which include sea salt and Himalayan salts. If half a teaspoon of salt is dissolved in half a glass of water and then a pH indicator solution is added, the dead salts demonstrate a neutral pH of 7. Himalayan and sea salt have an alkaline pH of 9, showing that the additional minerals fundamentally make these salts different and beneficial compared to the dead salts. The live salts contribute to your well-being. Beyond water balance, they contribute to the function of enzymes, hormones, and vitamins.

Hidden Sources of Sodium

If you have hypertension or kidney failure and you are sensitive to increased sodium, be aware of hidden sources of sodium. Restaurant food may be heavily salted to kick up the flavor or salted and spiced to disguise bad food. Water running through a water softener can increase its sodium content. A water softener works by passing water over plastic resin, where the contaminating metals in the water are exchanged for sodium carried by the resin. Water softeners are primarily used in private homes, with no quality checks.

Available Forms of Sodium

Common forms of sodium are table salt, sea salt, Celtic Sea Salt, Himalayan salt, and salted foods such as pretzels, potato chips, and preserved meats. Gatorade and sports drinks are designed to support high-stress activity and replace sodium with other electrolytes, such as potassium, chloride, and magnesium. Sodium chloride tablets are often used in hot environments where heat leads to dehydration and loss of salt. Return to normality requires not only water but also sodium so that the body can hold on to the replenished water.

Some inadvertent sources of sodium are medications that bring sodium into the body and others, like hormones, that influence the retention of sodium.

Strontium

Benefits of Strontium

- Improves bone strength
- Reduces sensitivity of teeth to hot and cold items and sweets

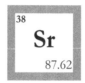

History of Strontium

Strontium is a trace element in the body; 98% of it is found in the bones. It is similar to calcium, shares many of its chemical properties, and supports the rigid strength of bones. Strontium has the symbol of **Sr,** it has an atomic number of 38 and a weight of 87.62, and it is in the alkaline earth metals group (IIA).

The most common stable isotopes are strontium-88, -87, -86, and -84, but the isotope most people associate with strontium is the atomic weight of 90. **Strontium-90** is produced from the detonation of an atomic bomb, when uranium undergoes fission, breaking down into strontium-90, iodine-132, and cesium-137, which are all radioactive. If radioactive strontium enters the body, it will enter the bone marrow and cause anemia and the inability of the blood to clot. The four other isotopes of strontium are not radioactive, and the most common isotope, strontium-88, improves bone strength, inhibiting fractures and vertebral compression.[301]

The mineral was first discovered in 1787, in the village of Strontian, Scotland, by a physician from Edinburgh, Dr. Adair Crawford. He discovered it at an old lead mine and called it strontianite. In 1791, Thomas Charles Hope, also from Edinburgh, tested it with a candle flame, and it burned red. Hope thought the sample looked like barium carbonate, which in the flame test would have burned green. The red flame proved to him that this was a new element. In 1808, Humphrey Davis isolated strontium by electrolysis, using a method similar to the one he used to isolate sodium and potassium.[302]

Strontium has several industrial applications:

- In the manufacture of television cathode ray tubes to block the X-rays the tubes created
- In the manufacture of road flares and fireworks to produce the crimson color
- To enhance ferrite ceramic magnets
- In the form of strontium oxide as a pottery glaze
- In the form of **strontium chloride hexahydrate** in toothpaste for sensitive teeth
- In the most accurate atomic clocks

Additionally, strontium-90 is a high-energy beta emitter for the treatment of cancer. Nonradioactive isotopes of strontium in concentrations below 0.4% in water are considered nontoxic.[303] In animals with chronic renal failure, a concentration greater than

---

[301] Stewart, D., "Strontium Element Facts," July 24, 2015, https://www.chemicool.com/elements/strontium.html.
[302] Weeks, M. A., *Discovery of the Elements*, 1933, Mack Printing Co., 1046.
[303] Yang, L., Harink, B., and Habibovic, P., "Calcium Phosphate Ceramics with Inorganic Additives," In Ducheyne, P., et al. (eds.), *Comprehensive Biomaterials*, 2011, 299–312.

0.34% of the chloride compounds causes the development of osteomalacia, a softening of the bones.

Functions of Strontium

Excessive bone reabsorption and loss is prevented with strontium. It functions similarly to calcium and has the same affinity to the protein of bone. In cell culture, it inhibits the function of osteoclasts that destroy bones. Strontium supports osteoblasts, which are the cells that make new bone, supporting the restoration of the skeleton and healthy bone. Many patented drugs, such as Boniva, Fosamax, and Reclast, do not produce healthy bone but produce poorly constructed bone that easily fractures. The most notorious example is osteonecrosis of the jawbone. So much of the bone is reabsorbed that there is not enough bone to support the teeth, with many of them falling out, and the jaw is subject to fracture.

Sr^{2+}
Strontium Citrate

The best form of strontium for a supplement is strontium citrate. A chelated form of strontium ranelate was removed from the market by the manufacturer because it promoted heart disease. It was felt that the ranelate molecule was the culprit. This does not occur with the citrate form.

Sensodyne toothpaste was originally manufactured with the citrate form to prevent sensitivity from hot, cold, or sweet food. Sensodyne toothpaste has been reformulated to the acetate form.

Strontium Acetate

The strontium from the toothpaste is taken up by the tubules in the exposed dentine of the tooth. The tubules are the sensory structures of the tooth and extend from the pulp in the center of the tooth to the enamel surface. If the enamel is worn away, the end of the tubule is exposed, transmitting the hot, cold, or sweet sensation to the nerve of the tooth. Strontium can plug the tubules, inhibiting the unpleasant sensations and giving relief.

Bone health is augmented by strontium and other minerals. I have used strontium in my office since 2008, with excellent results. Bone is primarily a protein structure that, by itself, is flexible; minerals are added, giving it rigidity. The primary element is calcium. But this is not the end of the story. Pure calcium is soft and flaky and does not hold up under pressure. Calcium is that soft white powder that precipitates on faucets and other plumbing fixtures. It is weak by itself and must be supported by other minerals such as magnesium, manganese, strontium, boron, and zinc, to name just a few. Certainly, calcium is the major mineral component, but it needs support from other minerals. The crystal lattice of calcium that is formed on the protein of the bone is given strength from other minerals of different atomic sizes. This is like adding supporting cross members to the structure—an analogy would be like adding trace minerals to iron to make steel. The steel amalgams are much stronger, more flexible, and more resistant to deterioration than iron. This is what happens to calcium when other minerals are added to bone.

Bone maintenance requires minerals, vitamins, and hormones. The vitamins and hormones not only support the metabolism of the bone but also help to direct the flow of minerals to the bone. The aging process directs minerals away from the bone to the soft tissues, such as calcium deposition on the arterial walls and in joint spaces. Calcium within the cell will displace magnesium and other minerals from enzymes, in effect turning them off. If the structure and function cannot be maintained, that is aging. The takeaway, as I like to tell my patients, is that **calcium is a marker of age**.

Strontium Supplements

The most common form of strontium supplement available is strontium citrate. Pure Encapsulations offers 227 mg capsules to be taken daily, and Life Extension offers doses of 750 mg, taken as three capsules a day.

The **formulations of strontium to avoid** are strontium ranelate[304] and strontium chloride. The ranelate form initiates blood clots, heart attacks, and dermatitis known as DRESS syndrome.[305] Strontium chloride causes an overload of the chloride (Cl^{-1}) ion, with symptoms of fatigue, muscle weakness, excessive thirst, dry mucous membranes, and high blood pressure.

There is criticism in the literature that because strontium functions much like calcium and deposits in the bone, DEXA scans[306] performed on bone show a false improvement in bone

---

[304] European Medicines Agency, "European Medicines Agency Recommends that Protelos/Osseor Remain Available but with Further Restrictions," press release, February 21, 2014, https://www.ema.europa.eu/en/news/european-medicines-agency-recommends-protelos-osseor-remain-available-further-restrictions.

[305] Choudhary, S., et al., "Drug Reaction with Eosinophilia and Systemic Symptoms (DRESS) Syndrome," *Journal of Clinical and Aesthetic Dermatology*, 2013, 6(6): 31–37.

[306] DEXA, or dual-energy X-ray absorption, determines the distribution of lean muscle, fat, water, and bone. This is accomplished by using two X-ray frequencies to differentiate the densities. The T score compares you to a 21-year-old of your

density because strontium is more dense on X-ray exams, as its atomic weight is higher than the atomic weight of calcium. In my medical experience, as a physician treating osteoporosis, this is not true. My patient Martha, an 83-year-old woman with pain from osteoarthritis and osteoporosis, was treated with my Bone Health formula for three years prior to a right hip replacement for pain from osteoarthritis. I received an unsolicited observation from the orthopedic surgeon who performed the surgery. He said that during the procedure, after he got past the arthritic bone, the deeper bone was of very strong quality and held the hardware very well. He went on to say that the bone quality was that of a much younger person. I have heard this operative report many times about patients on my Bone Health formula. My goal is clinical improvement. I will order a DEXA scan if the patient requests it, but there is no score that is better than another. The answer to any poor test, or for an older person, regardless of the score, is to increase bone density and to avoid falling.

---

sex, and the Z score compares you to people of your age group, sex, and, hopefully, weight and height.

Zinc

Benefits of Zinc

- Supports the immune system and cell-mediated and humoral immunity
- Shortens the duration of the common cold, pneumonia, and infectious diarrhea
- Promotes growth and wound healing
- Prevents dandruff and white spots in fingernail beds
- Improves sense of smell and taste
- Inhibits benign prostate hypertrophy
- Beneficial to the control of acne
- Needed for insulin production, secretion, and function
- Lowers the risk and progression of macular degeneration and blindness
- Improves resistance to infection
- Supports endocrine production of thyroxine, testosterone, and insulin
- Reduces hair loss
- Improves age-related macular degeneration and night blindness
- Prevents osteoporosis

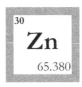

History of Zinc

The last essential trace mineral is zinc, **Zn**. It is a transitional element, usually bluish white in color, with a charge of +2. It often occurs as a metallic element or combined as a sulfide, carbonate, silicate, or oxide. Its atomic number is 30, and its atomic weight is 65.38. It is similar in chemical characteristics to magnesium. The body contains 2–3 g of zinc, mostly in the bones, teeth, hair, skin, liver, muscle, white cells, and testes. Dietary sources are beef, pork, liver, eggs, and oysters.

The first reference to a zinc deficiency in humans was a report by Ananda S. Prasad in the 1960s. It was observed that dwarfs in Iran did not live beyond 25 years of age; the usual cause of death was infection. Lacking effective analytical methods to measure trace elements and suspecting that zinc may be the cause, doctors developed a diet that increased the intake of zinc. In one year of treatment, corrections were noted in linear growth and sexual development, pubic hair appeared, anemia responded to iron, mental lethargy improved, and skin rashes cleared.[307]

Zinc deficiency was recognized in American medicine only recently, in the 1970s, by Dr. Graham, who observed that a patient with Crohn's disease who he was treating responded significantly to 220 mg of zinc twice a day.[308] Adding this essential trace element improved the patient's hair loss, vascular rash, and dermatitis.

---

[307] *The Merck Manual*, 17th edition, 1999.
[308] Hendricks, K. M., and Walker, W. A., "Zinc Deficiency in Inflammatory Bowel Disease," *Nutrition Reviews*, 1988, *46*(12), 401–408.

Additional patients with Crohn's disease and irritable bowel disease (IBD) were studied and showed improvements to such problems as retarded growth, arrested sexual development, acrodermatitis, depressed immune function, and night blindness with zinc.

These original findings were reported, but before and after treatment levels of serum zinc had not been recorded for all patients. In 1980, Sturniolo and colleagues reported their findings of a study involving patients with Crohn's disease compared to a healthy control group with before and after treatment levels of serum zinc.[309]

Zinc is now known to be absorbed in the distal small intestine; hence, zinc deficiency was first observed in patients with intestinal diseases such as Crohn's and IBS who have abnormal bowel function. Additional conditions were soon linked to zinc deficiency. Taste acuity and smell were added to the list, as was thymic atrophy, poor immunity and reduced T cell counts of CD4 cells, skin hypersensitivity, protein-calorie malnutrition, anemia, rough and dry skin, delayed wound healing, and baldness.

Zinc deficiency is often described in terms of marginal or severe, based on the intensity of symptoms. Marginal zinc deficiency is prevalent in the United States, usually caused by inadequate intake. The symptoms are skin changes, growth retardation, poor wound healing, and susceptibility to colds and flu. Severe deficiency is more often related to inborn defects of zinc absorption, liver disease, chronic renal disease, sickle-cell disease, and living in developing countries where there are limited food sources of meat and seafood.[310]

Simple forms of zinc are available for supplementation. The reduced metallic form is never used for health or medical conditions.

---

[309] Ibid.
[310] Song, Y., "Zinc Is Crucial for DNA Integrity and Prostate Health," *Linus Pauling Institute Research Newsletter*, Fall/Winter 2009.

Ionized zinc is positively charged and paired with a negatively charged anion such as chloride, sulphate, or glycinate.

$$Cl^- \quad Cl^-$$
$$Zn^{2+}$$

Zinc Chloride

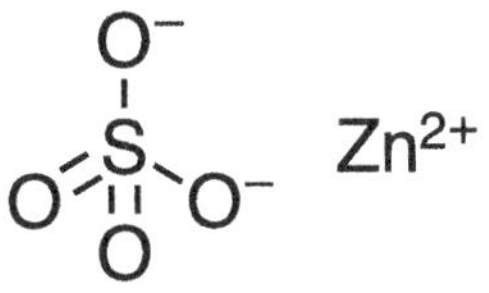

Zinc Sulfate

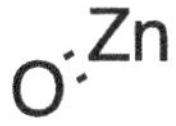

Zinc Oxide

The three forms above, zinc chloride, zinc sulfate, and zinc oxide, are considered inorganic forms. Below, zinc glycinate is considered an organic form, radially absorbed and utilized.

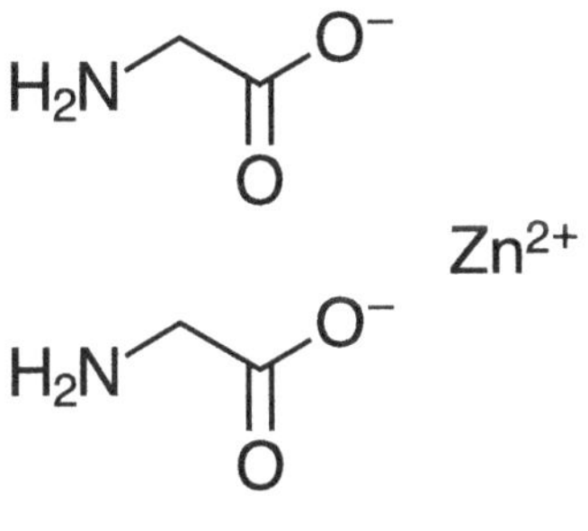

Zinc Glycinate

Functions of Zinc

The common cold, cold sores, and the flu are affected by zinc, as it boosts the immune system. Prasad showed that over a period of 12 months, the incidence of these infections decreased by 48% when patients were provided with zinc supplements.[311] Prasad, with a focus on the developing world, also reported beneficial effects in treating infantile diarrhea and respiratory infections with zinc through morbidity and mortality reports.

Zinc has an antioxidant effect in decreasing macular degeneration, as reported in a 10-year National Eye Institute (NHI) study.[312] Night blindness is caused by a depressed level of alcohol dehydrogenase in the retina that is also related to low levels of zinc.[313] Zinc is found in many of the vitamins packaged for eye health, with vitamin C, lutein, bilberry, and zeaxanthin.

Supplementation with zinc decreases proinflammatory cytokines and oxidative stress markers.[314] Collagen synthesis requires zinc; having normal levels promotes better wound healing and slows the sagging effects of time and gravity. Supplementation also improves T-lymphocyte function and testosterone levels.

Zinc is required for bone health and development. A fact that is seldom thought about is that a lack of zinc in the body causes many of the cases of osteoporosis. In discussions about osteoporosis, calcium is usually the first mineral people think about. Little thought is given to strontium, boron, and magnesium, and least of all to zinc. If foods are grown in soil depleted of zinc, they lack zinc. If zinc is lacking, the plants will, if it is present, take up cadmium. This cadmium will take the place of zinc in the enzymes in a person's cells, and the enzymes will not function. It is estimated that 20% of

---

[311] Prasad, A. S., "Zinc: Mechanisms of Host Defense," *Journal of Nutrition*, 2007, *137*(5), 1345–1349.
[312] Age-Related Eye Disease Study Research Group, "A Randomized Placebo-Controlled, Clinical Trial of High-Dose Supplementation with Vitamins C and E, Beta Carotene, and Zinc for Age-Related Macular Degeneration and Vision Loss: AREDS Report No. 8," *Archives of Ophthalmology*, 2001, *119*(10), 1417–1436.
[313] *The Merck Manual*, 17th edition, 1999.
[314] Prasad, A. S., "Zinc: Mechanisms of Host Defense," *Journal of Nutrition*, 2007, *137*(5), 1345–1349.

all osteoporosis is caused not only by inadequate zinc intake but also by toxins like cadmium making people prematurely old.[315]

Diabetes

Diabetes mellitus is a disease where the body cannot properly handle carbohydrates. Sugar is a prime source of energy that is broken down from complex carbohydrates in the intestines, absorbed into the blood, and transported to the body. For sugar to be transported across cell walls and into the cell, insulin is required. There are two major types of diabetes: **type 1, or insulin-dependent diabetes mellitus (IDDM)**, and **type 2, or non-insulin-dependent diabetes mellitus (NIDDM)**.

Type 1 diabetes is characterized as the pancreas being unable to produce sufficient insulin to help keep the blood sugar, specifically blood glucose, in the fasting range of 90 to 115 milligrams per deciliter (mg/dL). The pancreas does not respond to ingesting carbohydrates by producing insulin. The sugar remains in the blood at high levels, 200 mg/dL or 300 mg/dL, and, more importantly, unable to enter the cells. Sugar is abnormally elevated. At sustained high levels, sugar will attach to red blood cell membranes, making them stiff and not pliable. Glucose will attach to nerve cells and the walls of blood vessels and inhibit the immune system from functioning properly. The result is not only elevated blood sugar but also, over time, premature aging, the wearing out of body parts and systems. These harmful compounds are referred to as **advanced glycation end products (AGEs)**, and they are the primary cause of the end stages of diabetes: retinal hemorrhages and tears that lead to blindness, kidney failure, strokes, heart attacks, poor wound healing, and susceptibility to infections.

---

[315] Pizzorno, J., *The Toxin Solution: How Hidden Poisons in the Air, Water, Food, and Products We Use Are Destroying Our Health—And What We Can Do to Fix It*, 2017, HarperOne, 90.

Type 2 diabetes is the failure of the cells to respond to insulin in the blood. The result is that sugar remains elevated in the blood, with high levels of insulin. In this form of diabetes, the receiving cells that need the glucose do not respond to insulin. The theory is that the receptor sites on the cell are no longer responding to insulin or are missing.

Type 2 diabetes is also referred to as **adult-onset diabetes**, as it occurs later in life; type 1 is referred to as **juvenile diabetes**. However, these terms are inaccurate, and today, diabetes is classified according to the mechanism of either pancreatic failure (type 1) or the failure of the cells to respond to insulin (type 2). An older person can have juvenile diabetes, and a young person can have adult-onset diabetes.

People with diabetes who have been treated with zinc have shown improvements in both glucose levels and **glycosylated hemoglobin (hemoglobin A1C)**; the latter is an index used to determine the average blood sugar over the last six weeks.

Zinc takes part in the synthesis, storage, and release of insulin. It is part of the enzyme **carboxypeptidase B** that converts **proinsulin** to **insulin**, and a lack of zinc may play a role in the development of type 2 diabetes, but it is not the cause.[316] The pancreas removes zinc from the blood, stores some of it in storage sites called **extragranular fractions** in the pancreatic cells and eliminates it via the pancreatic duct. In general, women have lower zinc levels than men, those of people with type 1 diabetes are lower than those of people with type 2 diabetes, and the longer a person has diabetes, the lower their zinc level. As insulin is used, there is a

---

[316] Winterberg, B., et al., "Zinc in the Treatment of Diabetic Patients," *Trace Elements in Medicine*, 1989, 6(4), 173–177.

proportional loss of zinc.[317] Hemodialysis has little effect on zinc levels.

Insulin is the hormone that carries glucose into the cell. Its effects peak within one hour if given subcutaneously, just below the skin, or within 15 minutes if given intravenously. This is too fast and requires too many injections. In the mid-1950s, it was discovered that the rate of reaction of insulin could be slowed by mixing it with zinc, a protein called **protamine**, or both zinc and protamine. Zinc slows the onset of action of insulin and gives it a longer duration of action. Protamine slows the absorption of insulin at the injection site, adding to the delayed effect of injection. This gave rise to insulins with peak activity at different times from injection, such as medium- (2 hours), long- (7 hours), and ultralong-acting (12 hours) insulin. Fortunately, the fast-acting (1 hour) insulin can be mixed with any of the long-acting insulins to create multiple blends of activity and strengths.[318]

Chemosurgery with Zinc for Skin Cancer

Frederic E. Mohs, MD (1910–2002), is noted for the surgical technique he developed to remove skin cancer. He had the most success for basal cell cancer and squamous cell cancer and less for melanoma, but melanoma is the one he is noted for. He performed the first **Mohs surgery** in 1933.[319]

Mohs surgery involves excising or cutting out the cancer and examining the margins of the removed tissue to look for cancer cells. If any cancer cells are found by microscopic examination at the

---

[317] Jansen, J., Karges, W., and Rink, L., "Zinc and Diabetes—Clinical Links and Molecular Mechanisms," *Journal of Nutritional Biochemistry*, 2009, *20*(6), 399–417.

[318] Travis, R. H., and Sayers, G., "Insulin and Oral Hypoglycemic Drugs," In Goodman, L. S., and Gilman, A. (eds.), *The Pharmacological Basis of Therapeutics*, 4th edition, Macmillan, 1971, 1581–1603.

[319] Foreman, A., "The Quest to Understand Skin Cancer," *Wall Street Journal*, July 2–3, 2022, C5.

edges of the excised tissue, it indicates that the margins of the remaining tissue still contain cancer cells. The surgeon then must return to the wound and remove a wider piece of tissue until the margins are cancer free. This is usually performed while the surgical wound is still open. The surgical specimens are frozen and examined during the procedure, so the patient does not have to return on another day and have a second procedure. This technique was developed over many years.

Dr. Mohs performed his first surgical removal of skin cancer in 1933, while still a medical student. Fortunately, he worked under the guidance of Dr. Michael Guyer, his mentor and zoology professor. He was taught to examine the biopsied tissue under the microscope and to draw the cells that he was examining. This attention to detail would be the basis of the successful Mohs procedure. This procedure was called chemosurgery because, initially, before the lesion was approached with a scalpel, it was treated with **zinc chloride ($ZnCl_2$) paste**. This zinc compound would attack the malignant and dead tissue, producing a scar, or eschar, demarking the area to be removed.

This was the usual method of treating skin cancers before more aggressive treatment with knives. **Cansema**, or black salve, contains zinc chloride and was used for years.[320] It was previously sold as Z-Guard, but now it is sold as Remedy Zinc Paste.

In 1936, Dr. Mohs performed his first Mohs **micrographic surgery**, essentially the same procedure that is known today as Mohs surgery.[321]

---

[320] US Food and Drug Administration, "187 Fake Cancer 'Cures' Consumers Should Avoid," FDA, July 7, 2009.
[321] American College of Mohs Surgery, "History of Mohs Surgery," n.d., https://www.mohscollege.org/about-acms/history-of-mohs-surgery.

Zinc and Its Interactions

Zinc is necessary in most hormone systems. It has a similar effect on the thyroid as it has in insulin management in terms of production, delivery, and receptor function. Zinc is a cofactor in hormone production, is needed for the conversion of T4 to T3, and supports thyroid receptor function.[322] Many other hormone functions depend on zinc as a cofactor, coenzyme, or antioxidant. Some examples are ovulation, sperm production, testosterone production, the regulation of steroids from the adrenal gland, growth hormone, gonadal development, hair growth, and linear growth.

Industrial exposure to high levels of zinc oxide fumes causes neurological damage called **metal fume fever** and **zinc shakes**. Acute poisoning of zinc can occur from acidic foods stored in galvanized containers provoking vomiting and diarrhea.

Common Cold

In the 1990s, **Cold-EEZE** introduced its proprietary formula of **zinc gluconate glycine** to reduce the duration of the common cold by 42%. The manufacturer showed that the duration of the cold can be reduced from 7.6 days to 4.4 days if Cold-EEZE is started within 24 hours of the first symptoms of sneezing, coughing, stuffy nose, sore throat, postnasal drip, or hoarseness. One lozenge taken every two to four hours, dissolved, not chewed, releases 92% of the zinc to attach to the rhinovirus and inactivate it before the virus enters the cells and reproduces.[323]

---

[322] Pierini, C., "Test Uncovers a Common Deficiency," *Vitamin Research News*, 2009, *23*(10), 1–16.

[323] Mossad, S. B., et al., "Zinc Gluconate Lozenges for Treating the Common Cold. A Randomized, Double-Blind, Placebo-Controlled Study," *Annals of Internal Medicine*, 1996, *125*(2), 81–88; Cold-EEZE, "What Is Cold-EEZE?" accessed December 13, 2009, https://coldeeze.com/pages/faq.

Cold-EEZE lozenges, when taken, will reduce taste for a few hours, but taste will return. When taken according to instructions, it has a good safety profile. It is pleasant tasting, and I found it effective. Cheaper store brands are available, made with **zinc acetate**, and Zicam with **zinc gluconate** and homeopathic ingredients. On June 16, 2009, the FDA advised consumers to avoid Zicam Cold Remedy Nasal Gel, Zicam Cold Remedy Nasal Swabs, Zicam Cold Remedy Swabs, and Kids Size, as 130 Zicam users reported that it resulted in permanent loss of smell and taste.[324]

Loss of Smell and Taste

Anosmia, the medical term for loss of smell, and the loss of taste have been reported in the use of nasally applied zinc products, but this is not new. In the 1930s, in an attempt to prevent polio, zinc was applied to the nasal area, resulting in the loss of smell and taste.[325] The olfactory nerves are a part of the brain exposed to the outside world, and placing zinc on them can hurt them beyond repair. The damage from direct application of zinc will last longer than the cold. Keep to oral lozenges and be patient.

Male Health

Zinc is important for male health. High levels are found in the testes and higher levels in the prostate. Low levels of zinc in the prostate are associated with a higher incidence of prostate cancer, and higher levels of zinc with a lower incidence of prostate cancer. The higher levels of zinc also increase sperm count and testosterone.[326]

---

[324] "Zicam," *Wikipedia*, accessed December 13, 2009, http://en.wikipedia.org/wiki/Zicam.
[325] FDA, "Zicam: Loss of Taste," December 13, 2009.
[326] Ho, E., and Song, Y., "Zinc and Prostatic Cancer," *Current Opinion in Clinical Nutrition & Metabolic Care*, 2009, 640–645, https://doi.org/10.1097/mco.0b013e32833106ee.

Measuring Zinc Levels

Laboratory analysis of zinc is usually performed on the blood. The normal range of zinc in the serum is 68–161 micrograms per deciliter (mcg/dL). Special acid-washed tubes are used to collect the blood to avoid contamination from the glass test tube at these low concentrations. This is not a usual, routine test; it must be ordered as serum zinc by your doctor. Zinc is measured in hair analysis, but elevated zinc levels in the hair may reflect misdistribution of zinc from elevated cholesterol, malignancy, or liver dysfunction. Blood, cell, or urine zinc analyses are the tests of choice for zinc status.

I use the **red blood cell (RBC) zinc** test from blood. This test is considered a tissue test, as the zinc content of the RBC is measured and not the serum content. Tissue is a better measure of zinc stores in the body, as the serum and tissue amounts may vary. Zinc is needed for many enzymes to function; hence, the tissue measurement is more reflective of total body stores.

Zinc can also be measured in a 24-hour urine specimen; normal is 75–530 micrograms per liter (mcg/L). RBCs contain zinc in the range of 9.0–14.7 milligram per liter (mg/L). **Zinc protoporphyrin (ZPP)** accumulates in red cells from chronic lead absorption or in iron deficiency anemia. Its reference range is less than 100 mcg/dL.[327]

I would consider the above tests for zinc a direct measurement, as the element itself is being measured. Zinc protoporphyrin in blood, zinc measured in urine, and hair analysis may be subject to the misdirection of zinc, whereas RBC zinc may be a better reflection of zinc stored and available to participate in enzymatic reactions.

---

[327] Quest Diagnostics, "Directory of Services," 2009, https://testdirectory.questdiagnostics.com/test/home.

Indirect tests do not provide an assay of the metal itself but may indirectly suggest a low zinc level. Zinc interacts with almost all systems of the body through its enhancement of enzyme function.[328] A low serum zinc level can be suggested by low albumin, low alkaline phosphatase, or a depressed lymphocyte count.

Zinc is a metal; it is either there or not there. It does not convert to another element. Vitamin molecules can be cleaved into two pieces and produce two molecules that are unrelated to the first. This is not so for minerals. Although zinc does not engage in redox (reduction-oxidation) activity itself, it serves as a cofactor for many reactions that regulate redox reactions. Zinc is required for protein structure, RNA transcription, and DNA repair, and it is essential for more than 300 enzyme systems.

Zinc Deficiency

Zinc deficiency inhibits DNA repair, and this, if unchecked, will allow an accumulation of mutations to proceed to a cancer. This has been shown by Yang Song, PhD, in the laboratory at the Linus Pauling Institute. Moreover, a zinc deficiency increases oxidative stress by limiting the production of the zinc-containing antioxidant enzyme, for example, copper-zinc superoxide dismutase.[329] A deficiency in zinc may also lead to a deficiency of vitamin B_6 and magnesium.

The symptoms of zinc deficiency include growth retardation in stature and sexual development, baldness, skin rashes, night blindness, impaired taste and smell, poor wound healing, and a weak immune system. This can develop from poor food choices, a high-fiber diet, intravenous nutrition, increased growth demands, Crohn's

---

[328] Mocchegiani, E., Muzzioli, M., and Giacconi, R., "Zinc and Immunoresistance to Infection in Aging: New Biological Tools," *Trends in Pharmacological Sciences*, 2000, *21*(6), 205–208.
[329] Song, Y., "Zinc Is Crucial for DNA Integrity and Prostate Health," *Linus Pauling Institute Research Newsletter*, Fall/Winter 2009.

disease, irritable bowel syndrome (IBS), ulcerative colitis, bowel resection, fistula, and intestinal inflammation.

Zinc deficiency is also responsible for some conditions that are not readily apparent and are often overlooked in clinical medicine. Lack of zinc contributes to atrophy of thymic and lymphoid tissue. The thymus gland is located in the lower anterior neck and chest; it is responsible for the early development of immunologic function. After puberty, it begins to involute, or get smaller, and is replaced with fat. Zinc is required for the production of thymulin, a thymus hormone that affects T cell function.

Zinc Supplements

A Word of Warning: Zinc and Copper

If you are contemplating taking zinc, be intelligent. Know what your serum or blood zinc level is before treatment, and spot-check that it is between 60 micrograms per deciliter (mcg/dL) and 130 mcg/dL. The usual dose of zinc is 15–60 milligrams (mg) per day. Taking more than 100–150 mg per day may result in blocking the absorption of copper at the intestines.[330] Copper is required for the assimilation or incorporation of iron into hemoglobin. Too much zinc results in low copper levels and small red cell anemia. The iron is in the tissue but cannot be released because of the low copper. Additionally, the production of neutrophils, a type of white blood cell, is also reduced. To avoid this complication, I advise that if you take 30–60 mg of zinc per day, you should also take 2 mg of copper.

Available Supplements

This mineral comes in many useful forms for oral ingestion, such as tablets, capsules, lozenges, and liquid. For IV administration, the

---

[330] Hoffman, H. N., Phyliky, R. L., and Fleming, C. R., "Zinc-Induced Copper Deficiency," *Gastroenterology*, 1988, *94*(2), 508–512.

preparations of zinc chloride and zinc sulfate are most commonly used.

Soluble and insoluble forms of zinc are available for topical application. The soluble forms, such as **zinc sulfate ($ZnSO_4$)** and **zinc chloride ($ZnCl_2$)**, are used in eyewashes and in lotions to treat acne, poison ivy, impetigo, and lupus erythematous. In the early 20th century, it was known as **Cansema**, or **black salve**, with zinc chloride being the active ingredient. It is also used in nasal sprays to shrink nasal membranes. The insoluble forms are **zinc oxide (ZnO)** or zinc attached to a fatty acid of stearate or oleate as an ointment or paste. Topical **zinc pyrithione** 0.5% is used as a cream for psoriasis. **Calamine lotion** is 98% or more zinc oxide and less than 2% ferric oxide; it is the iron that gives calamine its pink color. Calamine is used to contain poison ivy and dry the skin after exposure. Zinc oxide has a mild astringent effect that constricts blood vessels and has an antiseptic action.

Several **over-the-counter (OTC)** oral zinc products are available. An OTC strength used in many hospitals is Zinc-220, the capsules so named because they contain 220 mg of zinc sulfate, providing 78.5 mg of elemental zinc. Other OTC oral forms are **zinc picolinate** and **zinc citrate**, both available in 15 mg and 30 mg strengths. The usual dose is 30–60 mg per day. **Zinc monomethionine**, an antioxidant, is available in 25 mg tablets, and it is a type of chelated zinc. Another form of **Zinc chelate** is zinc bound to the amino acid glycine to form zinc glycinate. This form is better absorbed orally than the ion form, such as zinc chloride. My favorite is the glycinate form, as it is an organic form and readily absorbed. It causes no stomach upset.

Injectable forms for either IV or intramuscular use are zinc chloride in a dose of 10 milligrams per milliliter (mg/mL), zinc citrate (1–10 mg/mL), zinc gluconate (7.5 mg/mL), and zinc sulfate (10 mg/mL).

Appendix

Water

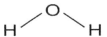

I decided to add this chapter on water not only because water is necessary for life but because it is a complex subject. I feel no book on nutrition is complete unless it addresses this most basic of substances. Knowing the many molecular forms of vitamins and minerals is important to selecting the best nutrients. Likewise, to understand water, what it is, where it comes from, what is in it, helps one to enjoy a better life. On second thought, the subject of water is probably the most complicated chapter in this book. It is neither a vital amine nor a mineral, but it deserves attention as its own neglected substance. Water. Cool, clear water.

The History of Water

Water is a simple compound made up of only three atoms: two hydrogen and one oxygen. Its molecular weight is 18, and 11.188% is hydrogen and 88.812% is oxygen. The bonding distance between the oxygen and hydrogen is 0.9584 angstroms, with the angle of the bonding between the two hydrogen atoms from the center of the oxygen atom being 104.45 degrees. At room temperature it is a clear, colorless, odorless, tasteless liquid that at sea level becomes a solid below 32 degrees Fahrenheit (0 degrees Celsius) and a gas above 212 degrees Fahrenheit (100 degrees Celsius). Chemically, the shorthand for denoting water is H_2O. Its weight by volume is a standard of measure.

Historically, the Greeks considered water one of the four elements. Not much more developed until about the time of the American Revolution. In the later years of the 1700s, our understanding of the physical world changed with new discoveries. An Englishman, Henry Cavendish, discovered hydrogen in 1766. This discovery was followed by that of another Englishman, Joseph Priestley, who discovered oxygen in 1772. Subsequently, Henry Cavendish continued his work but did not report until 1784 that water is made up of two volumes of hydrogen and one volume of oxygen. A Frenchman, Antoine Laurent Lavoisier, at the French Academy of Sciences on June 25, 1781, presented the idea that water is produced by the combination of oxygen and hydrogen. Lavoisier knew Cavendish and his work, but Cavendish being slow to report his findings may have allowed Lavoisier to present the idea first. Antoine Lavoisier is credited with the discovery of the composition of water, but Cavendish was the man with the experimental data.

Functions of Water

At first glance, water is a simple compound that we take for granted. The molecule is so simple it does not need a second thought. Just how complex can three atoms be?

Physically, it has special properties as it cools. Unlike other liquids, as it freezes to a solid, it expands, causing it to float on its warmer liquid state. As water precipitates in the atmosphere, depending on the temperature, it forms as rain, snow, or hail, remains as mist, or presents as virga, which is rain that evaporates before it reaches the ground.

Water is unique in that all life is dissolved in it. Without it there is no life. It is found in all animals and plants. It is necessary, in the proper proportions, in any life system. The amount of water in relation to the solids is narrow and critical to maintain a healthy system.

This molecule of water is unique in its properties of how each molecule of water reacts to each other, such as in the expansion of volume as water freezes. The oxygen is considered to be negatively charged because of its two extra electrons, and the hydrogen protons have a positive charge. This gives the molecule an unbalanced characteristic to the electric charge. The electric field of the molecule is not uniform; the two ends of the molecule are positive, and the center, where the oxygen is located, has a negative charge. To complicate the balance of the charge, the three atoms are not arranged in a line. The shape is like that of a boomerang. The angle of hydrogen bonding is 104.45 degrees. This angle of bonding adds to the uniqueness of how water molecules react to each other and to other substances. You only have to look at snowflakes to see physically how these molecules orient themselves to each other.

Water is more important to life than food. A person can live a month without food. A week without water is lethal. A loss of 5% of water from the normal body composition is significant, if not lethal, dehydration. The loss of total body water and sodium loss generally go together. The average body is 80–100 pounds of water. Forty percent of it is intracellular water—in other words, water within the cells. The first water to leave the body is the extracellular water. Incidentally, this is how a diuretic functions: It primarily promotes the loss of sodium at the kidneys, and as the sodium is eliminated, the water follows.

Dehydration

There are other factors, but for now let us look at the symptoms of dehydration. The skin shrinks, showing more wrinkles and less turgor because of less volume per cell; the mucous membranes become dry; and the axillary sweating decreases. In addition, the blood volume contracts, presenting with lower blood pressure and a faster pulse rate. Postural hypotension—that is, a drop of more than 10 mm of mercury (mmHg)—from the recumbent to sitting or sitting to standing positions occurs. If normal blood pressures cannot be maintained, this is called shock. As dehydration continues, urine output decreases and muscle strength dissipates.

Neurologically, the brain suffers because of the loss of sodium. Some of the remaining water enters the brain cells, resulting in brain swelling. The symptom progression begins with headache, lethargy, confusion, stupor, and coma. If dehydration is fast, the symptoms may present with hyperexcitability as muscle twitches, mental irritability, and convulsions. Most of these symptoms occur when the sodium concentration is less than 125 millimoles per liter (mmol/L). The normal range of sodium is 135–146 mmol/L.

Brownstein presented the concept that neurological functioning and homeostasis are improved when sodium levels are between 141 mmol/L and 146 mmol/L. This can be achieved by adding a quarter teaspoon of Celtic Sea Salt or Himalayan salt to a glass of water, provided there is no cardiac or renal problem.[331] If pure water, such as distilled water that contains no minerals, is used for replacement to correct dehydration, **water intoxication** develops because the sodium concentration falls.

Osmosis

To best understand how water functions in biological systems, we will take a moment to discuss the principle of osmosis. **Osmosis** is the transfer of a liquid, called the solvent, through a semipermeable membrane that does not permit dissolved solids to pass. This phenomenon is best demonstrated by a vessel that is separated into two compartments by a semipermeable membrane. Both compartments are filled with water to the same level. To one

---

[331] Brownstein, D., *Salt Your Way to Health*, 2nd edition, 2010, 68.

side is added a solute (e.g., dissolved solids such as sodium chloride); to the other side nothing is added. The pure water will pass to the chamber that contains the sodium chloride in an effort to equalize the concentration of the number of salt particles on both sides of the membrane. The level of the water in the chamber that contains the salt particles will rise as the pure water diffuses across the membrane. This elevation of the water is called the pressure of osmosis. The salt particles are too big to pass through the membrane; only the water molecules can pass through it.

The process of osmosis can be stopped if a pressure is applied to the chamber that contains the solute or the particles. If more pressure than the osmotic pressure is applied to the chamber that contains the particles, water will pass into the pure water chamber, leaving the particles behind. This is a mechanical means to purify water known as **reverse osmosis (RO)**.

The reverse osmosis process has been perfected since the late 1940s. It is a common practice to purify water by passing it through semipermeable membranes at high pressure to produce water that contains almost no particulate matter. Israel has a desalinization program where they take seawater, process it through RO, and produce potable water. The American military uses mobile RO units, and a unit mounted on a tractor trailer can service a 600-man unit for a month. This is significantly easier than carrying large quantities of water thousands of miles.

The cells in the body are small chambers; the cell wall is a semipermeable membrane. Intracellular water is the water contained in the cell; extracellular water is the water that surrounds and is between the cells. The cells contain 40% of the water in the body. Water passes into and out of the cells by osmosis. The body adjusts the pressures of osmosis by dialysis, transferring the particles or solute through the cell wall.

Living cells make this model even more complicated. The transfer of the solvent or solute in either osmosis or dialysis is a passive diffusion of molecules across a membrane. Living cells can perform the concentration of molecules either into or out of the cells through active transport. Active transport means the cell has an expenditure of energy and a mechanism to achieve that concentration. No matter what system the cell uses, either passive or active, water is in the equation somewhere.

Water Content

In most biological systems, water is important, but what is in the water, and how much of it is in the water, is very important. Pure distilled water has no organic or mineral content. It dilutes anything it is added to. The story of water becomes interesting when we consider the company it keeps. The molecule of water is simple H_2O. Most seventh graders know this. You do not need a chemical engineering degree to recognize the scientific shorthand. So what is it that makes one water better than another? What distinguishes a good water from a not-so-good water? It is what is in the water that makes all the difference. It is the dissolved minerals, gases, and sometimes organic material in the water that gives it a distinctive flavor, feel, and even wetness.

What is dissolved in water gives it a feel, a texture, and when drunk, a quality referred to as mouth feel. A drinking water can have a flavor. A flavor is generally made up of a taste, plus smell, plus mouth feel. Smell is an important component of taste. In fact, it may be the largest component. When drinking or eating something, pinching the nose will often reduce the taste or eliminate the detection of it altogether. I suggest this to children if they do not like the taste of medicine. Pinch the nose, swallow the medicine, and take a chaser of water or another beverage to wash it down. It does blind or confuse the senses. This is similar to having nasal congestion from a cold or sinusitis. Food and drink have almost no taste with impaired ability to smell.

The minerals dissolved in water give water its character. The taste can be unique. The blend of minerals gives it softness, hardness, or a sense of cleanliness that does not interfere with what else you would like to add to it. It is legend that breweries were located in various places because of the pureness of the water. Years ago, good towns for breweries were Newark, New Jersey; Milwaukee, Wisconsin; and Colorado Springs, Colorado. Tennessee is the home of iron-free water that makes good whiskey.

Mostly, when we think of water to drink, we want our water to be colorless, clear, cool, and tasteless. But water like that would be bland, uninteresting, and devoid of minerals; we would suspect that something about it meant it was not good to drink. The most popular waters contain dissolved minerals and even gases such as carbon dioxide. Some of the minerals dissolved in water give it terroir. This is its flavor from the ground and minerals, developed as it flowed to its source. This is the same term used to describe wine, as wine comes from a particular region and extracts its essence from the soil.

Settlements that became villages, towns, and cities all needed sources of good water to survive, which is why all major cities are located on streams, rivers, and lakes. The Tigris and Euphrates Rivers are believed to be the cradle of civilization. The Nile in Egypt runs as a main artery through that land, flooding its banks every June. The swift-rising water carries minerals from the river bottom up onto the banks. These minerals are incorporated into the wheat and other grains, adding to their good nutritional quality. Good-quality grain is just one thing Ceasar wanted from Egypt for his troops.

The Romans and Water

Rome became a city of over one million people that required plenty of water. The Tiber River that passes through the city could not handle all its needs for drinking, bathing, washing, and the carrying away of waste. A system of 11 aqueducts were constructed to carry water to the city. The most famous was spring water that was carried 14 miles by the Aqua Virgo to end at what is now the Trevi Fountain. Other important aqueducts included Aqua Marcia, Aqua Anio Novus, and Aqua Anio Vetus, coming from Tivoli.

The Romans were fortunate to have a selection of waters to choose from. They preferred clarity and taste derived from the minerals dissolved in it for drinking. I went to medical school at the University of Rome, and in that city, the water in the street fountains was suitable for drinking. While walking along, you needed to only partially occlude the spout of the fountain and the water would be directed upward though a hole on the upper surface, squirting cool, fresh water for easy access. My favorite was a small town 20 miles northwest of Rome, overlooking Lake Bracciano, called Anguillara. The fountains on the street poured out flavorful mineral water. On our many Sunday bus trips to Anguillara, my friend and I would take empty bottles to bring back the water because the taste was so good and the price was better.

For bathing, some Romans preferred the waters of the warm springs. Roman soldiers returning from battle needed a place to rest. Armies were not permitted in the walled city and frequently used the warm sulfur baths of Bulicame, Bagnaccio, Terme dei Papi, and Le Pozze di San Sisto outside Viterbo, northwest of Rome. The baths provided **sanus per aquam** ("healing through water"). The word **spa** is derived from the initials of the Latin phrase.

Water for Entertainment and Therapy

Swimming as we know it now, in the ocean, is a rather new phenomenon for humans. Venturing into the ocean for entertainment by aquatics started en masse only in the mid-1800s. The ocean is a dangerous place for a land animal to be, and as land animals, we are out of our natural habitat in the water. As a species, we are not fast swimmers, we are not capable of staying submerged for more than 20–30 seconds, and we have no attributes to protect us from harm from other animals. Nevertheless, we have developed the modern-day entertainment destinations of the Jersey Shore and Miami Beach or tubing down the Snake River in Wyoming and Idaho.

Water is necessary for life of any kind. The concentration of water for the homeostasis of life is very narrow. All the bodily chemical reactions occur in water. We drink water. We pass water. We expel water through our skin and breath. This last process is called **insensible loss** of water, and the loss is about 500–750 ml per day. The skin is mainly a barrier to water in both directions, but it is best equipped to actively pass water and some salts for evaporation and cooling.

Cold water or hot water is used for therapy. It is used to change the body temperature and to affect local blood flow. Hydrotherapy, where water is part of the treatment, has been used for massage, directed to the body surface under pressure. Bathing in water to transfer heat or cold to the body and soaking in water with dissolved minerals, oils, or fragrances have been standard treatments throughout the history of man. Adding compounds, such as **Epsom salt**, a solution of magnesium sulfate first prepared from the mineral springs of Epsom, south of London, in England, is frequently used today for muscular aches and strains.

The most famous mineral spring in the United States is Warm Springs, Georgia. These warm waters contain magnesium, and soaking in them reduced spasm and gave comfort to victims of poliomyelitis. Attention was drawn to this location by President Franklin Roosevelt, who was a victim of polio. The water not only had medicinal value but also provided a place where people with similar problems, while bathing, discussed their symptoms, inner feelings, disappointment, aspirations, and expectations.

Water is a social lubricant. Water dissolves the barrier we create to protect us from the risky unknown. It is difficult to say how or why we get this comfort, but every encounter changes us somehow. Touching water is a personal experience. One drop of rain grabs our attention. For instance, it makes us pause. The experience is instantly evaluated as a danger, a pleasure, something requiring immediate alteration of plans, or as of no consequence.

Water is mystical. It has healing powers. It can purify the soul. One drop can lead the way to heaven or eliminate a nasty witch. Water relieved Pontius Pilate of his culpability for the crucifixion of Christ as he washed his hands. John the Baptist gave the opportunity for eternal spiritual life with the help of water.

Water is defined not only as a molecule with physical properties—it is characterized by the substances dissolved in it, what is not dissolved in it, or what should be dissolved in it. Its description is often more about the impurities found in water than the molecule of water itself. Much discussion is directed at the smallest amounts of trace elements, the molecules that are outnumbered by the water molecules at a billion to one, which become most important when they should become more insignificant. Homeopaths dissolve many of the substances they use in water. The substance that is in the water is diluted so much that not even a single molecule of the substance is in the water; what is left in the fluid is an impression of the molecule. The fluid then becomes a ready receptacle for that molecule in the healing art of homeopathy.

The story of water is best told by describing the company it keeps, the processes it facilitates, and the life it supports. I find trying to accurately describe water most difficult; in fact, I find it can be slippery.

The Hydrologic Cycle

In our modern world, water somehow appears on the shelf in a plastic bottle or in a pitcher, or it flows from a faucet. Usually, we do not even question where it came from, nor do we know much about its composition. There are many sources of drinkable water, but the more important ones are spring water, artesian water, well water, rainwater, and iceberg, glacier, and deep-sea water. Water for most municipalities is drawn from rivers, streams, lakes, and, recently, sea water to be processed into a safe beverage or utility. The compositions are innumerable, and the flavors can be distinctive, sharp, subtle, or elusive. The physical characteristics in the liquid state can be cold, cool, tepid, warm, hot, or scalding, yet the feel to the skin or mouth could be robust, hard, soft, slippery, or wet. If the temperature is just right, the water may not even feel wet. It sounds strange, but we have all experienced this at the pool or shore when the water did not feel very wet. It is true there are no receptors for wetness. I don't know, but my best guess is that the wetness perception is the result of pressure and temperature change perceived together. If there is no change of temperature from being submerged to being in the air, wetness will not be perceived. In the rare condition of water and air having the same temperatures and sufficient humidity not adding or removing the slightest amount of heat, there is no wetness.

The **hydrologic cycle**, or the water cycle, is the process where water evaporates from rivers, lakes, streams, and oceans and passes into the atmosphere, leaving many impurities behind. Water is transported in the form of a cloud to another part of the earth to condense in the form of rain, snow, or hail. It runs off and into the ground, forming surface streams, rivers and lakes, an underground body of water, or an underground stream known as an aquifer.

The aquifer nearest the surface is referred to as the water table or groundwater. This first layer can be shallow or deep. Multiple layers of bodies of water may be stratified one below the other, separated by rocky layers of shale or limestone. The harder rock separates the layers, whereas the more porous layers may act as filters to purify the water, removing impurities and dissolving minerals into the water. Depending on which minerals are dissolved in the water, what bacteria are in the water, and the temperature, this process gives the water its own taste or personality.

All water started as natural rainwater that evaporated from a body of water somewhere in the world. Some water underwent a short cycle from the ocean to the cloud to the mountaintop and to a stream. This may be as short as a few days. Other water takes a much longer route, both in the length of the journey and in the time to complete one cycle. This could take hundreds or thousands of years if the water is delayed in a glacier or trapped in a slow-moving aquifer deep in the earth. Water with a longer cycle from the ocean to an acceptable source is referred to as having **vintage**. This is a quality often associated with better natural waters. Tap water and processed water are not usually referred to as vintage.

Spring Water

Spring water arrives at the earth's surface from the aquifer due to its own underground pressure. This water is considered pure, clean water, but it is usually far from it. It usually contains mineral contaminants that give it a distinctive taste associated with the aquifer. Besides minerals, other substances from the soil, including bacteria, may be found in the water; dissolved gases may make it effervescent. By definition, spring water must come to the surface naturally. If the minerals are beneficial, the bacteria are not disease producing (called nonpathogenic bacteria), the gases palatable, and the temperature steady, a pleasant-tasting water may be the end product.

In addition to the above characteristics of spring water, more so in Europe than the United States, there is a commercial definition of spring water. To advertise water as **spring water**, it must not be processed or must be processed as little as possible. The water in the bottle must be as close in taste as possible to the water at the spring source. And yes, it may contain small amounts of nonpathogenic bacteria.

Mineral spring water is popular in America again after many years of good, clean municipal water that does not contain pathogens. This fad of carting around and drinking from a water bottle began again in the mid-1970s, when Nestlé Waters North America initiated an advertising campaign to promote Perrier. Today, hundreds of spring waters are available in America, most of which became popular 100 to 150 years ago.

Around the time of the Civil War, the population was growing. Cities became bigger. Crowding was becoming an issue, with the need for sewage and clean water separation. Many recognized the value of clean water. The sources best protected from the industrialization of America were the springs. The water was carried and treated deep below the surface, far from any incidental contamination by civilization. Spring water was clean and free of harmful bacteria, and it became associated with health. "Taking the waters" became the slogan of American spas. Each spring had its own characteristic minerals and flavor, some still and a few with effervescences. The health benefits of spring water were promoted, and these waters served the nation well until they were eclipsed by plentiful, safe, pleasant-tasting municipal water.

Many American springs are still operating today, some under new names and definitely with more ornate spring heads. Some of the more recognized names are Deer Park Springs, Kansas; Mountain Valley Spring, Arkansas; Poland Spring, Maine; Saratoga Springs, New York; Seawright Springs, Virginia; Stone Clear Springs, Tennessee; Sunlight Springs, Wyoming; Mount Olympus, Utah; and the warmest spring head in America at 138 degrees Fahrenheit, Trinity Springs, Idaho.

Sources of Water

Water from Springs and Artesian Wells

A **spring** by definition is a source of water that reaches the surface from the aquifer by its own pressure to a natural opening. An **artesian well** is produced by digging a hole or placing a pipe in the ground, tapping into an aquifer, and having the water then rise by its own pressure to the surface.

Artesian water is of a similar quality as spring water, except it has to be directed to the surface. Many artesian sources do not have the legacy the spring wells have, but the porous rock filtering, the natural addition of minerals, and the long journey to perfection are similar. Artesian water with a confusing name is Eldorado Spring Water, captured in Eldorado Springs, Colorado. The water does not reach the surface on its own but gets its name from the geography.

Well Water

Well water is similar to both spring and artesian water, but the water must be pumped to the surface. There is much variability in the quality of the water—some is excellent and some bad. A high iron or sulfur content, which imparts an unpleasant taste, makes well water unsuitable for drinking.

Rainwater

Rainwater is exactly that. It is water collected from the rain on rooftops, like in Bermuda, where special canopies are erected to gather larger quantities for storage, or aboard sailing ships to supplement the fresh water supply. This water is considered young, of no vintage, and low in mineral content. It usually lacks taste and is pure if good collection methods are employed. Remember that water purity is not associated with a pleasant taste. The water molecule by itself does not have a taste.

Distilled Water

The purest of waters is distilled water. It does not taste good and is not friendly to biological systems. Pure water is harsh on cells, promoting a strong gradient to the semipermeable membranes that are the walls of cells. This water is hypotonic—that is, it contains little or no particulate matter. It has little osmotic pressure. The end result is that the water enters the cell to such a volume that the cell will burst.

Distilled water is heated above 212 degrees Fahrenheit to a gas and then condensed to a liquid. In the process of going from a liquid to a gas, the water leaves behind many minerals, solids, and liquids that boil at other temperatures. Sometimes vapors of organic compounds may carry over to the distillate, and the distilled water may not be truly pure.

Pure water from distillation or reverse osmosis becomes aggressive—that is, if it is exposed to the air, it seeks to replace the lost minerals with carbon dioxide. Carbon dioxide and water form carbonic acid, producing water that is slightly acidic.

Natural water

Natural water is the preferred drinking water. It has the right blend of minerals, gases, and elements to give water a pleasant taste, a friendly osmotic tension, and a feel and wetness that impart a blending and a unity to life. Drinking natural water is not offensive but compatible with every process, from hydration to digestion. It is an aid to heat loss and lubrication. Water remains in the stomach for only 15 minutes before it is absorbed and sent to every part of the body. It blends with us, becomes part of us, and passes from us like no other substance.

It is not only the molecule of water, of H_2O, that is important—what it contains, what it carries, to us and from us, are also important. If this chapter had been only about the molecule of water, it would be easy to present the details. Water is more than just two atoms of hydrogen and one of oxygen. It is about the company it keeps, how much company it keeps, and what it is not associated with. What it **is not** is just as important as what it **is**. No other molecule is defined like water: more by its associates than itself.

This article appeared in *Proceedings of the National Academy of Science USA*, October 1976, *73*(10), 3685–3689. It has been reprinted with the permission of the Linus Pauling Institute at Oregon State University and the Pauling family. The content is of such significance that I chose to not only reference this article but to reprint it in its entirety. Anyone who has cancer or is a professional who treats cancer should be aware of the information in this article.

Vitamin C and Cancer

Supplemental Ascorbate in the Supportive Treatment of Cancer: Prolongation of Survival Times in Terminal Human Cancer

EWAN CAMERON AND LINUS PAULING[332]

Vale of Leven District General Hospital, Loch Lomondside, G83 0UA, Scotland; and Linus Pauling Institute of Science and Medicine, 2700 Sand Hill Road, Menlo Park, California 94025

Contributed by Linus Pauling, August 10, 1976

Abstract

Ascorbic acid metabolism is associated with a number of mechanisms known to be involved in a host of resistance to malignant disease. Cancer patients are significantly depleted of ascorbic acid, and in our opinion this demonstrable biochemical characteristic indicates a substantially increased requirement and utilization of this substance to potentiate these various resistance factors.

The results of a clinical trial are presented in which 100 terminal cancer patients were given supplemental ascorbate as

---

[332] Publication no. 63 from the Linus Pauling Institute of Science and Medicine. This is part I of a series.

part of their routine management. Their progress is compared to that of 1,000 similar patients treated identically but who received no supplemental ascorbate. The mean survival time is more than 4.2 times as great for the ascorbate subjects (more than 210 days) as for the controls (50 days). Analysis of the survival-time curves indicate that the deaths occur for about 90% of the ascorbate-treated patient at one-third the rate for the controls and that the other 10% have a much greater survival time, averaging more than 20 times that for the controls.

The results clearly indicate that this simple and safe form of medication is of definite value in the treatment of patients with advanced cancer.

There is increasing awareness that the progress of human cancer is determined to some extent by the natural resistance of the patient to his disease. Consequently, there is growing recognition that improvement in the management of these patients could come from the development of practical supportive measures specifically designed to enhance host resistance to malignant invasive growth.

We have advanced arguments elsewhere indicating that one important factor in host resistance is the free availability of ascorbic acid (1–3). These arguments are based upon the demonstration that cancer patients have a much greater requirement for this substance than normal healthy individuals, on the realization that ascorbic acid metabolism can be implicated in a number of mechanisms known to be involved in host resistance, and finally, and most convincingly, on the published evidence that ascorbic acid can sometimes produce quite dramatic remissions in advanced human cancer (4, 5).

In this communication we present the results of a clinical trial in which 100 terminal cancer patients received supplemental ascorbate as their only definitive form of treatment and compare their progress with that of 1,000 matched patients managed by the same clinicians in the same hospital who did not receive any ascorbate supplementation or any other definitive form of specific anti-cancer treatment.

Protocol

The study involved a treated group of 100 patients with terminal cancer of various kinds and a control group of 1,000 untreated and matched patients. The treated group consists of 100 patients who began ascorbate treatment, as described by Cameron and Campbell (4) (usually 10 g/day, by intravenous infusion for about 10 days and orally thereafter), at the time in the progress of their disease when in the considered opinion of at least two independent clinicians the continuance of any conventional form of treatment would offer no further benefit. Fifty of the treated subjects are those described in ref. 4 and the other 50 were obtained by random selection from the alphabetical index of ascorbate-treated patients in the Vale of Leven District General Hospital, where treatment of some terminal cancer patients with ascorbate has been under clinical trial since November 1971. We believe that the ascorbate-treated patients represent a random selection of all of the terminal patients in this hospital, even though no formal randomization process was used. In the random selection three patients were excluded because supplemental ascorbate had been deliberately discontinued by order of another physician, and five were excluded because matching controls could not be found for them. Patients suspected or known to have voluntarily discontinued ascorbate treatment have been retained in the group, as have those who died from some cause other than their cancer. No patient was excluded because of short survival time. Eighteen patients, marked with a plus sign in Table 1, were still alive on 10 August 1976, 16 of them clinically "well." These 100 cancer patients, given ascorbate from the presentation date in their illness when their disease process was recognized to be "untreatable" by any conventional method, comprise the treated group.

The control group was obtained by a random search of the case record index of similar patients treated by the same clinicians in Vale of Leven Hospital over the last 10 years. For each treated patient, 10 controls were found of the same sex, within 5 years of the same age, and who had suffered from cancer of the same primary organ and histological tumor type. These 1,000 cancer patients comprise the control group.

The detailed case records of these 1,000 were then analyzed quite independently by Dr. Frances Meuli, M.B., Ch.B. (Otago, New Zealand), who established their presentation date of "untreatability" by such conventional standards as the establishment of inoperability at laparotomy, the abandonment of a definitive form of anti-cancer treatment, or the final date of admission for "terminal care." This presentation date of untreatability corresponds to the date when ascorbate supplementation was initiated in the treated group. Comparable survival times of the 10 matched controls could then be calculated. We accept that "the presentation date of untreatability" can be influenced by many factors in individual patients, but we contend that the use of 1,000 controls managed by the same clinicians in the same hospital over the last 10 years provides a sound basis for this comparative study. We record our thanks to Dr. Meuli for her unbiased and valuable contribution to this investigation.

Even though no formal process of randomization was carried out in the selection of our two groups, we believe that they come close to representing random subpopulations of the population of terminal cancer patients in Vale of Leven Hospital. There is some evidence in the data in Table 1 to support this conclusion.

A somewhat detailed description of the circumstances under which the study was made may be called for. Of the 375 beds in Vale of Leven Hospital, 100 are in the surgical unit, 50 in the medical unit, and 25 in the gynecological unit. The 100 beds in the surgical unit are in the administrative charge of Ewan Cameron, and 50 of them are in his complete clinical charge, the other 50 being in the charge of second Consultant Surgeon of the Hospital. The two Consultant Surgeons are assisted by a changing group of four Surgical Registrars, who are qualified surgeons on assignment for terms of 6 or 12 months from one of another of the Glasgow teaching hospitals. They are assisted by residents and interns. Although some of the cancer patients are initially treated in the medical or gynecological unit, there is a tendency for cases of advanced cancer of all kinds except leukemia and some rare childhood cancers, which are dealt with in a pediatric hospital in Glasgow, to gravitate into the surgical unit, in total probably 90% of all cases of cancer in the Loch Lomondside area.

All of the patients are treated initially in a perfectly conventional way, by operation, use of radiotherapy, and administration of hormones and cytotoxic substances. For example, all of the 11 breast-cancer patients in the ascorbate-treated group, with the exception of one who first presented in a grossly advanced state, had already had mastectomy and radiotherapy and all, including the exception, had been given hormones, sometimes with considerable benefit; but all had relapsed by the time ascorbate supplementation was commenced, and it seemed clear that their tumors were escaping from hormonal control. Similarly, all of the seven bladder-cancer patients in the ascorbate-treated group, with one exception because of her frailty, had received megavoltage irradiation and several had a partial cystectomy (one total) before ascorbate treatment was commenced when it seemed that these standard procedures had failed.

Treatment of terminal cancer patients with ascorbate was cautiously begun in November 1971, for reasons discussed in our earlier papers (1, 2) and has been continued because it seemed to have some value (4, 5). Once the practice had become locally established, the selection of a patient for treatment with ascorbate was often initiated by one of the younger surgeons (the Registrars), as they became familiar with the idea and convinced of its worth.

The suggestion that ascorbate treatment be tried was made by Registrars less often during the first part of their 6 to 12 months' service than during the second part. For strong ethical reasons, every patient in the ascorbate-treated group was examined and assessed independently by at least two physicians or surgeons (often more than two) who all agreed that the situation was "totally hopeless" and "quite untreatable" before ascorbate was commenced. More than 20 different Registrars were involved in this way in allocating patients to the ascorbate-treated group. No criterion was used, except agreed "untreatability."

As described above, selection of 10 matched patients for the control group for each patient of the ascorbate-treated group was made independently by Dr. Frances Meuli. For each ascorbate-treated patient she was given a sheet listing age, sex, primary tumor type, and a brief synopsis of the clinical state and extent of dissemination at the time ascorbate was commenced, but not the survival time. She searched for cases matching these cases as closely as possible, and assigned to each, from the case history, the time when the patient was classified as "untreatable." We believe that the procedure that was followed has not introduced any serious error, and that the ascorbate-treated group and the control group are in fact subpopulations of the population of "untreatable" patients selected in an essentially random manner. Two hundred of the 1,000 patients in the control group were completely contemporaneous with the ascorbate-treated patients. The mean survival time for these contemporaneous controls is 43.9 days, as compared with 52.4 days for the others (overlapping and historical). There has been no significant change in the treatment of patients with advanced cancer in Vale of Leven Hospital during the last 10 years, and the approximate equality of these values is not surprising.

DOTTORE CONOSCENTI TUTTI, MD

The Results of the Study

The results of the study are given in Table 1 and summarized in Table 2, in which values for different kinds of cancer represented by six or more patients treated with ascorbate (60 or more controls) are shown. For each of the nine categories the ratio of average days of survival (ascorbate/controls) is greater than unity, the range being from 2.1 to 7.6, with ratio 4.16 for all 100 patients. The ratios are somewhat uncertain; for example, omitting the patient with the longest survival in the colon group would decrease the ratio from 7.6 to 5.2. At the present time we cannot conclude that ascorbate has less value for one kind of cancer than for others. Our conclusion is that the administration of ascorbic acid in amounts of about 10 g/day to patients with advanced cancer leads to about a 4-fold increase in their life expectancy, in addition to an apparent improvement in the quality of life. This great increase in survival time results in part from the much larger numbers of ascorbate patients than the controls who live for long times, as shown in Fig. 1. Sixteen percent of the patients treated with ascorbic acid survived for more than a year, 50 times the value for the controls (0.3%).

Table 1. Comparison of time of survival of 100 cancer patients who received ascorbic acid and 1,000 matched patients with no treatment[a]

Case no.	Primary tumor type	Sex	Age	Survival time (days) Ten matched controls Individuals										Mean	Test case	Test case / mean control (%)
1	Stomach	F	61	12	41	5	29	85	124	8	54	21	36	38.5	121	314
2	Stomach	M	69	8	6	3	9	4	26	8	114	15	14	20.7	12	58
3	Stomach	F	62	15	1	72	19	19	27	35	99	76	111	47.4	9	19
4	Stomach	F	66	4	87	7	11	3	13	12	6	34	35	21.2	18	85
5	Stomach	M	42	8	1	74	358	9	84	14	16	16	128	70.8	258	368
6	Stomach	M	79	45	4	12	1	9	6	12	130	4	11	23.4	43	184
7	Stomach	M	76	22	19	12	9	14	7	15	3	5	14	12.0	142	1,183
8	Stomach	M	54	24	26	21	61	27	48	7	26	2	221	46.3	36	78
9	Stomach	M	62	14	23	13	89	4	11	4	4	36	27	22.5	149+	622
10	Stomach	F	69	6	19	55	2	21	8	53	11	103	17	29.5	182+	617
11	Stomach	M	45	17	24	7	57	128	16	44	64	110	78	54.5	82	150
12	Stomach	M	57	18	13	8	11	39	29	41	17	170	5	36.9	64	173
13	Bronchus	M	74	16	56	29	27	67	41	25	26	6	40	33.3	39	117
14	Bronchus	M	74	21	2	27	30	18	4	31	1	21	16	16.8	427	2,542
15	Bronchus	M	66	47	94	7	39	3	53	5	4	82	9	34.3	17	50
16	Bronchus	M	52	35	4	70	21	126	8	46	272	39	75	69.6	460	661
17	Bronchus	F	48	11	33	30	5	6	1	45	24	81	57	29.3	90	307
18	Bronchus	F	64	7	1	26	13	71	14	4	30	103	2	27.1	187	690
19	Bronchus	M	70	24	8	20	7	62	20	5	41	19	49	25.5	58	227
20	Bronchus	M	78	32	19	39	40	24	21	43	103	2	21	34.4	52	151
21	Bronchus	M	71	5	53	7	30	2	5	20	39	31	16	20.8	100	481

DOTTORE CONOSCENTI TUTTI, MD

22	Bronchus	M	70	3	2	33	24	25	35	25	62	2	63	27.4	200+	730
23	Bronchus	M	39	42	31	74	5	88	45	28	3	15	70	40.1	42	105
24	Bronchus	M	70	24	1	30	2	5	42	46	41	7	57	25.5	167	655
25	Bronchus	M	70	8	34	29	24	5	4	32	129	20	51	40.7	33	81
26	Esophagus	M	72	12	21	19	14	81	26	59	21	28	33	57.4	50	87
27	Esophagus	F	80	2	29	6	45	48	24	13	238	56	2	46.3	43	93
28	Colon	F	76	2	2	18	5	20	22	1	1	4	1	7.6	57	750
29	Colon	F	58	56	39	31	15	9	11	8	10	6	62	24.7	32	130
30	Colon	M	49	35	122	107	28	30	13	78	65	46	56	58.0	201	347
31	Colon	M	69	48	9	7	15	30	90	26	94	38	15	37.3	1,267	4,343
32	Colon	F	70	64	102	13	82	8	51	33	144	17	11	52.5	144	274
33	Colon	F	68	9	15	40	11	17	217	163	59	18	38	38.5	170	442
34	Colon	M	50	7	108	7	18	17	14	51	69	16	(32)	33.8	428	1,266
35	Colon	F	74	11	45	50	6	18	26	41	11	88	23	31.8	157+	494
36	Colon	M	66	13	7	224	31	72	11	1	4	11	14	38.8	58	149
37	Colon	F	76	23	129	8	63	60	21	28	3	15	70	43.8	123+	281
38	Colon	F	56	24	1	30	2	5	42	46	41	7	57	25.5	861	3,376
39	Rectum	F	56	51	406	74	36	41	106	30	82	82	98	100.6	62	62
40	Rectum	F	75	3	40	46	59	7	9	19	68	16	178	44.4	223	502
41	Rectum	M	56	3	18	52	36	34	7	49	3	6	(13)	22.2	18	81
42	Rectum	F	57	9	73	11	19	98	82	(184)	(97)	(89)	(47)	70.9	223	314
43	Rectum	M	68	11	11	91	47	18	23	4	13	79	84	38.1	140+	367
44	Rectum	M	54	52	36	10	127	18	98	6	73	11	19	45.0	198	440
45	Rectum	M	59	15	2	78	8	98	30	140	54	233	(14)	67.2	759	1,129
46	Ovary	F	49	36	5	117	29	31	22	101	140	94	73	64.8	226	349
47	Ovary	F	68	41	39	18	37	67	3	91	40	6	13	35.5	33	93
48	Ovary	F	49	53	15	38	122	68	33	841	18	21	40	124.9	183	146
49	Ovary	F	67	19	36	22	2	10	32	48	132	21	97	41.9	240+	573
50	Ovary	F	56	49	39	22	85	160	1	86	106	99	107	75.4	123+	163
51	Breast	F	56	1	65	26	6	2	15	19	102	71	131	43.8	4	9

THE FORGOTTEN AND HIDDEN FACTS OF VITAMINS & MINERALS

#	Type	Sex																
52	Breast	F	57	3	28	15	4	14	16	14	48	61	15	21.8	22	101
53	Breast	F	53	33	183	6	190	45	29	16	45	109	34	69.0	576	835
54	Breast	F	66	22	12	94	55	7	38	2	10	76	12	102.8	342	333
55	Breast	F	68	107	41	69	19	17	251	101	81	50	52	78.8	567	720
56	Breast	F	53	8	2	2	42	31	17	96	231	42	20	49.1	86	175
57	Breast	F	75	45	175	12	91	27	5	20	11	63	73	74.2	590	795
58	Breast	F	74	12	2	35	6	18	33	30	107	85	47	37.5	8	21
59	Breast	F	49	3	16	62	44	1	17	93	73	5	57	37.1	35	94
60	Breast	F	50	31	29	28	40	14	14	31	24	104	229	82.6	1,644+	1,990
61	Breast	F	53	105	73	193	159	8	127	126	167	71	42	107.1	173+	162
62	Bladder	M	93	17	47	21	12	2	18	21	46	133	48	36.5	241	660
63	Bladder	F	70	39	9	126	52	26	97	10	8	7	79	45.3	253	556
64	Bladder	F	73	1	23	52	30	38	38	25	13	45	24	28.9	110	381
65	Bladder	F	77	3	52	48	142	118	34	33	10	38	26	50.4	34	67
66	Bladder	M	44	6	9	36	48	10	21	8	52	42	16	24.8	34	137
67	Bladder	M	62	47	118	85	76	19	58	127	72	10	15	62.7	669+	1,067
68	Bladder	M	69	39	5	66	26	25	267	85	12	13	27	56.5	30	53
69	Gallbladder	F	71	7	8	56	22	91	44	30	22	47	14	34.1	22	64
70	Gallbladder	M	67	20	159	4	212	73	60	94	31	16	91	76.0	209	275
71	Kidney (Ca)	F	71	6	2	17	83	81	55	14	114	60	106	53.8	176	327
72	Kidney (Ca)	F	63	68	76	8	31	26	5	8	69	29	49	36.9	89	241
73	Kidney (Ca)	F	51	16	82	27	41	65	29	8	125	(95)	(117)	60.6	147	243
74	Kidney (Ca)	M	53	7	15	7	49	95	21	91	35	19	76	41.5	58	140
75	Kidney (Ca)	M	55	15	13	12	16	45	48	89	95	6	83	42.2	659	1,562
76	Kidney (Ca)	M	73	25	11	209	19	30	198	31	7	30	50	61.0	293	480
77	Kidney (Ca)	M	45	91	35	19	77	64	12	127	74	34	82	61.5	3	5
78	Kidney (Pap)	M	69	67	74	(24)	(37)	87[b]	43[b]	21[b]	82[b]	14[b]	41[b]	49.0	24	49
79	Kidney (Pap)	M	74	57	67	51	(491)	(127)	324	174	126[b]	179[b]	97[b]	169.3	1,554+	918
80	Lymphoma	M	40	144	41	53	29	16	20	41	279	302	103	102.8	1,016+	988
81	Lymphoma	M	65	28	68	51	56	117	138	10	36	51	142	69.7	82	118

449

DOTTORE CONOSCENTI TUTTI, MD

82	Prostate	M	47	24	14	22	23	101	53	157	123	16	80	82.3	166+	202
83	Uterus	F	56	25	11	7	67	130	126	30	18	185	61	66.0	68	103
84	Chondrosarcoma	M	63	20	25	3	17	136	17	31	23	19	157	44.8	9	20
85	"Brain"	M	49	1	85	56	(187)	57	24	13	29	1	95	54.8	37	67
86	Pancreas	M	77	11	25	19	38	91	78	13	41	40	94	45.0	317	704
87	Pancreas	M	67	112	6	55	36	256	25	91	76	67	52	77.6	21	27
88	Pancreas	F	60	11	42	23	49	57	69	122	253	78	59	77.4	16	21
89	Fibrosarcoma	F	54	13	1	171	10	30	64	(101)	(9)	(25)	(17)	44.1	22	50
90	Testicle	M	42	11	10	56	46	39	102	17	(19)	(29)	(87)	41.6	15	36
91	Pseudomyxoma	M	47	35	16	1	19	(37)	(27)	(12)	(15)	(87)	(162)	41.1	132	321
92	Carcinoid	F	68	19	12	45	8	31	12	18	15	82	(38)	28.0	162+	579
93	Leiomyosarcoma	F	32	31	74	66	(28)	(87)	(121)	[21]	[44]	[27]	[242]	74.1	456+	611
94	Leukemia	F	59	6	36	183	6	36	32	44	36	112	63	55.4	430+	776
95	Stomach	M	55	34	34	12	78	5	253	77	79	72	49	69.3	27	39
96	Ovary	F	51	128	13	76	31	65	216	62	140	62	40	83.3	82	98
97	Bronchus	M	69	92	30	90	160	43	147	32	20	135	125	87.4	31	35
98	Bronchus	F	67	93	2	29	90	97	68	185	8	37	26	65.3	138	211
99	Colon	M	77	8	69	80	14	30	9	57	68	14	21	37.0	15	40
100	Colon	M	38	3	41	78	17	58	40	66	98	42	(80)	52.3	152+	291

a The sign + following the survival time of the patients treated with ascorbic acid means that the patient was alive on August 10, 1976. Parentheses () indicate that the matched patient had the same sex, same kind of tumor, and same dissemination, but had an age difference greater than 5 years. Brackets [] indicate opposite sex, same tumor, same dissemination, age difference greater than 5 years. For kidney, Ca indicates carcinoma, Pap, papilloma.

b Diffuse urinary tract papillomatosis. The test cases (78 and 79) had lesions in both kidney and bladder. The nine control cases indicated had tumors of identical histology but their disease was confined to bladder mucosa.

Table 2. Ratios of average survival times for ascorbate patients and matched controls, with statistical significance

A	B (Days)	C (Days)	D	E (Days)	F (%)	G (%)	H	I
Bronchus (15)	136	38.5	3.53	47	47	8.7	24.5	<<0.0001
Colon (13)	282	37	7.61	59	54	20	7.63	<0.003
Stomach (13)	98.9	37.9	2.61	43	46	17	6.41	<0.006
Breast (11)	367	64	5.75	91	55	22	5.74	<0.026
Kidney (9)	333	64	5.21	88	67	22	8.35	<0.002
Bladder (7)	196	43.6	4.49	57	57	20	4.9	<0.028
Rectum (7)	226	55.5	4.1	71	86	33	7.57	<0.003
Ovary (6)	148	71	2.08	78	83	30	6.83	<0.005
Others (19)	172	56.8	3.03	67	53	27	5.28	<0.027
All (100)	209.6	50.4	4.16	65	60	25.7	55.02	<<0.0001

A, Type of cancer and, in parentheses, number of ascorbate patients. There are 10 matched controls for each ascorbic acid patient. B, Average days of survival for ascorbate patients. C, Average days of survival for controls. D, The ratio B/C. E, Average days of survival for all subjects in group. F, Percentage of ascorbate patients surviving longer than E. G, Percentage of controls surviving longer than E. H, Value of x2 for F and G (two-by-two calculation). I, Corresponding value of P (one-tailed).

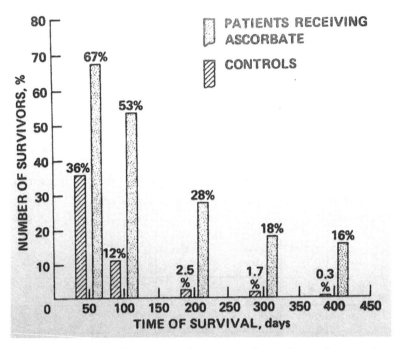

A, Type of cancer and, in parentheses, number of ascorbate patients. There are 10 matched controls for each ascorbic acid patient. B, Average days of survival for ascorbate patients. C, Average days of survival for controls. D, The ratio B/C. E, Average days of survival for all subjects in group. F, Percentage of ascorbate patients surviving longer than E. G, Percentage of controls surviving longer than E. H, Value of x^2 for F and G (two-by-two calculation). I, Corresponding value of P (one-tailed).

Fig. 1. The percentages of the 1,000 controls (matched cancer patients) and the 100 patients treated with ascorbic acid (other treatment identical) who survived by the indicated number of days after being deemed "untreatable." The values at 200, 300, and 400 days for the patients receiving ascorbate are minimum values, corresponding to the date August 10, 1976, when 18% of these patients were still alive (none of the controls).

Statical analysis shows that the null hypothesis that treatment with ascorbate has no benefit is to be rejected for each of the categories in Table 2. The result of a simple statistical test are given in the table. A reasonable dividing time, the average survival time for all subjects, is given in column E, and the percentages exceeding this value are given in columns F and G. Column H contains the value of x^2 obtained by a two-by-two calculation, and I gives the corresponding values of P (one-tailed). Similar values are obtained by nonparametric methods.

The fraction of survivors of the control group at time t is given to within about 2% by the exponential expression $\exp(-t/r)$. About 1.5% of the patients in this group live much longer than would be indicated by this expression. A very close approximation to the observed survival curve is given by the assumption that the control group consists of two populations. One consists of 985 patients with number of survivors at time t given by the expression $985 \exp(-t/r)$, in which r has the value of 45.5 days. This expression corresponds to a constant mortality rate for this subgroup, and its validity suggests that for them a single random process, occurring with a probability independent of time, leads to death. This probability is 2.2% per day. For the 14 of the 1,000 control patients the survival time is indicated to lie between 200 and 500 days. The distribution suggests that for this subgroup two random events lead to death, but the number of subjects is too small to permit this possibility to be tested thoroughly. One other patient, who survived 841 days, may constitute a third subgroup.

A similar analysis of the survival curve for the ascorbate-treated group shows that a considerably smaller fraction, 90%, constitutes the principal group, with number of survivors at time t equal to $90 \exp(-t/r)$, r equal to 125 days. For the remaining 10% the average survival time is greater than 970 days. (These numbers are uncertain because the number of ascorbate-treated patients is small, only 100, and 18 of them were alive on August 10, 1976, their survival times being greater than the value used in the calculation.) A simple interpretation of these facts is that the administration of ascorbate to the patients with terminal cancer has two effects. First, it increases the effectiveness of the natural mechanisms of resistance to such an extent as to lead to an increase by a factor of 2.7 in the average survival time for most of the patients; 2.7 is the ratio of the two values of r, 125 and 45.5 days. Second, it has another effect on about 10% of the patients, such as to cause them to live a much longer time. This effect might be such as to "cure" them; that is, to give then the life expectancy that they would have had if they had not developed cancer. On the other hand, it might only set them back one or more stages in the development of the cancer, in which case their life expectancy would be somewhat less than that corresponding to complete elimination of the effect of their having developed cancer. The uncertainty may be eliminated in the course of time, as the survival times of the 18 patients in the ascorbate-treated group who were still living on August 10, 1976, become known.

Conclusion

In this study the times of survival of 100 ascorbate-treated cancer patients in Scotland (measured from the day when the patient was pronounced to have cancer untreatable by conventional methods) have been discussed in comparison with those of 1,000 matched controls, 10 for each of the ascorbate-treated patients. The data indicated that deaths occur for about 90% of the ascorbate-treated patients at one third the rate of the controls, so that for this fraction there is a 3-fold increase in survival time, measured from the date when the cancer was pronounced untreatable. For the other 10% of the ascorbate-treated patients the survival time is not known with certainty, but it is indicated by the values in Table 1 to be more than 20 times the average for the untreated patients. The value of

4.16 (Table 2) for the ratio of average survival times expresses the resultant of these two effects.

We conclude that there is strong evidence that treatment of patients in Scotland with terminal (untreatable) cancer with about 10 g of ascorbate (ascorbic acid, vitamin C) per day increases the survival time by the factor of about 3 for most of them and by at least 20 for a few (about 10%). It is our opinion that a similar effect would be found for untreatable cancer patients in other countries. Larger amounts than 10 g/day might have a greater effect. Moreover, we surmise that the addition of ascorbate to the treatment of patients with cancer at an earlier stage of development might well have a similar effect, changing life expectancy after the stage when ascorbate treatment is begun from, for example, 5 years to 20 years.

This study was supported by research grants from the Secretary of State for Scotland and The Educational Foundation of America, and by contributions by private donors to the Linus Pauling Institute.

1. Cameron, E., and Pauling, L., "Ascorbic Acid and the Glycosaminoglycans: An Orthomolecular Approach to Cancer and Other Diseases," *Oncology*, 1973, *27*, 181–192.
2. Cameron, E., and Pauling, L., "The Orthomolecular Treatment of Cancer: I. The Role of Ascorbic Acid in Host Resistance," *Chemico-Biological Interactions*, 1974, *9*, 273–283.
3. Cameron, E., "Biological Function of Ascorbic Acid and the Pathogenesis of Scurvy: A Working Hypothesis," *Medical Hypotheses*, 1976, *3*, 154–163.
4. Cameron, E., and Campbell, A., "The Orthomolecular Treatment of Cancer: II. Clinical Trial of High-Dose Ascorbic Acid Supplements in Advanced Human Cancer," *Chemico-Biological Interactions*, 1974, *9*, 285–315.
5. Cameron, E., Campbell, A., and Jack, T., "The Orthomolecular Treatment of Cancer: III. Reticulum Cell

Sarcoma: Double Complete Regression Induced by High-Dose Ascorbic Acid Therapy," *Chemico-Biological Interactions*, 1975, *11*, 387–393.

Patient Handouts

Berberine

Benefits of Berberine

- Helps reduce blood sugar
- Lowers cholesterol
- Is effective in lowering blood pressure
- Relieves pain from first- and second-degree burns
- Can give relief from diarrhea

What Is Berberine?

Berberine is neither a vitamin nor a mineral—it is an herb. An herb is a plant that has micronutrient benefits, unlike foods, which are macronutrients and are eaten in larger quantities for calories and fats and to provide amino acids that will become proteins. Herbs have medicinal or beneficial life benefits when consumed or applied to the body. Herbs originate from the green leaf or the flower of a plant, not the woody stem; spices originate from dried seeds, bark, root, and fruits and are used as a seasoning.

Berberine

Berberine is a molecule produced by many plants. The first and most abundant source is from bayberry; other sources include

- the bark of philodendron,
- the Amur cork tree, Turmeric,
- goldenseal, and
- the Oregon grape.

The powder is bright yellow and easily stains fabrics and plastic surfaces. It is safe for adults, but it is not advised to be given to infants and pregnant women. It should not be given to transplant patients taking cyclosporine, because it inhibits the metabolism of cyclosporine.

Functions of Berberine

Berberine works very well in lowering the blood sugar. Metformin, sold as Glucophage, is an herb that lowers glucose and is an established treatment for diabetes. Unfortunately, large doses are needed to lower the blood sugar, and many people report that it makes them gassy and provokes diarrhea. Berberine, unlike metformin, does not provoke diarrhea, but can be used to treat diarrhea, and does not require a prescription. It is an over-the-counter product that is available from drugstores and vitamin shops.

My experience has been that a new diabetic with a blood sugar of 300 milligrams per deciliter (mg/dL) can attain a level in the 90–100 mg/dL range in about three to four weeks by taking 500 mg of berberine with each meal. If someone has three meals a day, that would be a dose of 500 mg three times a day, or if they eat only two meals a day, it would be a dose of 500 mg twice a day.

Berberine is not the cure-all for diabetes. If you have diabetes or any other medical condition, making berberine work will require effort on your part. No doctor or life coach can give you a pill and a pep talk. This is your disease. Own it. Take control. Get back the years of life this disease wants to take from you. Actuarial statistics show that a diabetic on insulin dies 15 years sooner that their nondiabetic friends. The Centers for Disease Control (CDC) estimates that the life expectancy of a type 1 diabetic is reduced by an average of 11.2 years—more for men and less for women. A type 2 diabetic loses 6 years compared to a healthy person. The intensity of your disease and how you manage it is a big variable in your quality of life and longevity.

Life span and quality of life are affected by berberine because it lowers blood sugar. Other major diabetic factors that it affects are cholesterol, blood pressure, BMI, waist circumference, and hemoglobin A1C.

A note of caution with berberine and diabetes: If you currently are on medication for diabetes, either insulin or hypoglycemic agents, monitor your glucose as you add berberine or transition from drugs to berberine. Berberine usually does not lower blood sugar to dangerous levels by itself, but when paired with traditional hypoglycemic medications, it may make the prescription drug too potent.

Monitoring Blood Sugar

Today, we have glucose monitors, such as the FreeStyle Libre 3 and Dexcom G7, that with one needle stick, remains in place for two weeks. You can scan the sensor with your monitor or your cell phone to get an instantaneous reading of your blood sugar. Readings can be taken before meals, after meals, one or two hours after eating, or as often as once every minute to guide you through food selections or the timing of medications. These instruments give you the power to take control of diabetes and monitor what you are eating and how long it affects you. These blood glucose monitors are not only for diabetics but are necessary for weight training, exercise, and participating in endurance marathons. You do not have to be a diabetic to benefit from the information.

Cholesterol

In my practice, it is very common to see a reduction of 30–40 mg or even a 50 mg reduction of **total cholesterol** with berberine. **High-density cholesterol**, referred to as **HDL cholesterol**, increases from 5 mg to 10 mg. This is the good cholesterol—I remember HDL cholesterol as the **H** being for healthy cholesterol. **Low-density cholesterol**, or **LDL cholesterol**, with the letter **L** I remember this as lethal cholesterol, is also reduced by berberine. Berberine lowers total cholesterol and LDL cholesterol and at the same time increases HDL cholesterol.

This is far better than statin drugs that cause muscle cramps, cognitive problems, and impotency, symptoms that may not go away when the statins are discontinued. A recent meta-analysis reported on in *The New York Times* asked this question about statins: "Do they prolong your life?" The short answer of several studies was NO.[333]

Berberine Supplements

Berberine is available in a capsule, in formulations in which it is the only ingredient, such as BerberPure by Whitaker Nutrition. The 500 milligram (mg) capsules are labeled "Clinical Grade Berberine 1,500 mg." Take three capsules daily—one before each meal.

---

[333] Parker-Pope, T., "Great Drug, but Does It Prolong Life?" *New York Times*, February 9, 2008, https://www.nytimes.com/2008/01/29/health/29iht-29well.9568465.html.

Whitaker Nutrition also offers Berberine GlucoGOLD+ for added diabetic control with chromium, cinnamon, and Banaba leaf extract. It contains the following:

- 133 micrograms (mcg) of Crominex 3+ (chromium), which aids in the utilization of insulin for better control of glucose and cholesterol
- 67 mg of cinnamon
- 16 mg of Banaba leaf extract, which is used for its antioxidant, cholesterol lowering, and anti-obesity effects[334]

Thorne makes a 500 mg capsule, and Luma Nutrition distributes a bottle marked 1,200 mg, but a closer reading of the label indicates that two 600 mg capsules make up a dose.

In the world of alternative medicine, you must do some investigations to know how much is in a tablet or capsule. If the dosage is two capsules, divide the amount by two; if the dosage is three capsules, divide the amount by three. I would prefer that they label the products in mg per capsule to avoid confusion.

February 14, 2022

---

[334] Lang, A., "What Are Banaba Leaves? All You Need to Know," Healthline, April 14, 2020, https://www.healthline.com/nutrition/banaba-leaf.

Bone Health

June 21, 2008, revised February 2022

The best treatment for aging bones is the substances that are provided by Mother Nature. Bones are not just a deposit of calcium but a structure made of a soft protein matrix on which is deposited a myriad of minerals, of which calcium is only one of many. Listening to the media, you might be led to think that eating calcium tablets and taking estrogen is all you need. Take a bone density test, find out how old your bones are, add a once-a-week or a once-a-month pill, avoid falling, and everything will be fine.

What Are Bones?

Bones are the stiff structures that give us form by providing a frame to attach our muscles. Bones are basically a protein matrix on which is deposited calcium and the additional elements of magnesium, strontium, boron, and manganese to make the protein less flexible and more rigid so that it can withstand the stress of standing erect and moving about. To help facilitate the transport of these elements into the bone matrix, the body uses hormones and vitamins such as calcitonin, parathyroid hormone, progesterone, vitamin D, and vitamin K. The problem is not that the body lacks calcium. The problem is that it lacks the substances that cause calcium to be absorbed and transported to the bones and that these substances become less abundant as we age. A low blood calcium level is a rare find in medicine. Taking more calcium and adding estrogen, as was done in the early 1980s, has not prevented osteoporosis. The aging process goes on, the dwindles accelerate, and the skeleton becomes fragile, with bones easily broken after a simple fall.

Measuring Bone Density

A bone scan, often referred to as a **DEXA** scan, documents the bone density only in comparison to an earlier age. The test itself does not reverse the aging process. It is not a preventative procedure for osteoporosis. It is only a snapshot in time of the density of your bones. Do you need a test to tell you you are getting older? I think not. The simplest and cheapest test of bone density is still the ruler. Measure your height and keep your own records. Any loss of height indicates the onset of osteoporosis.

Enhancing Bone Density

The real question, and what you would like to know, is what can be done to slow the process. If bones can be restored, this is truly a bonus. The best course of action is to promote and provide the substances that enhance bone density. Calcium is not required. You already get 1.5 grams per day in the food you eat and the water you drink.

This is the short list of what you need to enhance bone density:

- **Vitamin D_3**, starting at 5,000 units daily to maintain blood level of at least 60 nanomoles per liter (nmol/L)
- **Vitamin K_2**, 1 milligram (mg) as a combination of MK4 and MK7 (Life Extension Super K)
- **DHEA**, 10–25 mg daily
- **Magnesium glycinate**, 200–400 mg daily
- **Strontium citrate**, 200 mg daily
- **Boron glycinate**, 3 mg daily
- **Manganese**, 8 mg daily

- **Zinc**, 15 mg, and **Copper**, 2 mg, daily
- **Hormone replacement**—biest for women and testosterone for men

DHEA Hormone Replacement

Dehydroepiandrosterone (DHEA) is a hormone that controls much of the sex hormone production, influences mental state, and stimulates the immune system, and its production is related to a person's biological age. As we grow and develop as children, the level constantly increases. DHEA levels seem to peak at 25 years of age for both sexes. After 25, the level is almost a straight line to zero at the age of the 80s or so.

No other laboratory test relates better to a person's age, and the lack of DHEA correlates to problems that appear with aging, such as declining energy levels, depression, memory loss, loss of lean muscle mass, ability to cope with stress, increasing cholesterol levels, and the accumulation of fat.

DHEA, Dehydroepiandrosterone

Functions of DHEA

DHEA is the precursor to testosterone and the estrogens, and it has its own biological effects. It was isolated at about the same time as testosterone, the estrogens, and progesterone in the 1920s. It did not draw much attention, as it was not noted to be as active as the other sex hormones. But it was still produced, leading to sex hormone production.

All sex hormones derive from cholesterol. Cholesterol is a complex made of four rings of carbon atoms, three 6-carbon rings and one 5-carbon ring. It is the backbone of all the sex hormones. Changing the side chains of cholesterol, with methyl groups, oxygen, hydrogen, or hydroxyl groups, or removing them makes a new compound—in this case, a hormone.

The body starts with cholesterol, and through a series of changes, it transforms the cholesterol molecule into pregnenolone, a new compound. This pregnenolone acts in the body much like prednisone—to reduce inflammation and reduce allergic reactions—but it does not have many of the side effects of prednisone, such as water retention, muscle wasting, and the promotion of osteoporosis. Next, the body uses pregnenolone to manufacture DHEA by altering its side chains. To carry this a step further, DHEA is transformed to androstenedione by changing its side chains. Androstenedione is acted upon and basically transformed into testosterone, a hormone that has significant biological activity.

This cascade of one molecule of cholesterol becoming pregnenolone, becoming DHEA, becoming androstenedione, and becoming testosterone does not stop there. Much of the testosterone is transformed into estrogen. There is a factor that controls the rate of transformation of testosterone to estrogen. This is important. If you are a man, you want a slow conversion of the testosterone to estrogen so the testosterone has more time to influence your secondary sexual characteristics. If you are a woman, you probably prefer a faster conversion of testosterone to estrogen to help develop your secondary characteristics.

As you can see from this example, not all cholesterol is bad. In fact, cholesterol is required for healthy, appropriate development. It is required for this cascade of hormones to be produced. And it is required for proper brain development, cell wall integrity, and the production of other hormones and vitamin D.

Measuring DHEA Levels

DHEA is not only a compound in a chemical pathway from cholesterol to the sex hormones—it is a hormone that affects other systems. It was not studied as well as the sex hormones because its effect is measured in weeks and months and not hours and days. In fact, the effect is so slow that the US Food and Drug Administration (FDA) permits it to be sold over the counter without a prescription. During the period the FDA studied it, researchers could see no effect. DHEA levels peak at 25 years of age, dropping to near zero when someone is about 80 years old. In other words, if we plot DHEA levels, it is essentially a straight line down from 25 years old to death. In practical terms, this is too long a period to study the hormone. FDA drug studies usually last six weeks. This is much too short a period to see the effects of DHEA.

If blood levels of DHEA are taken to evaluate DHEA levels after taking it either orally or topically, it will take at least three months for the new blood level to stabilize. Saliva levels register a boost in about a week, but again, it would take weeks to arrive at a new cellular functioning level. Biologically, someone may have to take the compound for at least six weeks before they feel any effects. After two to three months, they may feel an increase in muscle strength and stamina, but to see the full effects on the body, to take on a more youthful appearance, may take six to nine months.

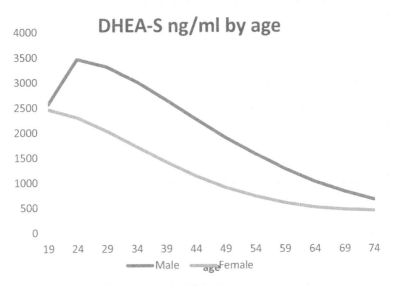

DHEA Levels Over the Lifetime

Normally, DHEA blood levels are reported by laboratories through decades of life. The highest level is reported for 20- to 30-year-olds, slightly lower for 30- to 40-year-olds, lower again for 40- to 50-year-olds, and so on.[335] It is nearly a straight line down from the early 20s to death. So what should your DHEA level be? The best answer I ever heard was from the late Dr. Robert Atkins. He said that you should try to attain the blood level of a 35-year-old. This level of DHEA does not overload the system and has not been found to overstimulate the body by exaggerating the cascade of hormones to produce too much testosterone or estrogen.

---

[335] Cherniske, S., *The DHEA Breakthrough: Look Younger, Live Longer, Feel Better*, Ballantine Books, 1996.

Immune System Support

DHEA supports the immune system. It is a well-known fact that young people have better immune systems than the elderly. They generally suffer fewer infections and show better vitality. This fits with the fact that after the age of 25, the DHEA level declines.

Cortisol and DHEA are produced in the adrenal glands. Pregnenolone is converted to either cortisol or DHEA, and there is an inverse relationship to production. The more cortisol the body makes, the less DHEA is produced; the less cortisol, the more DHEA is produced. Stress causes cortisol production to go up and DHEA to go down. This appears to weaken the immune system, lowering the T4 cell count and decreasing the libido or sex drive.

Peter Casson of the University of Tennessee found that DHEA increases the number of natural killer cells that fight cancer. Additionally, it has been shown that if DHEA is added to the diet of laboratory animals in which it has been easy to induce cancer in the past, it becomes more difficult to induce cancer to grow.

Heart Attack and Stroke

DHEA is better than aspirin to prevent a heart attack or stroke. Platelets in the blood begin the clotting process to stop bleeding after a cut or an injury to the vessel. The development of a clot in a blood vessel produces a stroke or heart attack by blocking the flow of blood carrying oxygen to the heart or brain. There is an inverse relationship between the aggregation, or stickiness, of platelets and DHEA. The more DHEA in the body, the less sticky the platelets become. As the level of DHEA falls with age, the stickier the platelets are, and the formation of a clot to block a blood vessel is more likely. It is not common for a 25-year-old to have a stroke. In fact, it is rare. With every decade of life, the level of DHEA in the blood falls to a lower value and the chance of a heart attack or stroke goes up.

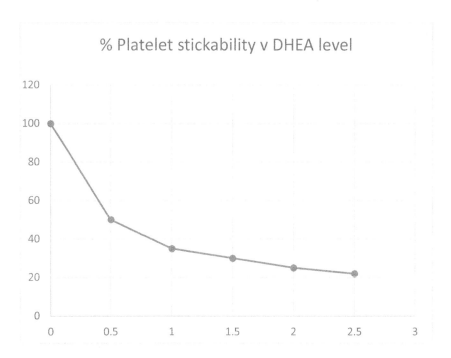

% Platelet stickability v DHEA level

Reducing the stickability of the platelets with aspirin to avert a heart attack or stroke has been the fashion in cardiology. I have not used aspirin in my practice to reduce the clumping of platelets—I use DHEA. Having an elevated DHEA level is Mother Nature's way to maintain fluidity of the blood without stomach irritation, bleeding, and bruising to the skin. This is how the body regulates blood flow without interfering with normal coagulation.

The takeaway: An anecdotal observation in my practice is that in the last six years of prescribing DHEA to reduce clotting, I have not had either one heart attack or one stroke in any patient who followed my recommendation. I feel this is a great accomplishment and a major benefit to my patients.[336]

---

[336] This paragraph was added to the patient information sheet in this book to inform you of the powerful results I have obtained over my years of use of DHEA.

DHEA Supplements

There are side effects of DHEA, but fortunately they are all reversible by reducing the dose or stopping it altogether. The most common are breast tenderness or swelling, menstrual changes, deepening of the voice, and facial hair. I have not seen any liver function changes in my patients. For women, I usually use one-half to one-quarter of the dose I use for men. I follow all with DHEA sulfate (DHEAS) blood tests before and while on treatment, and I have not encountered any problems. I like to start with a baseline blood level, maintaining women in the range of 30–100 micrograms per deciliter (mcg/dL) and men in the range of 60–150 mcg/dL.

Treatment typically starts with the following oral dosages for men, reduced for women:

- Age **40**—25 mg a day for men and 5 mg a day for women
- Age **50**—50 mg a day for men and 10 mg a day for women
- Age **65**—75 mg a day for men and 20 mg a day for women

The added boost to well-being that you receive will benefit you in many ways: better weight distribution, better immune function with fewer colds and infections, and better sex with more stamina, moisture, and endurance. Psychologically, you will feel less fear and more courage; your outlook on life will be brighter. Exercise will be easier. Take advantage of this new energy and get the double benefit of exercise and DHEA. You may not be 35 years old again, but you will be younger than you are now.

October 20, 2005

Estrogen Metabolite Ratios

The 2/16α estrogen metabolite ratio (EMR) refers to the ratio of the two estrogen metabolites **2-hydroxyestrone (2OHE1)** and *16α-hydroxyestrone (16αOHE1)*. The normal ratio is 2 or greater. A high ratio in the urine is a healthy ratio, and a lower ratio is found to promote breast cancer. In a person who is not undergoing hormone treatment for either menopause or andropause, this is a healthy situation. Cancer risk has been found to be elevated in people with a ratio of less than 2. This holds true for people with no hormone treatment and with hormone treatment.

The treatment for an imbalance in the 2/16α EMR is **indole-3-carbinol (I3C)** or its metabolite **diindolylmethane (DIM)**. These two compounds are derived from cruciferous vegetables such as broccoli. The supplements cause more of the 2-hydroxyestrone to be formed instead of the 16α-hydroxyestrone and are more effective than the raw vegetables themselves. With microscopic examination and tissue staining, it was found that healthy normal tissue contains, in the cytoplasm, 2-hydroxyestrone and more in the urine; in breast cancer tissue there is 16α-hydroxyestrone in the tissue, and its levels are higher in the urine. The urine is a good place to find these hormone metabolites, and we have a tool to make that ratio more favorable for health.

Prostate tissue reacts the same as breast tissue to hormone stimulation, and urine testing is also effective in men; therefore, treatment schedules are the same.

This ratio applies to other conditions such as **human papilloma virus (HPV)**, which causes cervical cancer, and recurrent

respiratory papillomatosis (RRP). In both these conditions, HPV and RRP viruses will be reduced with DIM or I3C.[337]

For DIM, the dosage is 200 milligrams (mg) a day. If you take indole-3-carbinol, the dosage is 400 mg per day.

This ratio can easily be obtained and monitored using urine samples. The value is calculated by dividing the 2-hydroxyestrone value by the 16α-hydroxyestrone value; for example:

2OHE1/16OHE1 = 1.7 mcg/g ÷ 0.7 mcg/g = 2.4

Anything above 2.0 is considered healthy.

May 5, 2017

Author's Note

This handout was put in circulation in my practice on May 5, 2017. Polyps are large papilloma. This thought led to the idea that colon polyps might also be reduced by DIM. A patient of mine, Joe (that is his real name—he wanted to be recorded in this book), complained that at his last coloscopy he had 11 polyps. Generally, people who have colonic polyps have more at each subsequent colonoscopy. Joe volunteered to take DIM daily and monitor how many polyps he had at the next scoping. I am aware that this report is an anecdotal observation, but all studies originate from someone observing something that others did not see.

Joe reported that at his next colonoscopy, he only had one polyp. It is too early to know whether this application of DIM influences all cases of polyps or not, but Joe thought it was a big deal, and I thought it was a big deal, although Joe's gastroenterologist was not impressed. Because Joe and I were impressed, he continues to take DIM, and I now recommend it to my patients if polyps are found on colonoscopy or a family history of polyps exist.

---

[337] Klug, T. L., "Response to Dr. Jacob Schor's Article 'Estrogen Metabolite Ratios: Time for Us to Let Go,'" *Townsend Letter*, April 2013.

I take it myself. I am not waiting for big studies to be done. I take it now as a preventive measure for colon cancer. I cannot find any contraindications or side effects. This is better than doing nothing before or after finding polyps. It is better to avoid polyps. What did your gastroenterologist recommend?

Fish Oils

The Benefits of Fish Oils

- Helps raise good HDL cholesterol and lower total cholesterol
- Lowers triglycerides
- Reduces blood pressure
- Supports healthy brain tissue and calms seizures
- Lowers inflammation of arthritis and bowel disease
- Prevents macular degeneration

Fatty Acids

Fatty acids are neither vitamins nor minerals but long chains of carbon atoms terminated on one end with a carboxyl acid configuration and a methyl group on the other. The chains of atoms are of differing lengths of carbon and may be connected with either single or double bonds. Most fatty acids are fats and are a store of energy or are involved with the structure of the cell wall. Many types of fats and fatty acids align to form the cell wall. Oil and water do not mix, and the cell wall is a barrier that partitions the water and water-soluble substances in the cell from the extracellular fluids.

Polyunsaturated fatty acids (PUFA) refer to the extent that all or some of the bonds between the carbons are attached to each other with either single or double bonds. Fatty acids are classified as **short chain**, with 2 to 4 carbons; **medium chain**, with 6 to 10 carbons; and **long chain**, with 12 to 26 carbons. Further classification is the **omega-6** or **omega-3** designation. The *6* and *3* refer to the carbon location from the methyl end of the molecule where the first double bond appears. Medically, this is significant because omega-3 fatty acids are anti-inflammatory and omega-6 fatty acids are proinflammatory.

Industrialization of Food Production

The industrialization of food growing, gathering, processing, and transporting developed along with advances in manufacturing and the standardization of products. The mechanization of harvesting, irrigation, and transporting changed farms from small plots of land to consolidated, larger tracts of land to benefit from the economies of scale. This industrialization included the redirection of water, the genetic engineering of plants, and the application of chemicals for not only plant growth but also to inhibit unwanted weeds, pests, and mold, which led to the loss of beneficial bacteria and minerals. The gain of increased production was offset by decreased nutritional quality, the depletion of minerals in the soil, and the contamination of runoff water.

The most significant changes occurred in the latter half of the 1800s and into the 1900s. Processing methods also changed. For example, the milling of grain progressed from simply grinding the grains into a powder to a process that separated the germ, or the part of the seed that is the new **embryo** of the plant, from the carbohydrate portion of the seed, or the **endosperm**—that is, the new plant's food until the seed sprouts and photosynthesis supports the growth of the plant. The wheat germ contains the oils, of which vitamin E is one. Vitamin E becomes rancid over time with exposure to air, so separating the wheat germ prolonged the shelf life of the flour, but the nutrient value of vitamin E in the wheat was discarded. This nutrient loss promoted heart attacks, strokes, and abnormal clotting of the blood.

At the turn of the century, lard from pigs was the primary cooking oil. More abundant, cheap supplies of cooking oils could be derived from cottonseed, rapeseed, peanuts, corn, grape seed, soy, safflower, and sunflower. These oils could be hydrogenated to give them more of a semisolid texture—for example, peanut oil to peanut butter and corn oil to margarine. Hydrogenation is the process of adding hydrogen to the double bond of a series of carbon atoms in a fatty acid. Through this process, polyunsaturated oil turns into saturated oil that contains no double bonds between carbon atoms.

Ethylene + HH ⇒ Ethane

Chemically, the molecule is changed, giving it new chemical qualities, and physically, it changes from a liquid to a semisolid state at room temperature. The melting point increases, but more importantly, the chemical characteristics and the reactions with other substances are altered.

The first oil to be commercially produced was **Crisco**, in June 1911 by Proctor and Gamble, from cotton seed oil. In 2002 the product was sold to the J. M. Smucker Company. It is now a mixture of partially and fully hydrogenated soybean oil, hydrogenated palm oil, palm oil, monoglycerides, and diglycerides; t**ertiary B**utylhydroqu**inone (TBHQ)**, a fat antioxidant; and citric acid. Eighty-seven percent of animal fats have been replaced by vegetable fats in the diet.[338]

---

[338] Shallenberger, F., "How to Eliminate Macular Degeneration," *Dr. Frank Shallenberger's Second Opinion*, 2024, *XXXIV*(1), 4.

Macular Degeneration Promoted by Vegetable Oils

Recent research by Nicolas Bazan, MD, shows that the amount of **docosahexaenoic acid, an omega-3 oil** derived from fish, is greatly reduced in the periphery of the retina of the eye, leading to damage and death of the **rod photoreceptor** cells. This progresses to the **macula** of the eye, the area of color perception by the **cone photoreceptors** and where central vision and the area responsible for eye-to-eye contact is located.

The foods we eat have changed a great deal since 1900. The fat that was consumed was nearly all animal fats, namely omega-3s. The industrialization of food processing has shifted the human diet to the incorporation of plant-based oils such as omega-6. One hundred years ago, **the ratio** of **omega-6** to **omega-3** was **4:1**. Today that ratio has changed to approximately 20:1.

EPA is eicosapentaenoic acid, a 20-carbon fatty acid. **DHA is docosahexaenoic acid**, a 22-carbon fatty acid. These are natural products found in cold-water fish such as mackerel, salmon, and herring and nuts such as walnuts and Brazil nuts.

DHA, Docosahexaenoic Acid, a 22-carbon fatty acid

EPA, Eicosapentaenoic Acid, a 20-carbon fatty acid

Fish oils are referred to as **omega-3** fatty acids. This is a chemical designation that means the double bonds begin at the third carbon from the tail of the chain, known as the methyl end. In the group of structures represented here, they are on the right side of the page.

In the Paleolithic era, millions of years ago, to the early 1900s, fish was the main source of EPA and DHA. People consumed 600 to 14,250 milligrams (mg) of oil per day. Today the intake of EPA/DHA is estimated to be 100 to 200 mg/day. The omega-6 consumption from plant sources has increased. An interesting side note is that fish do not produce omega-3 oils but accumulate it from the algae they eat, and then we eat the fish to get the omega-3s.

The primary **omega-6 oil** is **arachidonic acid**, obtained from safflower, sunflower, rapeseed, soybean, cottonseed, and corn oil.

Arachidonic Acid, $C_{22}H_{32}O_2$

Omega-6 indicates that the double bonds begin with the sixth carbon atom from the methyl end of the molecule, on the right side of the structure on this page.

The omega-3 oils EPA/DHA are anti-inflammatory, whereas the **omega-6 oils are proinflammatory**. Corn oil has an omega 6:3 ratio of 60:1 and safflower has a ratio of 77:1. This is certainly a factor driving chronic autoimmune diseases—allergies, arthritis, and asthma. Farm-raised fish are grown in ponds and fed corn as the principal food. These fish contain very large amounts of omega-6 oils, unlike wild-caught fish that have an omega-6:3 ratio of 4:1. This is similar to cows that are fed corn products in feed lots and are not permitted to eat grass, producing beef that is high in omega-6 instead of the natural 4:1 ratio of omega-6 to omega-3. Omega-6 fats are proinflammatory and are potent mediators of vasoconstriction and platelet aggregation, which is a recipe for clot formation.[339]

Too Much Information

This definitely is more technical information than is needed to understand fish oils, but I present it for clarity and completeness of the topic. In nature, fish oils are connected to a 3-carbon glycerin molecule in differing combinations—**EPA, DHA**, and maybe **ALA (alpha-linolenic acid)**, an 18-carbon chain acid—and are attached to glycerol. Glycerol is the alcohol form of glycerin with the **hydroxyl (-OH)** radical attached to each one of the three carbon atoms. A fish oil supplement sold in the store is usually the components of the individual fatty acids. In nature, fish oil is the complex of EPA, DHA fatty acids, and glycerol connected together. This chemical structure is a triglyceride.

A Fish Oil Triglyceride of DHA, EPA, and ALA Attached to a Glycerol Molecule

I will now try to give some clarity to the term *triglycerides*. This is the description of a group of chemicals and how these molecules are put together: three fatty acids attached to an alcohol called glycerol. The physical structure of the triglyceride molecule is similar to the letter *E*. The vertical line of the letter represents the glycerol

---

[339] https://ods.od.nih.gov/factsheet/Omega-3FattyAcids-HealtProfessional/

molecule, and the three horizontal lines represent the three fatty acids. This is a triglyceride.

The type of fatty acids that are attached to the glycerol determines its chemistry and its function. Triglycerides are of great concern in the fields of cardiology, cardiovascular disease, and ophthalmology. These triglycerides are different in that the fatty acids are of short- and medium-chain length. Remember, the short-chain fatty acids have 2 to 4 carbon atoms, and the medium-chain fatty acids have 6 to 10 carbon atoms. These are primarily the molecules involved with coronary and peripheral vascular plaque obstruction, diabetes, obesity, and metabolic syndrome. Long-chain fatty acids have 12 to 26 carbon atoms, and fish oils are a subgroup of the long-chain fatty acids with 18 to 22 carbon atoms. Fish oils and fish oil triglycerides are involved with structure, such as becoming part of the cell wall or a precursor molecule to hormones.

Krill oil is harvested from crustaceans in the waters of Antarctica. Fishing is limited to 60,000 pounds a year in the area between the tip of South America and the continent of Antarctica. It is a product similar to fish oil in that it has EPA and DHA attached to the glycerin molecule, but in the third position it has a **phosphate group** with **choline**. This phosphate and choline combination is also called **phosphatidylcholine**, or **lecithin**. The phosphate group enhances the anti-inflammatory effects of EPA and DHA, but with the phosphate group, it becomes a structural component of biologic membranes—in simple terms, the cell wall.

Krill Oil: DHA, EPA, and Phosphatidylcholine Attached to Glycerol

There are two things about the **cell wall** I would like to bring to your attention. The first is that the wall is a fatty or lipid structure. You know that oil and water do not mix. The function of the wall is to partition the **intracellular** watery contents of the cell from the **extracellular** watery fluids. The concentration of sodium is low in the cell and high in the external cell fluid; the concentration of potassium is high in the cell and much lower in the extracellular fluid. The second concept that I want to bring to your attention is that the cell wall is a functioning part, or organelle, of the cell. The cell wall regulates what goes into the cell or exits the cell. It controls the flow of minerals in and out of the cell with hormones such as insulin or mediators of inflammation. The integrity of the cell wall is very dependent on adequate fatty acids.

Erroneous Reference Ranges

Modern laboratories have the ability to measure arachidonic acid, EPA, and DHA. They also give a reference range for these substances and the ratio of omega-6 to omega-3. I do not question the absolute amount of these oils, but I do question the ratio of omega-6 to omega-3. A laboratory develops a reference range by producing a bell curve based on the results of measuring levels in 10,000 people and then trimming the results by removing 5% off the low and high ends of the curve. BioReference Laboratories reports the omega-6 to omega-3 ratio to be 5.7 to 21.3. No doubt, these are their findings, but the range is open to interpretation. The laboratory is measuring levels in Americans who are eating a diet that contains much more omega-6 than Americans ate 100 years ago. It would be informative to measure the levels in a population that is not eating modern processed food. It would also be helpful to perform a study that compares diets, health, longevity, and omega ratios. This basic information would be beneficial to anyone wanting a healthier and longer life.

Some researchers have reported that an omega-6:3 ratio higher than a 7 often accompanies the beginning of **macular degeneration**. Macular degeneration is not something you develop at the age of 60 or 70—it has been developing throughout your adult life. Once the condition deteriorates to where the periphery and the macula are involved, it is already a major problem. Avoid this problem. Clean up your diet and have your omega-6:3 ratio checked to be sure that it is, in fact, 4:1 or better.

Predominant Sources of Fatty Acids

Food sources are a blend of fatty acids. No one food is totally omega-3 or omega-6. One food may have a predominant amount of one or the other, but it does not have one form to the exclusion of the other. The tables below list foods that contain predominantly omega-3 and omega-6.[340] When it comes to balancing fatty acids, this issue is related more closely to nutrition than to taking the proper supplement.

---

[340] DiNicolantonio, J. J., and O'Keefe, J., "The Importance of Maintaining a Low Omega-6/Omega-3 Ratio for Reducing the Risk of Autoimmune Diseases, Asthma, and Allergies," *Missouri Medicine*, 2021, *118*(5), 453–459.

Dietary Sources of Omega-3	
Food Source	**Grams of EPA/DHA per 3 oz. serving**
Salmon roe	2.7
Halibut	2.21
Herring	1.7–1.8
Salmon (wild)	1.0–3.0
Sardines	1.0–1.74
Trout	1.0
Oysters	4.5–1.15
Mackerel	0.3–1.80
Tuna	0.25–1.30

Dietary Sources of Omega-6	
Food Source	Grams of total omega-6 per 1 oz. serving
Walnuts	10.8
Pine nuts	9.5
Sunflower seeds	6.5
Sesame seeds	6.0
Brazil nuts	5.8
Pumpkin seeds	5.8
Pecans	5.8
Pistachios	3.7
Almonds	3.4

Recommended amounts of fish oil are gleaned only from observational data of what is observed as healthy in 50% of the population. The only data that is somewhat clear is that breast-fed infants, from birth to 12 months of age, receive about 0.5 grams per day. After that, the diet is so varied in terms of the amounts of DHA, EPA, and ALA that the **Academy of Medicine** does not issue a **recommended daily allowance (RDA)** but provides an **adequate intake (AI)**. They present the following table of grams per day.[341]

---

[341] The Academy of Medicine, NIH.gov.

Recommended Adequate Intake (AI) for Omega-3s (Grams/Day)				
Age	Male	Female	Pregnancy	Lactation
0–12 months	0.5	0.5		
1–3 years	0.7	0.7		
4–8 years	0.9	0.9		
9–13 years	1.2	1.0		
14–50 years	1.6	1.1	1.4	1.3
51+ years	1.6	1.1		

Drug Warning

Natural fatty acids are difficult enough to understand. The molecules are long, the names seem to be even longer, and there are so many of them. If this is confusing, take a look at how Big Pharma added to the confusion of the fatty acid market. The fish oils, DHA and EPA, have long been known to be heart healthy, to protect the nerves, and to preserve brain function and structure. Big Pharma approached the molecules like they had in the past: by physically altering the molecule. In this instance, they altered the molecules by producing an ester at the acid end of the molecule. This in effect creates a new molecule that is unlike the original. The new molecule is a new invention and is patentable so that it can be owned, advertised, and sold for the life of the patent. Hopefully, the physiological effect is similar to that of the original molecule, but it never is an exact duplicate. There is always a difference in the amount and effect, and sometimes the effect is detrimental.

These two synthetic molecules have terrible effects. The Vascepa and Lovaza molecules are pictured below. These two synthetic products, produced by adding a two-carbon substance, either an acetyl group or ethane, to the acid terminus, have the potential to produce allergic reactions and significant heart problems such as atrial fibrillation and atrial flutter, leading to lightheadedness, dizziness, shortness of breath, and chest pain. Bleeding can ensue, along with joint and muscle pain, edema of the extremities, constipation, and gout. The real effects are opposite to the intended objective.

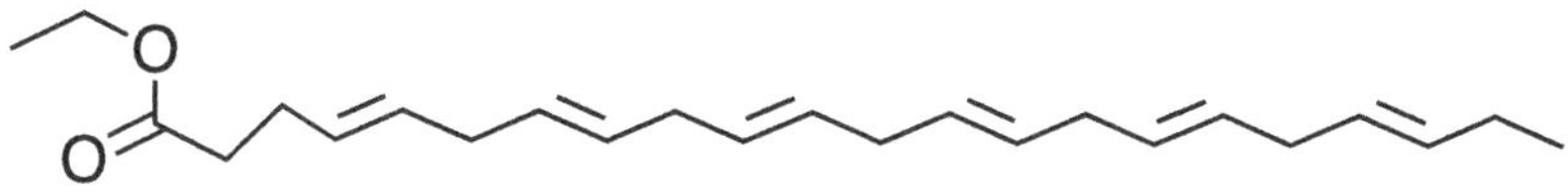

Vascepa, Icosapent Ethyl, an Adulterated DHA

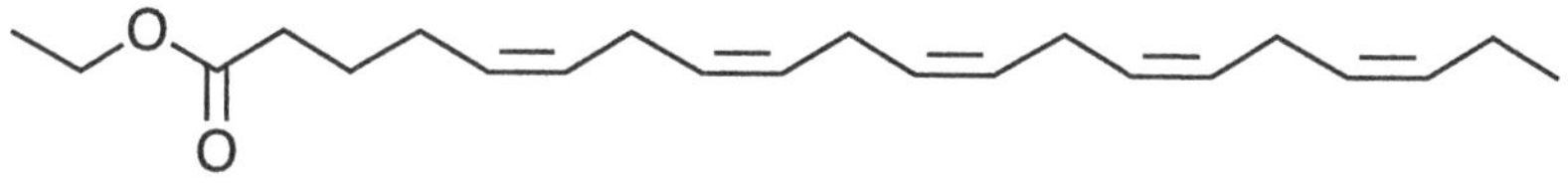

Lovaza, Omega-3-Acid Ethyl Ester, an Adulterated EPA

The synthetic molecules may be cheaper after paying for them with your prescription insurance card or a coupon from GoodRx, but you will pay the price of poor health. This is not a bargain. My advice is to stay with Mother Nature's molecules.

Available Forms of Fish Oil

There are many purveyors of fish oil and many sources. The best oils are sourced from cold-water fish such as salmon, herring, and sardines. The smaller fish are free of mercury, dioxins, and PCBs. Vegan sources are from algae and the conversion of flax seed to EPA and DHA. The conversion is not very efficient and does not yield sufficient therapeutic doses. I like **Nordic Naturals** from

Arctic cod fish and algae. The oils are processed under nitrogen, and the gel caps are packed in bottles infused with nitrogen. This avoids long exposure to oxygen. Oxygen causes the oils to go rancid and smell bad. This process avoids the fishy burp. I would avoid any brand that smells fishy. Oxidized oils have no benefit and should be avoided. Nordic's best is **Ultra Omega 2X** with 1,175 mg of EPA and 875 mg of DHA from anchovies and sardines. **Pure Encapsulations** sells **EPA/DHA essentials** from anchovies, sardines, and mackerel; a 1,000 mg gel cap provides 300 mg of EPA and 200 mg of DHA.

Often, you will see the term **fish oil concentrate**. Many brands extract the oils through chemical processes that result in only two or three fatty acids in the product and possibly some chemical residue or contaminant. Natural fish oil complexes contain up to 50 different fatty acids, are less prone to oxidation, and offer more of the benefits, like eating fish. Fish oil concentrates may be a step backward. Generally, most systems in the body do not lack one ingredient but respond to a blend of substances.

Dr. Mercola sells **Antarctic krill oil** and emphasizes that its omega-3s are bound to phospholipids and that one capsule also contains 1 mg of astaxanthin. The packaging of the bottle I bought claims that the krill were caught in the Antarctic at 64° 18S, 61° 21W, observing the **Marine Stewardship Council (MSC.org)** guidelines for sustainable fishing.

Do not want to take anymore capsules? Eat cold-water fish two or three times a week. Remember, farm-raised fish are grown in ponds and fed corn. Corn has 60 times more omega-6 oil than omega-3 oil. The industrial farming of fish eliminates the nutritional benefit of the omega-3 oils found in wild fish. All farm-raised fish are inferior to fish raised by Mother Nature. Fish farming is an industrial process designed to raise fish production, not to increase the nutritional value of the fish.

QR Code for Updates

Use this QR code to receive new patient handouts as new, timely applications of vitamins and minerals are developed. During the writing of this book, new information was discovered about vitamins. Two chapters that I had completed required substantial additions as new information became known. Other chapters required minor rewrites because of new applications of vitamins or minerals to current problems.

This book is not only a historical record—it is current medical knowledge about and applications of vitamins and minerals. Using a QR code helps keep the information in these pages current.

This book can never be completed because information is forever accumulating, and new protocols will be developed for old and new medical conditions. Thus, there will never be a final draft and certainly no final copy.

Made in the USA
Middletown, DE
22 June 2025

77315249R00275